Lippincott's Guide to Infectious Diseases

Diseases

REMOVED
FROM
STOCK

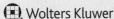

Wolters Kluwer | Lippincott Williams & Wilkins
Health

Philadelphia · Baltimore · New York · London
Buenos Aires · Hong Kong · Sydney · Tokyo

Staff

Publisher
Chris Burghardt

Clinical Director
Joan Robinson, RN, MSN

Clinical Project Manager
Lucia Kubik, RN, BSN

Clinical Editors
Kate Stout, RN, MSN, CCRN
Collette Hendler, RN, MS, CIC, CCRN
Joanne Bartelmo, RN, MSN

Product Director
David Moreau

Product Manager
Rosanne Hallowell

Editor
Maureen McKinney

Copy Editor
Jerry Altobelli

Editorial Assistants
Megan L. Aldinger, Karen J. Kirk,
Jeri O'Shea, Linda K. Ruhf

Art Director
Elaine Kasmer

Cover Designer
Joseph DePinho

Design Assistant
Kate Zulak

Vendor Manager
Cynthia Rudy

Manufacturing Manager
Beth J. Welsh

Production Services
Aptara, Inc.

Library of Congress Cataloging-in-Publication Data
Lippincott's guide to infectious diseases.
    p. ; cm.
    Includes bibliographical references and index.
    ISBN 978-1-60547-975-0 (alk. paper)
    1. Communicable diseases. 2. Communicable diseases–Nursing.
    [DNLM: 1. Communicable Diseases–nursing–Handbooks. WY 49]
    RC111.L73 2012
    616.90231–dc22
                       2010026298

Contents

Contributors and consultants

Dorothy Borton, RN, BSN, CIC
Infection Preventionist
Albert Einstein Healthcare Network
Philadelphia, Pennsylvania

Vicki Brinsko, RN, BSN, CIC
Director, Infection Control and Prevention
Vanderbilt University Medical Center
Nashville, Tennessee

Gayle K. Gilmore, RN, MA, MIS, CIC
Consultant
Duluth, Minnesota

Collette Bishop Hendler, RN, MS, CCRN, CIC
Infection Control Nurse
Abington Memorial Hospital
Abington, Pennsylvania

Irena L. Kenneley, PhD, APRN-BC, CIC
Assistant Professor
Case Western Reserve University
Frances Payne Bolton School of Nursing
Cleveland, Ohio

Catherine Lopez, RN, MEd, CIC
Assistant Dean for Student Services
Louisiana State University Health Sciences
    Center—School of Nursing
New Orleans, Lousiana

Patricia J. McBride, RN, MSN, CIC
Infection Preventionist
Bryn Mawr Hospital
Bryn Mawr, Pennsylvania

Barbara Wyand Walker, RN, BSN, CIC
Infection Control/Employee Health
    Coordinator
Greenbrier Valley Medical Center
Ronceverte, West Virginia

Foreword

As an infection preventionist for more than 30 years, I have led numerous educational sessions on infections and infectious diseases. These sessions have described the responsible organism, the signs and symptoms of the infection or infectious disease, the means of transmission, and practices to use to prevent the spread of the infection or infectious disease to other individuals, including the caregiver. As a registered nurse, my favorite audiences have included bedside nurses.

The bedside nurse devotes many hours to patient care and assumes much of the responsibility for patient and family education. This education is an important component of the plan of care for patients with infections or infectious diseases. Patients and family members must understand the disease process and the treatment required in order to ensure compliance with therapy and to prevent both complications and transmission of infection to others. The nurse is the predominant member of the health care team whom patients and family members approach with questions about the infection or infectious disease. The nurse must keep his or her knowledge of infections and infectious diseases current not only to answer questions accurately for patients and family members but also to provide appropriate nursing care.

Lippincott's Guide to Infectious Diseases focuses on the essential information needed to deliver quality care to the patient with an infection or infectious disease. It has a unique visual design that helps the reader navigate through the book in a quick and logical manner.

The book is divided into two sections. Part I, Understanding and Preventing Infectious Diseases, provides a refresher course for the nurse by covering the fundamentals of disease transmission and prevention. Part II, Managing Infectious Diseases, provides a brief overview of more than 150 infections and infectious diseases ranging from otitis media and the common cold to serious health care–associated infections (HAIs) caused by such current organisms as *Acinetobacter, Clostridium difficile,* and *methicillin-resistant Staphylococcus aureus* (MRSA).

Part II offers a general description of the distinguishing characteristics of each infection or infectious disease, a short description of the responsible organism(s), the complications associated with the infection or disease, diagnostic approaches, treatment, applicable nursing interventions, and information to include in patient and family teaching. This section of the book is a nurse's dream. Each entry provides useful information to help the nurse plan the patient's individualized care, adequately assess the patient throughout the delivery of care, provide the necessary services, and evaluate the patient's progress toward established goals. Everything the nurse needs to provide safe, quality nursing care is covered.

Lippincott's Guide to Infectious Diseases is a treasure for nurses at all levels. It is an excellent reference for specific nursing care for the patient with an infection or infectious disease. It comes at a perfect time: when health care providers, patients, and third-party payers are concerned about the consequences of HAIs, including cost as well as morbidity and mortality. Hospitals are implementing various approaches to reduce the incidence of HAIs to zero. This book will help the nurse play an important role in that effort.

Fran Feltovich, MBA, RN, CIC, CPHQ
The Methodist Hospital
Houston, Texas
Past President, the Association for Professionals
in Infection Control and Epidemiology, Inc.
(APIC)
Past President, APIC-Houston
Past President, the Texas Gulf Coast Association
for Healthcare Quality
2010 President, the Certification Board of
Infection Control and Epidemiology, Inc.

Part I

Understanding and Preventing Infectious Diseases

Despite improved treatment and prevention strategies, including powerful antibiotics, complex vaccines, and modern sanitation practices, infection continues to cause a great deal of serious illness throughout the world—even in highly industrialized countries. In developing countries, infection remains a critical health problem.

Normal microbial flora

Large numbers of microorganisms exist in the air we breathe, on the surfaces we touch, and on and within our bodies. Microorganisms naturally found on and within the body are called *normal flora*—they concentrate in certain body regions, such as the skin, mouth, and GI tract. The skin harbors more than 10,000 microorganisms/cm². Scrapings from the surface of the teeth or gums may show millions of organisms per milligram of tissue.

The human body and its normal flora coexist in a sort of ecosystem whose equilibrium is essential to good health. Under normal circumstances, these microorganisms are nonpathogenic and harmless. In fact, they may aid the body by competing for nutrients with disease-producing microorganisms or by performing special tasks. For example, the lumen of the bowel contains microorganisms that carry out many chemical functions. Moreover, disruption of the normal ecology of the microbial flora can pose substantial risks to the host. (See *Where normal flora live.*)

Relatively few of the many species of microorganisms that exist become adapted to the unique environments of various body tissue. Thus, to a certain degree, the flora of a given species—even of specific body tissue—is predictable.

What is infection?

Infection is the invasion and multiplication in or on body tissue of microorganisms that

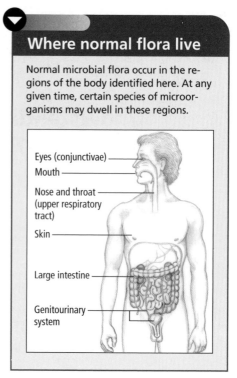

Where normal flora live

Normal microbial flora occur in the regions of the body identified here. At any given time, certain species of microorganisms may dwell in these regions.

Eyes (conjunctivae)
Mouth
Nose and throat (upper respiratory tract)
Skin
Large intestine
Genitourinary system

produce signs and symptoms along with an immune response. Such reproduction injures the host either by causing cellular damage from microorganism-produced toxins or intracellular multiplication or by competing with host metabolism. The host's own immune response may increase tissue damage, which may be localized (as in infected pressure ulcers) or systemic. The very young and the very old are most susceptible to infections.

Microorganisms that cause infectious diseases are difficult to overcome for many reasons:

▶ Some bacteria develop a resistance to antibiotics.

▶ Some microorganisms, such as human immunodeficiency virus (HIV), include many different strains, and a single vaccine can't provide protection against them all.

▶ Most viruses resist antiviral drugs.

▶ Some microorganisms localize in areas that make treatment difficult, such as the central nervous system and bone.

▶ New infectious agents, such as HIV and severe acute respiratory syndrome–coronavirus, occasionally arise.

▶ Opportunistic microorganisms can cause infections in immunocompromised patients.

▶ Much of the world's ever-growing population has not received immunizations.

▶ Increased air travel by the world's population can speed a virulent microorganism to a heavily populated urban area within hours.

▶ Biological warfare and bioterrorism with organisms such as anthrax, plague, and smallpox are an increasing threat to public health and safety throughout the world.

▶ Invasive procedures and the expanded use of immunosuppressive drugs increase the risk of infection for many. (See *When microorganisms grow resistant*, page 4.)

Also, certain factors that normally contribute to improved health, such as good nutrition, clean living conditions, and advanced medical care, can actually lead to increased risk for infection. For example, travel can expose people to diseases against which they have little natural immunity. The increased use of immunosuppressants, as well as surgery and other invasive procedures, also heighten the risk for infection. (See *Sporadic, epidemic, or endemic*, page 5.)

TYPES OF INFECTION

Microorganisms responsible for infectious diseases include bacteria, viruses, fungi (yeasts and molds), and parasites.

Bacteria are single-cell microorganisms with well-defined cell walls that can grow independently on artificial media without the need for other cells. Bacteria inhabit the intestines of humans and other animals as normal flora used in the digestion of food. Also found in soil, bacteria are vital to soil fertility. These microorganisms break down dead tissue, which allows the tissue to be used by other organisms.

Despite the many types of known bacteria, only a small number are harmful to humans. In developing countries, where poor sanitation increases the risk of infection, bacterial diseases commonly cause death and

disability. In industrialized countries, bacterial infections are the most common fatal infectious diseases.

Bacteria are classified by shape. Spherical bacterial cells are called cocci; rod-shaped bacteria, bacilli; and spiral-shaped bacteria, spirilla. Bacteria are also classified according to their response to staining (gram-positive, gram-negative, or acid-fast bacteria); their motility (motile or nonmotile bacteria); their tendency toward encapsulation (encapsulated or nonencapsulated bacteria); and their capacity to form spores (sporulating or nonsporulating bacteria). (See *Comparing bacterial shapes*, page 6.) Viruses are subcellular organisms made up only of a ribonucleic acid or a deoxyribonucleic acid nucleus covered with proteins. They're the smallest known organisms, so tiny they're visible only through an electron microscope. Viruses can't replicate independent of host cells. Rather, they invade a host cell and stimulate it to participate in the formation of additional virus particles. The estimated 400 viruses that infect humans are classified according to their size, shape (spherical, rod-shaped, or cubic), or means of transmission (respiratory, fecal, oral, or sexual). (See *Viral infection of a host cell*, page 7.)

Fungi are single-cell organisms whose nuclei are enveloped by nuclear membranes. They have rigid cell walls like plant cells but lack chlorophyll, the green matter necessary for photosynthesis. They also show relatively little cellular specialization. Fungi occur as yeasts (single-cell, oval-shaped organisms) or molds (organisms with hyphae, or branching filaments). Depending on the environment, some fungi may occur in both forms. Fungal diseases in humans are called *mycoses*.

Parasites are unicellular or multicellular organisms that live in or on their hosts and are dependent on the host for nourishment. They usually only take the nutrients they need and rarely kill their hosts, although they can cause harm. Parasites are divided into two types, depending on their relationship with the host: Endoparasites live inside the

When microorganisms grow resistant

Over the past few decades, many microorganisms have developed resistant strains—those that won't succumb to the antibiotics normally used to combat them. Resistant strains pose serious problems for health care facilities and for the general population because the infections are becoming increasingly more difficult to treat.

Reasons for resistant strains
Practices by health care professionals, patients, and certain industries have contributed to the emergence of resistant bacterial strains. Such practices include:
• Unnecessary use of antibiotics
• Inappropriate prescribing of antibiotics (such as prescribing a drug that doesn't specifically combat the infecting organism)
• Patient failure to complete the full prescribed course of antibiotics
• Use of antibiotics in animal feed
  Contributing to the problem are easy access to over-the-counter antibiotics (in some countries) and symptomless carriers who harbor and spread resistant microorganisms.

From adaptation to resistance
A microorganism develops resistance by continuously adapting to its changing environment in an effort to survive. Through adaptation, some microorganisms have developed the ability to enzymatically destroy an antibiotic, such as by inducing cellular or metabolic changes in target areas. Some bacteria decrease cellular intake of a drug. Others have receptor sites on the bacteria that have less attraction for a drug. New strains of gonococci emerging during the past 25 years are resistant to the antibiotics typically recommended for treating gonorrhea. Penicillin was the drug of choice until a resistant strain developed in 1976; tetracycline-resistant *Neisseria gonorrhoeae*

emerged in 1986. Consequently, eradicating endemic antibiotic-resistant gonorrhea is now difficult.

Hereditary resistance
Hereditary drug resistance is commonly carried by extrachromosomal genetic elements with cell resistance factors. These factors can be transferred among bacterial cells in a population and between different, but closely related, bacterial populations.

Effects of hospitalization
Lengthy hospital stays and frequent hospitalization place some patients at special risk for drug-resistant infections. Most vulnerable are the very young, the very old, the seriously ill, and those requiring invasive equipment. Many of these patients already have weakened immune systems, making them even more susceptible.

Antibiotic therapy
Persons already taking antibiotics are at an increased risk of infection by resistant microorganisms because the antibiotic kills off susceptible microorganisms, allowing resistant strains to take hold.

Striking back
When an outbreak of a resistant microorganism occurs, researchers use molecular typing techniques to identify the microorganism, track it to the source, and contain it. Medicine has managed to stay just ahead of resistant microorganisms. Recently, however, some microorganisms have emerged that are resistant to all antibiotics. Some experts even fear that most infections may eventually result from drug-resistant microorganisms.

host (for example, protozoans, worms, flukes, and amoebae), while ectoparasites live on the host's skin (such as fleas, ticks, and lice).

HOW INFECTION OCCURS

Whether or not an infection develops hinges on variables relating to three crucial factors:

▶ An infectious organism (pathogen)
▶ A host (any organism that can support the nutritional and physical growth of another organism)
▶ A favorable environment
  As long as one of these factors is missing, infection does not occur. However, if an

Sporadic, epidemic, or endemic?

To determine whether an infection problem exists in a particular health care facility or geographic area, investigators study the current incidence of the disease in that facility or area and compare it with past incidence rates.

Sporadic diseases

If investigators find cases occurring occasionally and irregularly with no specific pattern, they classify the infection as sporadic. Examples of diseases that typically occur sporadically are tetanus and gas gangrene.

Epidemic diseases

If a greater-than-expected number of cases of a given disease arise suddenly in a specific area over a specific period, investigators label it an epidemic. A highly publicized epidemic occurred during an American Legion convention in Philadelphia in 1976, resulting in the naming of a new illness, Legionnaire's disease.

A *pandemic* is an epidemic that affects several countries or continents. A current example is the H1N1 influenza pandemic.

Endemic diseases

Endemic diseases are those that are present in a population or community at all times. They usually involve relatively few people during a specified time. Hepatitis B, for example, is endemic in certain Asian cultures.

Herd immunity

When a high proportion of a population has developed immunity to a specific infectious agent, herd immunity exists. For example, thanks to the measles vaccine, the population of the United States has herd immunity to measles, and most Americans are able to resist it.

---

imbalance develops—for example, if a patient's immune system is suppressed and can't fight off pathogens—the potential for infection increases.

Infection starts when a microorganism invades body tissue. Once the microorganism breaches the patient's immune defenses and enters the body, it multiplies and causes harmful effects. The severity of the infection depends on such factors as microbial characteristics, the number of microorganisms present, and the way in which the microorganisms enter the body and spread. (See *The fragile chain of infection*, pages 8–9.)

THE INFLAMMATORY RESPONSE

The body reacts to microbial invasion by producing an inflammatory response. The five classic signs and symptoms of inflammation are as follows:

▶ Redness—Caused by dilation of arterioles and increased circulation to the site; a localized blush caused by filling of previously empty or partially distended capillaries

▶ Pain—Results from stimulation of pain receptors by swollen tissue, local pH changes, and chemicals excreted during the inflammatory process

▶ Heat—Caused by local vasodilation, fluid leakage into the interstitial spaces, and increased blood flow to the area

▶ Swelling—Caused by local vasodilation, leakage of fluid into interstitial spaces, and blockage of lymphatic drainage

▶ Loss of function—Results primarily from pain and edema

Other manifestations of the inflammatory response include fever, malaise, nausea, vomiting, and purulent discharge from wounds.

Not all infections are apparent or symptomatic. With subclinical, or asymptomatic, infection, the infectious microorganism is present and an immune system response is initiated, but the person shows no signs or symptoms of the disease. (See *Types of infection*, page 10.)

Comparing bacterial shapes

Bacteria exist in three basic shapes: rods (bacilli), spheres (cocci), and spirals (spirilla).

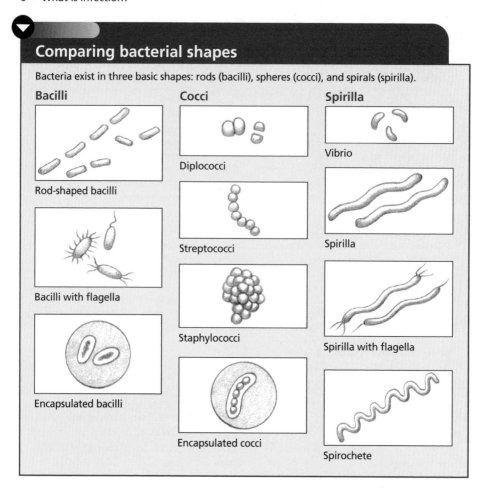

Bacilli

Rod-shaped bacilli

Bacilli with flagella

Encapsulated bacilli

Cocci

Diplococci

Streptococci

Staphylococci

Encapsulated cocci

Spirilla

Vibrio

Spirilla

Spirilla with flagella

Spirochete

ENDOGENOUS AND EXOGENOUS MICROORGANISMS

Microorganisms may be endogenous or exogenous. Endogenous microorganisms are those found on the skin and in such body substances as saliva, feces, and sputum. They can cause disease in a susceptible individual.

Exogenous microorganisms originate from sources outside the body. Humans and exogenous microorganisms usually live together in harmony. However, if something disrupts this harmonious relationship, the microorganisms may cause infection.

INVASION AND COLONIZATION

The presence of microorganisms in or on an individual is called *colonization*. Colonized microorganisms grow and multiply but may not invade tissue and thus don't produce cellular injury. In cases of colonization, tissue culture results are positive but the patient lacks evidence of infection.

However, some people who are colonized with bacteria do develop localized signs and symptoms of infection—tenderness, swelling, redness, and pus—because the bacteria has invaded the tissue, producing cellular injury. A culture of the pus typically elicits the microorganism. Colonized bacteria may also cause systemic infection, producing fever, an elevated white blood cell count, and possibly shock.

PATHOGENICITY

Pathogenicity refers to a microorganism's ability to cause pathogenic changes, or disease. An example of a highly pathogenic microorganism is the rabies virus, which always causes clinical disease in the host. In contrast, alpha-hemolytic streptococci have low pathogenicity; although they commonly colonize humans, they rarely produce clinical disease. Factors affecting pathogenicity include the microorganism's mode of action, virulence, dose, invasiveness, toxigenicity, specificity, viability, and antigenicity.

MODE OF ACTION. The means by which a microorganism produces disease is called its *mode of action.* Viruses, for example, cause infection by invading host cells and interfering with cell metabolism. Other modes of microbial action include:

▶ Evasion or destruction of host defenses by preventing host phagocytes (scavenger cells) from engulfing and digesting them (used by *Klebsiella pneumoniae*)
▶ Secretion of enzymes or toxins, which allows the microorganism to penetrate and spread through host tissue (used by the measles virus)
▶ Production of toxins that interfere with intercellular responses (used by tetanus bacilli)
▶ Stimulation of a pathologic immune response (used by group A beta-hemolytic streptococci)
▶ Destruction of T-helper lymphocytes (used by HIV). (See *Stages of infection,* page 11.)

VIRULENCE. Virulence refers to the degree of a microorganism's pathogenicity. Virulence can vary with the condition of the body's defenses. For instance, *Mycobacterium avium-intracellulare,* bacteria commonly found in water and soil, can cause severe pulmonary and systemic disease in patients with acquired immunodeficiency syndrome but typically do not cause illness in those with a normal immune system. Virulence can be enhanced by several factors:

▶ Toxins produced by bacteria such as *Streptococcus* and *Clostridium*
▶ The ability of microorganisms to elude host defenses (such as *Pneumococcus* with its polysaccharide capsule)

Viral infection of a host cell

The virion becomes attached to receptors on the host cell's plasma membrane and releases enzymes that weaken the membrane, allowing the virion to penetrate the cell.

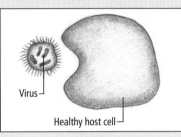

Virus
Healthy host cell

The virion uncoats itself and replicates within the host cell.

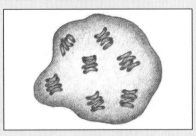

New virus particles mature within the cell and escape by budding from the plasma membrane. The viruses then infect other host cells.

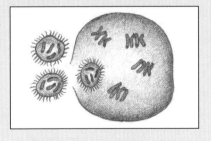

▶ Persistence in the environment (spores and cysts)
▶ Genetic variation (influenza)

DOSE. A microorganism must be present in a sufficient dose to cause human disease. The size of the pathogenic dose varies from one

The fragile chain of infection

An infection can occur only if the six components described here are present. Breaking any of the links in this chain can prevent the infection.

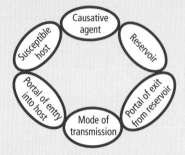

Causative agent

The causative agent for infection is any microorganism that is capable of producing disease. Forms of microorganism responsible for infectious diseases include bacteria, viruses, fungi (yeasts and molds), and parasites.

Reservoir

The reservoir of infection is the environment or object in or on which a microorganism can survive and, in some cases, multiply. Inanimate objects, humans, and other animals can all serve as reservoirs, providing the essential requirements for a microorganism to survive at specific stages in its life cycle. Infectious reservoirs abound in health care settings and may include everything from patients, visitors, and staff members to furniture, medical equipment, medications, food, water, and blood.

Portal of exit from reservoir

The portal of exit is the way the infectious agent leaves its reservoir. Usually, this portal is the site where the microorganism grows. Common portals of exit associated with human reservoirs include the respiratory, genitourinary, and GI tracts; the skin and mucous membranes; and the placenta (in transplacental disease transmission from mother to fetus). Blood, sputum, emesis, stool, urine, wound drainage, and genital secretions also serve as portals of exit.

The portal of exit varies from one infectious agent to the next. For example, the respiratory tract is the portal for the microorganisms that cause tuberculosis and the common cold; the GI tract is the portal for microorganisms that produce typhoid fever.

Mode of transmission

The mode of transmission is the means by which the infectious agent passes from the portal of exit in the reservoir to the susceptible host. Most infectious diseases are transmitted in one of four ways:

• In contact transmission, the susceptible host comes into direct contact (with, for example, blood or body fluids) or indirect contact (with contaminated inanimate objects or by close-range spread of respiratory droplets) with the source. The most common method of contact transmission is contaminated hands.
• Airborne transmission results from the inhalation of contaminated aerosolized droplet nuclei (as in pulmonary tuberculosis).
• Vector-borne transmission occurs when an intermediate carrier (vector), such as a flea, mosquito, or other animal, transfers an organism.
• A vehicle is a substance that maintains the life of the microorganism until it's ingested or inoculated into the susceptible host. The vehicle itself isn't harmful but may harbor pathogenic microorganisms and thus serve as an agent of disease transmission.

Many actions can be taken to prevent the transmission of infectious diseases, including the following:
• Comprehensive immunization (including required immunization of travelers to, or emigrants from, endemic areas)
• Drug prophylaxis
• Good nutrition, healthy living conditions, and proper sanitation
• Correction of environmental factors
• Widespread disease tracking

Immunizations can now control many diseases, including diphtheria, pertussis, measles, rubella, some forms of meningitis, poliovirus, hepatitis B, pneumococcal pneumonia, influenza, rabies, and tetanus. Smallpox (variola)—which has killed and disfigured millions—was believed to have been

The fragile chain of infection *(continued)*

successfully eradicated by a comprehensive World Health Organization program of surveillance and immunization. However, in light of recent concerns regarding bioterrorism, smallpox is now considered a viable terror threat. Health care personnel must recognize potential cases of smallpox and initiate appropriate precautions as well as notify health department officials. Smallpox vaccination may be appropriate for certain emergency and first-response health care providers.

Although preventive antibiotic therapy may thwart certain diseases, the risk of super-infection and the emergence of drug-resistant strains may outweigh the benefits. Therefore, preventive antibiotics are usually reserved for patients at high risk for exposure to dangerous infections. Antibiotic-resistant bacteria are on the rise mainly because antibiotics have been misused and overused. Some bacteria, such as enterococci, have developed mutant strains that don't respond to antibiotic therapy.

Portal of entry into host
The portal of entry refers to the way a microorganism invades a susceptible person.

The portal of entry is usually the same as the portal of exit. Typical portals of entry for specific microorganisms include the following:
• The microorganisms that cause tuberculosis, common colds, diphtheria, influenza, and whooping cough enter through the respiratory tract.
• Hepatitis B virus and HIV enter through the bloodstream or body fluids.
• *Salmonella* enters through the GI tract.
• The microorganisms responsible for gonorrhea and syphilis enter through the mucous membranes (usually those of the genitourinary tract).
• Rabies virus and *Clostridium tetani* (the microorganism that causes tetanus) enter the body through puncture wounds.

Susceptible host
The human body has many defenses against the entry and multiplication of microorganisms. When these defenses function normally, infection does not occur. However, in a weakened host, a microorganism is more likely to be successful in invading the body and launching an infectious disease.

---

microorganism to the next and from person to person and may be affected by the mode of transmission. The patient's immune system also plays an important role in the pathogenic dose requirement.

In order to cause diarrhea, the infective dose of *Shigella* is approximately 10 microorganisms, whereas the infective dose of *Salmonella* required to cause typhoid fever is 1,000 microorganisms. A lower infective dose does not necessarily imply that the organism causes more severe immediate disease.

INVASIVENESS. Invasiveness (sometimes called infectivity) refers to the ability of a microorganism to invade tissue. Some microorganisms can enter the human body through intact skin; others can penetrate only through a break in the skin or mucous

membranes. *Leptospira interrogans* usually enters the body through a minor skin abrasion; *Clostridium tetani*, through a deep puncture wound. The invasiveness of some microorganisms is increased by the enzymes they produce.

TOXIGENICITY. Toxigenicity, which is related to virulence, refers to a microorganism's potential to damage host tissue by producing and releasing toxins. Some bacteria, such as diphtheria and tetanus, release exotoxins that are quickly disseminated in the blood, causing systemic and neurologic manifestations. Other bacteria, such as *Shigella*, release endotoxins that can cause diarrhea and shock.

SPECIFICITY. Specificity refers to the attraction of a microorganism to a specific host or range of hosts. For example, the flavivirus that causes St. Louis encephalitis has a

Types of infection

A laboratory-verified infection that causes no signs or symptoms is called a *subclinical, silent,* or *asymptomatic infection.* A multiplication of microorganisms that produces no signs, symptoms, or immune response is called a *colonization.* A person with a subclinical infection or colonization may be a carrier and transmit infection to others.

A *latent infection* occurs after a microorganism has been dormant in the host, sometimes for years. An *exogenous infection* results from environmental pathogens; an *endogenous infection,* from the host's normal flora (for instance, *Escherichia coli* displaced from the colon may cause urinary tract infection).

number of hosts, including birds and humans; whereas rubeola, the virus that causes measles, is carried only by humans.

VIABILITY. Viability refers to the ability of a microorganism to survive outside the host. Microorganisms can live and multiply in a reservoir, which provides what the microorganisms need to survive. The microorganisms can then be transmitted from the reservoir to another person.

ANTIGENICITY. Antigenicity, the degree to which a microorganism can induce a specific immune response, varies among microorganisms. Those that invade and localize in tissue initially stimulate a cellular response, whereas those that disseminate more quickly generate an antibody response.

Defense mechanisms

There are two kinds of defense mechanisms against infection: first-line and second-line.

FIRST-LINE DEFENSES

External and mechanical barriers (such as the skin, other body organs, and secretions) function as the body's first line of defense.

Intact skin and mucous membranes, certain chemical substances, specialized structures such as cilia, and normal microbial flora can prevent pathogens from establishing themselves in the body. The gag and cough reflexes and GI tract peristalsis work to remove pathogens before they can establish a foothold. Chemical substances that help prevent infection or inhibit microbial growth include secretions such as saliva, perspiration, and GI and vaginal secretions.

Microbial antagonism is a mechanism by which normal flora controls the growth of potential pathogens. In this mechanism, the normal flora uses nutrients that pathogens need for growth, competes with pathogens for sites on tissue receptors, and secretes naturally occurring antibiotics to kill the pathogens. When microbial antagonism is disrupted, an infection may develop; for example, antibiotic therapy may destroy the normal flora of the mouth, leading to overgrowth of *Candida albicans* and the development of thrush.

SECOND-LINE DEFENSES

If a microorganism gets past the first line of defense, the body reacts by producing an inflammatory response. These responses are called "nonspecific" because they respond to any type of injury.

The main function of the inflammatory response is to bring phagocytic cells (neutrophils and monocytes) to the inflamed area to destroy the invading microorganisms and remove the dead and dying cells from tissue spaces so that tissue repair can take place. Inflammation produces five primary signs and symptoms: redness, swelling, pain, heat, and loss of function. The first three result from local vasodilation, fluid leakage into extravascular spaces, and blockage of lymphatic drainage. Pain results from tissue space distention caused by swelling and pressure and from chemical irritation of nociceptors (pain receptors). Pain and edema lead to loss of function.

By raising the body's temperature, fever defends against infection by enabling host defenses to inhibit the growth of pathogens. Certain microorganisms, such as *Cryptococcus*, are unable to replicate at body temperatures above 100.4° F (38.7° C).

If a pathogen gets past the body's nonspecific defenses, it then confronts specific immune responses in the form of cell-mediated immunity or humoral immunity. Cell-mediated immunity involves T cells (a type of white blood cell). Some T cells synthesize and secrete lymphokines, whereas others become killer (cytotoxic) cells, hunting down infected body cells. Once the infection is under control, suppressor T cells bring the immune response to a close.

Humoral immunity, which is mediated by antibodies, involves the action of B lymphocytes in conjunction with helper T cells. Antibodies produced in response to the infectious agent help fight the infection. In response to the effects of suppressor T-cell activity, antibody production then diminishes.

WHEN DEFENSES ARE IMPAIRED

Impaired host defenses can invite infection. Conditions that may weaken a person's defenses include poor hygiene, malnutrition, extremes of age, climate, inadequate physical barriers, inherited and acquired immune deficiencies, emotional and physical stressors, chronic disease, medical and surgical treatments, and inadequate immunization.

HYGIENE. Poor hygiene increases the risk of infection because untended skin is more likely to crack and break, allowing microorganisms to enter. Also, dirty skin harbors transient microorganisms, and microbial colonization of the skin increases.

Good hygiene promotes normal host defenses. Washing (and using topical moisturizers, if necessary) lubricates the skin and protects the epidermis against breaks. Removing microbial buildup on clothing through frequent laundering is another important step in controlling infection.

NUTRITION. The body produces antibodies from proteins, which are obtained through nutritional intake. With inadequate protein, a malnourished person lacks the energy to

Stages of infection

Stage I: Incubation
• Duration can range from instantaneous to several years.
• Pathogen is replicating, and the infected person becomes contagious, thus capable of transmitting the disease.

Stage II: Prodromal stage
• Host makes vague complaints of feeling unwell.
• Host is still contagious.

Stage III: Acute illness
• Microorganisms actively destroy host cells and affect specific host systems.
• Patient recognizes which area of the body is affected.
• Complaints are more specific.

Stage IV: Convalescence
• Begins when the body's defense mechanisms have contained the microorganisms.
• Damaged tissue is healing.

mount an adequate attack against invading organisms. In addition, many nutrients (such as zinc, selenium, and vitamins A and E) are necessary for an optimal immune system response.

AGE. The very young and the very old are at higher risk for infection. The immune system doesn't fully develop until about age 6 months. During the infant's first exposure to an infectious agent, the infection usually wins out—especially if it's an upper respiratory infection, the most common type among infants and toddlers. Also, toddlers tend to put toys and other objects in their mouths, play in the dirt, or soil their clothes with urine and feces, bringing further exposure to microorganisms.

Exposure to communicable diseases continues throughout childhood. Preschoolers are exposed in day-care facilities; school-age children are exposed in school. Skin diseases, such as impetigo and lice (scabies), commonly travel from one child to the next.

Childhood accidents, such as abrasions, lacerations, and fractures, may also allow microorganisms to enter the body.

Lack of immunization contributes to childhood infection. Measles, virtually eradicated in the United States by the measles vaccine several decades ago, resurfaced in community outbreaks in 2008. Its revival has been linked to unvaccinated individuals, many of whom were children whose parents chose not to have them vaccinated. Most cases of measles occurring in the United States are imported from endemic areas.

At the opposite end of the age spectrum, advancing age is associated with weakened immune system function as well as with chronic diseases that reduce host defenses. What's more, the increased use of long-term care facilities, such as nursing homes and personal care units, has added to the risk of disease transmission among the elderly.

Infection in health care facilities

In health care facilities, patients of all ages stand a higher chance of developing an infection. Invasive procedures and devices, drugs that suppress the immune system, increased use of blood products, and inhalation therapy add to the potential threat. Heroic techniques such as massive radical surgery with prolonged anesthesia and organ transplants also place tremendous stress on the patient's immune system. Likewise, poor aseptic technique by health care providers also increases the risk of infection.

CLASSIFICATION

Infections among patients in health care facilities are classified as health care–associated, community-acquired, or iatrogenic infections.

▶ A *health care–associated infection* is an infection that develops during the patient's hospital stay and was not present or incubating at the time of admission. Most health

care–associated infections appear before the patient is discharged, although some (such as hepatitis B and surgical wound infections) typically are incubating at discharge but don't become apparent until later. Health care–associated infections can also occur in patients who undergo outpatient procedures.

▶ A *community-acquired infection* is one that is present or incubating at the time of encounter with the health care system in a patient who has no history of being treated in the same facility.

▶ An *iatrogenic infection* is caused by the actions or treatments of a health care provider. Such an infection may also represent a secondary condition caused by treatment of a primary condition. Depending on when an iatrogenic infection develops, it may be health care associated or community acquired.

HEALTH CARE–ASSOCIATED INFECTIONS

Every year, 5% to 10% of hospitalized patients in the United States develop health care–associated infections. Health care–associated infections are estimated to more than double the mortality and morbidity risks of any admitted patient and probably result in as many as 90,000 deaths per year in the United States. Costs for diagnosing and treating these infections reach billions of dollars annually. The longer a patient remains in the hospital, the greater his or her chance will be for developing a health care–associated infection.

The microorganisms that flourish in health care settings, along with patients' weakened defense mechanisms, help set the stage for health care–associated infections. The microorganisms responsible for health care–associated infections may be either endogenous (from normal flora) or exogenous (from external sources). (See *A dangerous combination.*)

Invasion sites

Health care–associated infections most commonly invade the body through the urinary tract. Other common portals of entry include surgical wounds, the respiratory tract, and the bloodstream.

URINARY TRACT. Urinary tract infections (UTIs) are the most common health care–associated infections in the United States, accounting for 35% to 45% of reported cases and affecting an estimated 600,000 patients each year. Of these infections, 80% follow introduction of instrumentation into the urinary tract, primarily indwelling urinary catheters. Health care–associated UTIs may lengthen a patient's hospital stay and are costly to treat. It is estimated that the annual cost of health care–associated UTIs in the United States ranges from $424 to $451 million.

Normal bowel flora is also implicated in UTIs. These microorganisms can gain access to the urinary tract through the use of contaminated equipment or irrigant solutions, through inadequate cleaning at the time of catheter insertion, or from the unwashed hands of health care providers.

RESPIRATORY SYSTEM. Most respiratory health care–associated infections are linked to respiratory devices used to aid breathing or administer medications. Pneumonia is the second most common health care–associated infection in the United States. It is also the most dangerous, causing more deaths than any other type of health care–associated infection. For those who become infected while in the intensive care unit, pneumonia is the primary cause of death. Respiratory system–related infections typically lengthen a patient's hospital stay by 1 to 2 weeks and add billions to U.S. health care costs every year.

Health care–associated pneumonia most commonly stems from gram-negative bacteria, although it can also result from other bacteria, fungi, and viruses. Typically, the pathogen invades the lower respiratory tract by one of three routes:

▶ Aspiration of oropharyngeal organisms
▶ Colonization of the aerodigestive tract
▶ Use of contaminated equipment or medications

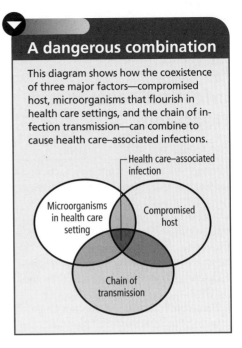

A dangerous combination

This diagram shows how the coexistence of three major factors—compromised host, microorganisms that flourish in health care settings, and the chain of infection transmission—can combine to cause health care–associated infections.

Health care–associated infection

Microorganisms in health care setting

Compromised host

Chain of transmission

SURGICAL WOUNDS. The third most common type of health care–associated infection, accounting for about 25% of cases, are surgical wound infections. Occurring in about 2% to 5% of surgical patients, these infections lengthen hospital stays by about 6 days.

Surgical wound infections can occur in the incision as well as in the deep tissue of a wound. Most are thought to originate from bacteria that enter the wound during surgery.

BLOODSTREAM. Called bacteremia, health care–associated infections of the bloodstream account for about 6% of health care–associated infections, although this number is decreasing due to recent initiatives. Bacteria and fungi are common culprits. Although local infections outside the bloodstream are sometimes the source of the infection, more than 75% of bacteremias seen in hospitals are related to intravascular devices such as I.V. catheters. Microorganisms can move from the patient's skin to the catheter tip and along the outer surface of the catheter and then enter the bloodstream. The sicker a patient is, the more central and peripheral lines he or she is likely to have, bringing more opportunities for microorganisms to invade the bloodstream.

Infection control and treatment

BREAKING THE WEAKEST LINK

The best way to control infections is to break the weakest link in the chain of infection (usually the mode of transmission). Many strategies exist to prevent or control the transmission of infectious agents, and they fall into four general categories:
▶ Control or elimination of infectious agents by appropriate sanitation, disinfection, and sterilization
▶ Control of transmission through proper hand hygiene, effective ventilation, and aseptic technique
▶ Reservoir control. In health care settings, a number of interventions are directed at controlling or destroying infectious reservoirs:
- Using disposable equipment and supplies whenever possible
- Disinfecting or sterilizing equipment as soon as possible after use
- Using appropriate equipment for each patient
- Handling and disposing of patient secretions, excretions, and exudates properly
- Helping to identify and treat persons who are infection carriers. To help reduce the number of reservoirs in both the community and the health care setting, patients should be encouraged to obtain active and passive immunizations, to practice positive health behaviors, to avoid high-risk behavior, and to maintain first-line defenses.
▶ Isolating infected patients, according to Centers for Disease Control and Prevention (CDC) recommendations, to limit the chance that they will transmit the infection

TREATMENT

Treatment for infections can vary widely. Vaccines may be administered to induce a primary immune response under conditions that won't cause disease. If infection occurs, treatment is tailored to the specific microorganism causing the infection. Drug therapy should only be used when appropriate. Supportive therapy can play an important role in fighting infections.
▶ Antibiotics work in a variety of ways, depending on the class of drug used. Antibiotic action is either bactericidal or bacteriostatic. Antibiotics may inhibit cell wall synthesis, protein synthesis, bacterial metabolism, or nucleic acid synthesis or activity, or they may increase cell membrane permeability.
▶ Antifungal drugs destroy the invading microorganism by increasing cell membrane permeability. The antifungal binds sterols in the cell membrane, resulting in leakage of intracellular contents, such as potassium, sodium, and nutrients.
▶ Antiviral drugs stop viral replication by interfering with DNA synthesis.

Bacterial resistance

Certain gram-positive microorganisms have become resistant to many of the antimicrobial drugs previously used to treat them. Resistant microbial strains that pose a serious challenge to health care facilities (especially acute-care hospitals and long-term care facilities) include methicillin-resistant *Staphylococcus aureus* (MRSA), resistant *Streptococcus pneumoniae*, and vancomycin-resistant *Enterococcus* (VRE). These strains, which are rapidly becoming part of the flora in many health care facilities, must be controlled to prevent health care–associated infections. (See *Mechanisms of resistance*.)

RESISTANT *S. AUREUS* INFECTIONS

S. aureus commonly occurs on the skin without producing any disease, but it can produce a variety of signs and symptoms ranging from a skin pustule to bloodstream infections to death. It's also a frequent cause of pneumonia, septicemia, and surgical site infections in hospitalized patients. Disease can also be caused by community-associated infections.

Methicillin is an antibiotic commonly used to treat staphylococcal (staph) infections. Although methicillin is very effective in treating most staph infections, some staph bacteria have developed resistance to methicillin and can no longer be killed by this antibiotic. According to the CDC, MRSA infections accounted for 2% of all staph infections in 1974, 22% in 1995, and 63% in 2004.

The antibiotic used to treat MRSA infections is vancomycin. However, in 1996, an infection caused by a strain of *S. aureus* with reduced susceptibility to vancomycin was diagnosed in a patient in Japan. This strain of *S. aureus* was referred to as vancomycin-intermediate-resistant *S. aureus* (VISA). Since then, several more infections with VISA have been identified.

A great concern among infectious disease experts is the emergence of a strain of *S. aureus* with full resistance to vancomycin. This could leave doctors with no antibiotics for the treatment of *S. aureus* infections.

Some persons are asymptomatic carriers of resistant *S. aureus*, with colonies in the nose and on the skin. The infection spreads from patient to patient, mainly on the hands of health care providers as they become contaminated during patient care. Appropriate control measures to prevent the spread of MRSA and VISA include strict hand hygiene, barrier protection (gloves, gowns, and masks), and contact precautions.

RESISTANT *S. PNEUMONIAE* INFECTIONS

S. pneumoniae is the most common cause of bacterial pneumonia in the United States and is a major cause of ear infections, sinusitis, bloodstream infections, and meningitis. Until 2000, *S. pneumoniae* infections caused 100,000 to 135,000 hospitalizations for pneumonia, 6 million cases of otitis media, and 60,000 cases of invasive disease, including 3,300 cases of meningitis. Disease figures

Mechanisms of resistance

Bacteria become resistant to antibiotics through several known mechanisms.

Natural resistance
Within a bacterial population, some microorganisms may have a natural resistance to a certain antibiotic. If so, the antibiotic will eliminate the sensitive microorganism, leaving the resistant ones to proliferate. This is especially likely to occur in health care facilities.

Mutant resistance
Within a population of bacteria, resistant mutants may arise spontaneously and then proliferate as described above.

Genetic resistance
Drug resistance may be transferred from one microorganism to another through the exchange of genes, called plasmids, that confer such resistance.

are now decreasing due to the introduction of a conjugate vaccine.

The emergence of drug-resistant *S. pneumoniae* has complicated the treatment of these infections. Infections involving these microorganisms may eventually necessitate treatment with costly broad-spectrum antibiotics.

VRE INFECTIONS

Enterococci exist as part of the normal flora of the GI tract and female genital tract. Most enterococcal infections can be traced to endogenous sources. However, in the health care setting, patient-to-patient transmission of *Enterococcus* can occur through direct contact with the hands of health care workers or indirectly through contaminated surfaces. This highlights the need for strict adherence to infection control measures such as hand hygiene and the use of gowns, gloves, and disinfectants.

Responsible for a rising number of health care–associated infections over the past 5 years, VRE is of great concern among infectious disease specialists today. Doctors lack effective antibiotics to treat these infections; most VRE microorganisms also resist other drugs used against enterococcal infections. Also, there's a possibility that vancomycin-resistant genes present in the microorganisms may be transferred to other gram-positive microorganisms such as *S. aureus.*

The risk of VRE colonization and infection is associated with the following conditions:

▶ Previous vancomycin therapy, multiple antimicrobial therapy, or both
▶ Severe underlying disease
▶ Immunosuppression
▶ Intra-abdominal or cardiac surgery

COMBATING RESISTANT ORGANISMS

In the past, medicine has been able to stay a step ahead of resistant strains thanks to the development of new drugs. Today, however, we may be losing the battle. This makes education—of both health care professionals and the public at large—the best weapon against the spread of resistant bacteria. (See *CDC Hand Hygiene Guidelines Fact Sheet.*)

Teaching efforts should center on proper antibiotic use as well as on hand hygiene and other measures that reduce the risk of transmission.

USING ANTIBIOTICS PROPERLY. Not all bacterial infections warrant antibiotics. Doctors and other professionals with prescribing power must prescribe antibiotics only when warranted. Also, whenever possible, an exact bacteriologic or antigenic diagnosis should be made before antibiotic treatment begins to avoid inappropriate drug therapy, which promotes drug resistance.

PROMOTING PATIENT COMPLIANCE. If your patient has been prescribed antibiotics, emphasize the importance of completing the entire course of therapy exactly as prescribed, even if the patient feels better. Caution against storing antibiotics in medicine cabinets, where they could deteriorate from heat, and warn patients never to take antibiotics that have been prescribed for another person.

REDUCING THE TRANSMISSION RISK. Keep in mind that MRSA is usually carried on the hands. *Enterococcus* species are present in the bowel, and VRE lives on bed rails and equipment. Because these organisms can be spread to patients from your hands, wash your hands thoroughly and frequently—not just between patients but also between care activities involving the same patient.

BARRIER PRECAUTIONS. Besides handwashing, precautions that reduce the risk of transmission include use of protective gear when appropriate. Gloves provide a physical barrier between the hands and the patient's skin and mucous membranes.

To avoid transferring an organism from one site to another on the same patient, always use a clean pair of gloves for each patient care activity. To protect yourself, be sure to wash your hands after removing gloves.

Gowns and aprons protect your clothing while providing a barrier against organisms. A mask and protective eyewear guard your face against anticipated splashes of blood and body fluids.

CDC Hand Hygiene Guidelines Fact Sheet

The CDC has released these guidelines to improve adherence to hand hygiene in health care settings.

• Improved adherence to hand hygiene (that is, handwashing or use of alcohol-based hand rubs) has been shown to terminate infection outbreaks in health care facilities, reduce transmission of antimicrobial-resistant organisms, such as MRSA, and reduce overall infection rates.

• In addition to traditional handwashing with soap and water, the CDC recommends the use of alcohol-based hand rubs by health care personnel for patient care because these products address some of the obstacles that health care professionals face when caring for patients.

• Handwashing with soap and water remains a sensible strategy for hand hygiene in non–health care settings and is recommended by the CDC and other experts.

• Health care personnel should wash with soap and water when their hands are visibly soiled.

• The use of gloves does not eliminate the need for hand hygiene. Likewise, the use of hand hygiene does not eliminate the need for gloves. Gloves reduce hand contamination by 70% to 80%, prevent cross-contamination, and protect patients and health care personnel from infection. Hand rubs should be used before and after contact with each patient just as gloves should be changed before and after contact with each patient.

• When using an alcohol-based hand rub, the product should be applied to the palm of one hand. The hands and fingers should then be rubbed together, covering all surfaces, until hands are dry. Note that the volume needed to reduce the number of bacteria on hands varies by product.

• Alcohol-based hand rubs significantly reduce the number of microorganisms on the skin, are fast acting, and are less likely to cause skin irritation.

• Health care personnel who care for patients who are at high risk of acquiring infections, such as those in intensive care units or in transplant units, should avoid wearing artificial nails and keep natural nails less than a quarter-inch long. When evaluating hand hygiene products for potential use in health care facilities, administrators or product selection committees should consider the relative efficacy of antiseptic agents against various pathogens and the acceptability of hand hygiene products by personnel. Characteristics of a product that can affect acceptance and therefore usage include its smell, consistency, and color as well as its effect on the skin, particularly skin dryness.

• As part of its recommendations, the CDC is asking health care facilities to develop and implement a system for measuring improvements in adherence to these hand hygiene guidelines. Some of the suggested performance indicators include periodic monitoring of hand hygiene adherence and providing feedback to personnel regarding their performance, monitoring the volume of alcohol-based hand rub used per 1,000 patient-days, monitoring adherence to policies dealing with wearing artificial nails, and diligently assessing the adequacy of health care personnel hand hygiene when outbreaks of infection occur.

• Allergic contact dermatitis due to alcohol hand rubs is very uncommon. However, with increasing use of such products by health care personnel, it is likely that true allergic reactions will occasionally be encountered.

• Cleansing with alcohol-based hand rubs takes less time than traditional handwashing. In an 8-hour shift, an estimated 1 hour of an ICU nurse's time will be saved by using an alcohol-based hand rub.

• The guidelines should not be construed to legalize product claims that are not allowed by a Food and Drug Administration (FDA) product approval according to the FDA's *Over-the-Counter Drug Review*, nor are they intended to apply to consumer use of the products discussed.

Source: Centers for Disease Control and Prevention. (October 25, 2002). Hand hygiene fact sheet. Office of Communication, Division of Media Relations. http://cdc.gov/media/pressrel/fs021025.htm

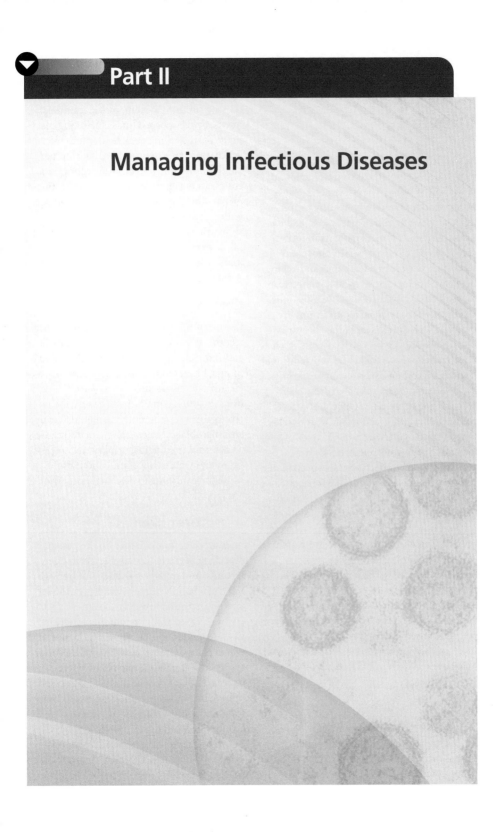

Part II

Managing Infectious Diseases

CONTACT PRECAUTIONS

Acinetobacter Infection

Acinetobacter is a group of gram-negative, nonmotile bacteria most commonly found in the soil or water. The bacteria have also been found on the skin of healthy people—especially health care providers. *Acinetobacter* most often colonizes patients in intensive care units (ICUs), particularly those with devices such as endotracheal tubes, indwelling urinary catheters, intravascular catheters, or surgical drains. It can also cause infections. Outbreaks of *Acinetobacter* infections are typically seen in ICUs and other health care settings that house very sick patients, such as hospice facilities, as well as in nontraditional health care settings, such as nursing homes. *Acinetobacter* infections have rarely been seen outside these areas. Once the bacteria are introduced in a facility, serial or overlapping outbreaks often occur as a result of various multidrug-resistant strains.

Acinetobacter infections have been clinically prominent in hot, humid areas, such as tropical regions, and are a recurrent problem during times of war and natural disaster. Recently, *Acinetobacter* infection has been reported in Europe, Asia, and North America, including among U.S. military members injured in the Middle East. There are at least 25 types of *Acinetobacter*, all of which can cause disease in humans. However, these bacteria cause little risk to healthy people. Those with weakened immune systems, chronic lung disease, or diabetes may be more susceptible to *Acinetobacter* infection.

CAUSES

Acinetobacter infections are rapidly emerging health care–associated infections. The microorganism is often cultured from the sputum, wounds, and urine of hospitalized individuals who have been either colonized or infected. It also can be a source of contamination of irrigating solutions and I.V. solutions. Risk factors include advanced age, serious underlying conditions, a suppressed immune system, major trauma or burns, invasive procedures (including placement of indwelling catheters), mechanical ventilation, an extended hospital stay, parenteral nutrition, and administration of a course of antibiotics. *Acinetobacter* is spread by person-to-person contact or by contact with a contaminated surface. Research shows that outbreaks occur more frequently in the summer months. *Acinetobacter baumannii* accounts for about 80% of reported *Acinetobacter* infections.

COMPLICATIONS

Colonization with *Acinetobacter* precedes infection. The respiratory system is the most common site for infection, including pneumonia, bronchiolitis, and tracheobronchitis. Health care–associated *Acinetobacter* infections are often complicated because the microorganism is inherently resistant to many antimicrobials. *Acinetobacter* can also cause bacteremia, meningitis, urinary tract infections, and wound infections, and it can cause or contribute to death in those who are very ill.

ASSESSMENT FINDINGS

Acinetobacter may colonize on the patient, especially at tracheostomy sites or in open wounds, and in the urine and sputum without causing infection or symptoms. However, this microorganism can also cause a variety of diseases, from pneumonia to serious wound and blood infections. The symptoms will depend on the system involved. Typical symptoms of pneumonia include fever, chills, cough, or change in oxygenation requirements. A wound infection might cause fever and redness, increasing pain, and pus around the wound.

According to the National Nosocomial Infection Surveillance System, *Acinetobacter* species caused 7% of ICU-related health care–associated pneumonias in 2003 compared with 4% in 1986.

DIAGNOSTIC TESTS

▶ *Acinetobacter* will grow in cultures from respiratory secretions, wounds, or urine. In order to differentiate between colonization and infection, culture results must be evaluated in conjunction with signs and symptoms.

▶ Chest radiography, magnetic resonance imaging, and computed tomography may define the extent of pneumonia.

▶ Cerebrospinal fluid culture is necessary if *Acinetobacter*-associated meningitis is suspected. A positive result will reveal *Acinetobacter*.

TREATMENT

Consultation with an infectious disease specialist is recommended to differentiate between bacterial colonization and infection as well as for antibiotic recommendations if an infection is present. In general, *Acinetobacter* strains are often resistant to many commonly prescribed antibiotics, making infection difficult to treat. Finding an effective treatment can be a formidable challenge; therefore, treatment decisions should be made on an individual basis.

Traditionally, imipenem (Primaxin) has been used, although outbreaks of imipenem-resistant *Acinetobacter* infections have occurred. The combination of ampicillin and sulbactam (Unasyn) has also been used effectively in many multidrug-resistant strains of *Acinetobacter*, but it is becoming less effective as the microorganism develops new mechanisms of resistance. Polymyxins are proving to be a promising new group in the treatment of *Acinetobacter* infection. Other antimicrobials may include meropenem (Merrem), amikacin (Amikin), or tigecycline (Tygacil). Treatment with one drug may be effective for mild to moderate infections; however, more serious infections will need to be treated with combination therapy. Bactericidal synergy has been witnessed when several antimicrobials are combined with an aminoglycoside.

If the infection is present in localized cellulitis or phlebitis associated with a foreign body, it may be sufficient to remove the foreign body and treat the infection locally. Pulmonary hygiene alone may resolve tracheobronchitis after endotracheal intubation.

NURSING CONSIDERATIONS

 Contact precautions should be used to prevent the spread of the microorganism, particularly in the ICU setting.

▶ Although *Acinetobacter* colonization does not necessarily lead to infection, it does precede infection. Colonization in one patient may lead to infection in another. Colonized patients should be isolated to prevent colonization in other patients.

▶ When possible, group colonized or infected patients together.

▶ Practice aseptic care of vascular and endotracheal tubes, and remove tubes as soon as they are no longer clinically indicated.

▶ Ensure proper cleaning and disinfection of equipment (especially mechanical ventilators and other respiratory equipment) between patient uses.

▶ Ensure frequent environmental cleaning of high-touch surfaces in patient rooms.

 SAFETY An alcohol-based hand sanitizer is more effective in killing bacteria than is handwashing with soap and water. Wash with soap and water if hands are obviously soiled.

Patient teaching

▶ Because *Acinetobacter* is spread by direct contact, teach the patient good handwashing technique to prevent transmission.

▶ Instruct the patient about good environmental cleaning to prevent the spread of *Acinetobacter* because the microorganisms can live in the environment for several days.

▶ Avoid touching bed rails, bedside tables, I.V. pumps, and other equipment when visiting an infected patient.

SAFETY Because *Acinetobacter* can live on skin and dry surfaces for several days, proper hand hygiene and environmental cleaning can reduce the risk of transmission.

Actinomycosis

Actinomycosis is a subacute-chronic bacterial infection primarily caused by the gram-positive anaerobic bacillus *Actinomyces israelii*, which produces granulomatous and suppurative lesions with multiple abscesses. Common sites for infection are the head, neck, thorax, and abdomen, but it can spread to contiguous tissue as well, causing multiple draining sinuses that may discharge sulfur granules.

CAUSES

A. israelii occurs as part of the normal anaerobic flora of the throat, tonsillar crypts, and mouth (particularly around carious teeth). *Actinomyces* may also be found in the membranes lining the intestines and vagina. Infection results from introduction of the bacteria into body tissue by a break in the integrity of the mucous membranes or weakened tissue of deeper body structures.

In cervicofacial actinomycosis ("lumpy jaw"), dental extraction or trauma to the mouth, poor dental hygiene, or periodontal disease may cause infection. Neoplasms or osteonecrosis of the jaw from radiation treatments may also be a cause. The infection may spread to the brain or bloodstream if left untreated. Cervicofacial actinomycosis is the most common type of *Actinomyces* infection, comprising 50% to 70% of reported cases. (See *Cervicofacial actinomycosis.*)

Pulmonary actinomycosis is typically caused by aspiration of bacteria from the mouth into areas of the lungs that are already anaerobic from infection or atelectasis.

In GI actinomycosis, intestinal mucosa disruption (usually by bowel surgery), ingestion of foreign bodies such as chicken bones, and inflammatory bowel conditions such as appendicitis are the most common causes of infection. Sometimes, esophageal perforation can result in infection with *Actinomyces.* Eventually, empyema follows, a sinus forms through the chest wall, and septicemia may occur.

COMPLICATIONS

The complications of actinomycosis vary, depending on the site of infection. Cervicofacial actinomycosis may progress to involve sinus and maxillofacial subcutaneous tissue. Abscesses and fistulas of the brain may also result. When the respiratory system is affected, the patient may develop pneumonia and empyema. Septicemia may occur if the infection is left untreated. Endocarditis is another reported complication, as is osteomyelitis of the jaw, ribs, and vertebrae.

ASSESSMENT FINDINGS

Symptoms appear days to months after injury and may vary, depending on the site.

In cervicofacial actinomycosis, painful, indurated swellings appear in the mouth or neck, making chewing difficult and causing a fever. The swellings gradually enlarge and form fistulas that open onto the skin. The skin overlying the swelling becomes reddish or bluish. Adjacent tissue becomes infected over time. Sulfur granules (yellowish gray masses that are actually colonies of *A. israelii*) appear in the exudate.

Pulmonary actinomycosis produces a fever and a cough that becomes productive and occasionally causes hemoptysis. The patient may have chest pain and shortness of breath. Abnormal lung sounds, weight loss, and fatigue would be expected.

GI actinomycosis produces abdominal discomfort, fever, a palpable mass, and an external sinus. Symptoms reflect the organ involved but usually are similar to those of a slow-growing tumor.

Rare sites of actinomycotic infection are the bones, brain, liver, kidneys, and female reproductive organs.

DIAGNOSTIC TESTS

▶ Culture of the tissue or aspirated exudate will grow *A. israelii* (the specimen must be collected and transported anaerobically).

Cervicofacial actinomycosis

Cervicofacial actinomycosis is an infection that most commonly affects the head and neck and occurs more frequently in adult men. *Actinomyces* are part of the normal flora of the mouth. Infection is characterized by painful swellings in the mouth or on the neck. Eventually, these areas swell to the point of fistula formation. These fistulas then open onto the skin.

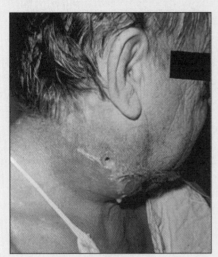

Initial presentation as a large fluctuant mass at the angle of the jaw.

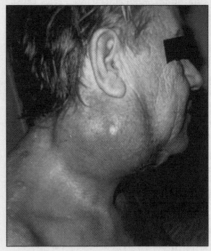

The same mass with induration and a sinus tract.

▶ Chest radiography or computed tomography may reveal a poorly defined masslike lesion or abscess.

▶ A complete blood count may reveal anemia and mild leukocytosis, elevated erythrocyte sedimentation rate and C-reactive protein, and normal chemistries with the exception of an elevated phosphatase level in the presence of hepatic actinomycosis.

 ALERT Proper collection of specimens and prompt transport to the laboratory, preferably in an anaerobic transport device, are imperative for optimal isolation of the microorganism.

TREATMENT

In most cases, antibiotic therapy is the only treatment required. Treatment is long term, with 1 to 2 months of penicillin I.V. followed by 6 to 12 months of penicillin taken by mouth. Occasionally, surgical drainage of the lesion may be required.

NURSING CONSIDERATIONS

▶ Dispose of all dressings in a sealed plastic bag to prevent the spread of infection.

▶ Provide proper aseptic wound management following surgical procedures.

▶ Administer antibiotics as ordered. Watch for hypersensitivity reactions.

Patient teaching

▶ The regimen of antibiotics must be taken as prescribed and until it is finished.

▶ If surgical drainage was necessary, teach the patient and the patient's family how to properly care for the wound.

▶ Explain to the patient the importance of good oral hygiene.

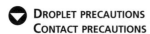

▼ DROPLET PRECAUTIONS
CONTACT PRECAUTIONS

Adenovirus Infection

Adenoviruses are a group of viruses that infect the tissue lining the respiratory tract, eyes, intestines, and urinary tract. They cause acute, self-limiting, febrile infections, with inflammation of the respiratory or ocular mucous membranes, or both. Infants and young children are affected much more frequently than adults, with adenoviral respiratory tract infections most common in the late winter, spring, and early summer. Pharyngoconjunctival fever and conjunctivitis caused by adenovirus typically affect older children mostly in the summer months. Adenoviral GI infections occur year round.

CAUSES

There are 49 known serotypes of adenoviruses; they cause 5 major infections, all of which occur in epidemics. These organisms are common and can remain latent for years; they infect almost everyone early in life, although maternal antibodies offer some protection during the first 6 months of life.

Adenovirus infections are highly contagious. The types of adenovirus that cause respiratory and intestinal infections spread via respiratory droplets, such as coughing or sneezing, or by fecal contamination. Direct transmission can result from poor hand hygiene between using the bathroom and eating or preparing food, or from poor hygiene after handling diapers. Indirect transmission can occur through exposure to contaminated surfaces or items such as soiled tissues. The virus can live on inanimate objects for several hours. The types that cause conjunctivitis can be transmitted by water, such as swimming pools, by touch, or by sharing contaminated objects, such as towels.

 SAFETY Always perform proper hand hygiene after using the bathroom; after coming into contact with oral, nasal, or eye secretions; before preparing food; and before eating.

COMPLICATIONS

Although the complications associated with adenovirus vary with the area that is infected, the most common complications are acute conjunctivitis, sinusitis, pharyngitis, bronchiolitis, and pneumonia. Acute respiratory disease can be caused by adenovirus during conditions of stress and crowding. Intussusception has occurred in infants with the GI form of infection.

Patients with a compromised immune system or with underlying respiratory or cardiac disease are especially susceptible to severe complications of adenovirus.

ASSESSMENT FINDINGS

The incubation period—usually lasting less than 1 week—is followed by acute illness that lasts less than 5 days. Clinical features vary, depending on the type of infection. Prolonged asymptomatic reinfection may occur.

Infection of the respiratory tract will often manifest with flu-like symptoms and can include fever, pharyngitis, rhinitis, cough, and swollen lymph nodes. It can also lead to otitis media. Adenovirus can also affect the lower respiratory tract, causing bronchiolitis, croup, or viral pneumonia. This virus can produce a dry, harsh cough that sounds like whooping cough (pertussis). Young children with respiratory infections such as bronchiolitis or pneumonia should be maintained with droplet and contact precautions. Older children or adults can be managed with droplet precautions alone.

When the infection affects the eyes, symptoms include red eyes, discharge, tearing, and a foreign-body sensation. Keratoconjunctivitis is a more severe infection that involves the conjunctiva and cornea. This type of adenoviral infection is extremely contagious and is most often seen in older children and young adults. Symptoms include red eyes, photophobia, tearing, and pain. Contact precautions should be used for acute hemorrhagic conjunctivitis.

Pharyngoconjunctival fever typically occurs in small outbreaks among school-age children. Symptoms of pharyngoconjunctival fever include red eyes, a very sore throat, fever, rhinitis, and swollen lymph nodes. Contact precautions should be used.

If the virus infects the GI tract, the most common findings will be watery diarrhea, vomiting, fever, and abdominal cramps.

Urinary tract infections can cause urinary frequency, burning, pain, and hematuria.

DIAGNOSTIC TESTS

▶ Laboratory tests may reveal leukocytosis.
▶ Culture of respiratory secretions by nasopharyngeal swab will grow adenovirus. (See *Obtaining a nasopharyngeal specimen*.)
▶ Stool samples may be positive for adenovirus.
▶ Serum antibody titer with a fourfold increase indicates recent adenoviral infection.

TREATMENT

Supportive treatment includes rest, antipyretics, and analgesics. Ocular infections may require corticosteroids and direct supervision by an ophthalmologist. Bronchodilators may be used to improve ventilation. Hospitalization is required in cases of pneumonia (in infants) to prevent death and in epidemic keratoconjunctivitis to prevent blindness.

NURSING CONSIDERATIONS

▶ During acute illness, monitor respiratory status as well as intake and output. Give analgesics and antipyretics as needed. Stress the need for rest and increased fluids.
◆ Enforce and practice droplet and contact precautions as recommended.

   PREVENTION There is no way to completely prevent adenoviral infection. Primary prevention includes good hand hygiene and thorough environmental cleaning. Vaccines developed for adenovirus serotypes 4 and 7 are available only for preventing acute respiratory disease among the military.

▶ Epidemic keratoconjunctivitis can be prevented by sterilization of ophthalmic instruments, adequate chlorination in swimming

Obtaining a nasopharyngeal specimen

When the swab passes into the nasopharynx, gently but quickly rotate it to collect a specimen. Then remove the swab, taking care not to injure the nasal mucous membrane.

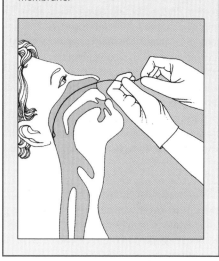

pools, and avoidance of swimming pools during epidemics. A killed virus vaccine (not widely available) or a live oral virus vaccine can prevent adenoviral infection and is recommended for high-risk groups.

Patient teaching

▶ Teach the patient and family the importance of both proper hand hygiene, including covering the mouth when coughing or sneezing, and good environmental cleaning.
▶ Instruct patients who have pools to maintain adequate levels of chlorination.
▶ A cool mist humidifier may help loosen congestion. Instruct the patient or family to clean and dry the humidifier thoroughly every day to prevent contamination.
▶ Warm compresses on the eyes may help to relieve the symptoms of conjunctivitis.

Amebiasis

Amebiasis, also known as amebic dysentery or intestinal amebiasis, is an acute or chronic protozoal infection caused by *Entamoeba histolytica*. This infection produces varying degrees of illness, from no symptoms at all or mild diarrhea to fulminant dysentery. Extraintestinal amebiasis can induce hepatic abscess and infections of the lungs, pleural cavity, pericardium, peritoneum and, rarely, the brain. Ninety percent of people with amebiasis do not have symptoms.

The prognosis is generally good, although complications can increase mortality. Brain abscess, a rare complication, is usually fatal.

CAUSES

E. histolytica exists in two forms: a cyst (which can survive outside the body) and a trophozoite (which can't survive outside the body). Transmission occurs through ingestion of feces-contaminated food or water. The ingested cysts pass through the intestine, where digestive secretions break down the cysts and liberate the motile trophozoites within. The trophozoites multiply and either invade and ulcerate the mucosa of the large intestine (causing colitis, or chronic diarrhea) or simply feed on intestinal bacteria. As the trophozoites are carried slowly toward the rectum, they are encysted and then excreted in feces. Humans are the principal reservoir of infection.

Amebiasis occurs worldwide but is most common in the tropics, subtropics, and other areas with crowded living conditions and poor sanitation and health practices. People with suppressed immune systems are at increased risk for severe amebiasis, as are those suffering from alcoholism, cancer, or malnutrition. In addition, advanced age, pregnancy, and recent travel to a tropical area increase the risk of infection. In the United States, amebiasis is most common among immigrants from developing countries, people who live in institutions, and people who have anal intercourse.

COMPLICATIONS

Complications associated with amebiasis affect the GI system and include chronic diarrhea, abdominal pain, extraintestinal abscesses, ameboma, megacolon, intussusception, intestinal strictures, intestinal hemorrhage, and intestinal perforation. The parasite can spread through the blood to the liver, lungs, or brain.

ASSESSMENT FINDINGS

The clinical effects of amebiasis vary with the severity of the infestation. Acute amebic dysentery causes a sudden high temperature of 104° to 105° F (40° to 40.6° C) accompanied by chills and abdominal cramping; profuse, bloody, mucoid diarrhea with tenesmus; excessive flatulence; and diffuse abdominal tenderness due to extensive rectosigmoid ulcers.

Chronic amebic dysentery produces intermittent diarrhea that lasts for 1 to 4 weeks and recurs several times a year. Such diarrhea produces 4 to 8 (or, in severe diarrhea, up to 18) foul-smelling, mucus- and blood-tinged stools daily in a patient with a mild fever, vague abdominal cramps, possible weight loss, tenderness over the cecum and ascending colon and, occasionally, hepatomegaly. Amebic granuloma (ameboma), commonly mistaken for cancer, can be a complication of the chronic infection. Amebic granuloma produces blood and mucus in the stool and, when granulomatous tissue covers the entire circumference of the bowel, causes partial or complete obstruction.

Parasitic and bacterial invasion of the appendix may produce typical signs of subacute appendicitis (abdominal pain and tenderness). Occasionally, *E. histolytica* perforates the intestinal wall and spreads to the liver. When it perforates the liver and diaphragm, it spreads to the lungs, pleural cavity, peritoneum and, rarely, the brain.

ALERT Up to 90% of infected people have no symptoms.

DIAGNOSTIC TESTS

 ALERT In patients with amebiasis, exploratory surgery is hazardous; it can lead to peritonitis, perforation, and pericecal abscess.

▶ Ultrasound or computed tomography can rule out liver abscesses.

▶ Stool examination for amoebae may require more than one sample obtained on different days.

▶ Aspirate or biopsy can identify *E. histolytica*.

▶ An indirect hemagglutination test will be positive with a current or previous infection.

▶ Complement fixation is usually positive only during the active phase.

▶ Barium studies can be used to rule out nonamebic causes of diarrhea.

▶ Sigmoidoscopy may detect rectosigmoid ulceration.

 ALERT Patients with amebiasis shouldn't have preparatory enemas because enemas may remove exudates and destroy the trophozoites, thus interfering with test results.

TREATMENT

Drugs used to treat amebic dysentery include metronidazole (Flagyl), an amebicide at intestinal and extraintestinal sites; chloroquine (Aralen) for liver abscesses, not intestinal infections; and tetracycline (Sumycin; in combination with emetine hydrochloride, metronidazole, or paromomycin), which supports the antiamebic effect by destroying intestinal bacteria on which the amoebae normally feed.

When nausea and vomiting are present, I.V. therapy may be necessary until medications are tolerated by mouth.

NURSING CONSIDERATIONS

▶ Enforce and practice standard precautions.

▶ Tell patients with amebiasis to avoid drinking alcohol when taking metronidazole. The combination may cause nausea, vomiting, and headache.

▶ Antidiarrheals should not be prescribed and can make the condition worse.

▶ After treatment, stools should be rechecked to make sure the infection has been cleared.

Patient teaching

▶ Instruct the patient to employ safer sex measures, such as using condoms during intercourse and dental dams for any anal contact.

▶ Teach the patient and family about the importance of proper hand hygiene after using the bathroom, changing diapers, and handling food.

▶ Patients who have amebiasis-associated diarrhea should not attend school or work but can return when they are feeling better and their stools are normal.

 PREVENTION Instruct patients who are traveling to tropical countries with poor sanitation to drink only bottled, purified, or boiled water and/or carbonated drinks from a can or bottle and not to eat any uncooked vegetables or unpeeled fruit. Instruct them to not drink any fountain drinks or anything with ice cubes.

Anthrax

Anthrax, also called wool-sorter's disease or ragpicker's disease, is an acute bacterial infection that occurs most commonly in hoofed animals, such as cattle, sheep, goats, and horses. It can also affect people who come in contact with contaminated animals or the hides, bones, fur, hair, or wool of contaminated animals. Anthrax is also used as an agent for bioterrorism and biological warfare.

Anthrax occurs worldwide, but is most common in developing countries. In humans, anthrax occurs in three forms, depending on the mode of transmission: cutaneous, inhalational, and GI.

At least 17 nations are thought to have a biological weapons program, but it is not known how many nations or groups are currently working with anthrax. Bioterrorism experts believe it is difficult to use anthrax effectively as a weapon on a large scale.

CAUSES

Anthrax is caused by the bacteria *Bacillus anthracis*, which exists in the soil as spores that can live for years. Transmission to humans usually occurs through exposure to or handling of infected animals or animal products. Anthrax spores can enter the body through abraded or broken skin (cutaneous anthrax), by inhalation (inhalational anthrax), or through ingestion of undercooked meat from an infected animal (GI anthrax). Anthrax is rarely spread from person to person.

COMPLICATIONS

Cutaneous anthrax can spread to the bloodstream, causing septicemia. Inhalational anthrax can cause hemorrhagic meningitis, pleural effusions, mediastinitis, shock, and acute respiratory distress syndrome. GI anthrax can cause hemorrhage and shock. All three forms of anthrax can lead to death in cases of severe or untreated infection.

ASSESSMENT FINDINGS

Signs and symptoms of infection usually occur within 1 to 7 days after exposure but may take as long as 60 days to appear. The signs and symptoms of anthrax depend on the form that is acquired.

Cutaneous anthrax is the most common form, with 95% of infections occurring when the spore enters a break in the skin. Skin infection may begin as a small, elevated, itchy lesion that develops into a vesicle in 1 to 2 days and ultimately becomes a small, painless ulcer with a necrotic center. A scab usually develops and then drops off within 2 weeks (although complete healing may take longer). Enlarged lymph glands in the surrounding area are common. Without treatment, mortality from cutaneous anthrax is 20%. (See *Cutaneous anthrax infection.*)

With inhalational anthrax, the patient may initially report flu-like signs and symptoms, such as malaise, fever, headache, cough, shortness of breath, chest pain, myalgia, and chills. These mild signs and symptoms may progress to severe respiratory difficulties, such as dyspnea, stridor, chest pain, and cyanosis, followed by the onset of shock. Even with treatment, inhalational anthrax is usually fatal.

With GI anthrax, ingestion of anthrax spores can cause acute inflammation of the intestinal tract. The patient may present with nausea, vomiting, decreased appetite, and fever, which then progress to abdominal pain, vomiting blood, and severe diarrhea. The prognosis for GI anthrax is also poor, as the majority of people die from this form of the disease.

DIAGNOSTIC TESTS

▶ Gram stain of tissue or fluid may show gram-positive bacilli characteristic of *B. anthracis*.
▶ Blood cultures may grow *B. anthracis*.
▶ Culture of skin lesions may identify *B. anthracis*.
▶ Sputum culture may identify *B. anthracis*.

▶ Chest radiography may show fluid surrounding the lungs or widening of the mediastinum.

▶ Cerebrospinal fluid culture may grow *B. anthracis*.

▶ Tissue or fluid specimens may be sent to reference labs for specific testing for *B. anthracis*.

TREATMENT

Initiation of treatment as soon as exposure to anthrax is suspected is essential to prevent infection; early treatment may also help prevent death. Many antibiotics are effective against anthrax. The most widely used are penicillin, ciprofloxacin (Cipro), and doxycycline (Doryx). The length of treatment for inhalational anthrax is typically about 60 days, since it may take that long for anthrax spores to grow. Treatment for cutaneous anthrax is oral antibiotics for 7 to 10 days. The length of treatment for GI anthrax is 60 days, but safety has not been evaluated beyond 14 days.

NURSING CONSIDERATIONS

▶ Obtain culture specimens before starting antibiotic therapy.

▶ Supportive measures are geared toward the type of anthrax exposure.

▶ An anthrax vaccine is available, but, due to limited supplies, it is currently administered only to U.S. military personnel and isn't for routine civilian use.

▶ Report all cases of anthrax to the state health department or the Centers for Disease Control and Prevention (CDC).

 SAFETY According to the CDC, person-to-person transmission of anthrax is extremely unlikely. It has only been reported with cutaneous anthrax, in which discharge from skin lesions is thought to be potentially infectious.

Cutaneous anthrax infection

Cutaneous anthrax occurs when a spore of the bacteria *B. anthracis* enters a break in the skin. Within 2 days of exposure, an itchy sore (similar to an insect bite) develops. The sore may blister and form a black, painless ulcer, usually surrounded by a large amount of swelling. The ulcer may then form a scab, which dries and falls off within about 2 weeks, although complete healing of the sore may take longer.

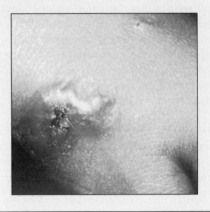

Patient teaching

▶ Teach the patient and family that anyone who has been exposed to anthrax must see a doctor immediately.

▶ Instruct the patient to take the antibiotics as prescribed and until completed.

▶ Instruct the patient with cutaneous anthrax not to scratch at the lesions.

▶ Alcohol-based hand sanitizers do not kill anthrax spores; wash hands with soap and water.

 PREVENTION There are two main ways to prevent anthrax: antibiotics in people who have been exposed to anthrax and the anthrax vaccine, which is given in a series of six doses.

Aspergillosis

Aspergillosis is an opportunistic infection caused by fungi of the genus *Aspergillus*, usually *A. fumigatus*, *A. flavus*, and *A. niger*. Aspergillosis occurs in four major forms: aspergilloma, which produces a fungus ball in the lungs (called a mycetoma); allergic bronchopulmonary aspergillosis, a hypersensitive asthmatic reaction to *Aspergillus* antigens; aspergillosis endophthalmitis, an infection of the anterior and posterior chambers of the eye that can lead to blindness; and invasive aspergillosis, an acute infection that produces septicemia, thrombosis, and infarction of virtually any organ, but especially the heart, lungs, brain, and kidneys.

Aspergillus may cause infection of the ear (otomycosis), cornea (mycotic keratitis), and prosthetic heart valves (endocarditis); pneumonia (especially in patients receiving immunosuppressants, such as antineoplastic agents or high-dose steroids); sinusitis; and brain abscesses.

The prognosis varies with each form. Occasionally, aspergilloma causes fatal hemoptysis.

CAUSES

Aspergillus is found worldwide, commonly in decaying vegetation, such as dead leaves, stored grain, compost piles, and damp hay. It can also be found in household dust, building materials, and some food items. Transmission is by inhalation of fungal spores or, in aspergillosis endophthalmitis, by the invasion of spores through a wound or other tissue injury. It's a common laboratory contaminant. (See *Aspergillus infection*.)

Aspergillus produces clinical infection only in people who become especially vulnerable to it. Such vulnerability can result from excessive or prolonged use of antibiotics, glucocorticoids, or other immunosuppressive agents; from radiation; from such conditions as acquired immunodeficiency

Aspergillus infection

After the *Aspergillus* spores are inhaled, they cause mucus buildup in the lungs, which in turn leads to wheezing, dyspnea, cough with some sputum production, hemoptysis, pleural pain, and fever.

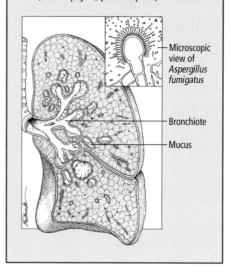

Microscopic view of *Aspergillus fumigatus*

Bronchiote

Mucus

syndrome, Hodgkin's disease, leukemia, azotemia, alcoholism, sarcoidosis, bronchitis, or bronchiectasis; from organ transplants; and, in aspergilloma, from tuberculosis or another cavitary lung disease.

COMPLICATIONS

Invasive *Aspergillus* in the lungs can cause massive bleeding. If it does not respond to treatment, infection can result in respiratory failure and death. An *Aspergillus* infection of the sinuses can cause destruction of the facial bones. Aspergillosis can spread to other body parts, especially the brain, heart, and kidneys.

ASSESSMENT FINDINGS

The incubation period in aspergillosis ranges from a few days to weeks. In aspergilloma, colonization of the bronchial tree with *Aspergillus* produces plugs and atelectasis and forms a tangled ball of hyphae (fungal filaments), fibrin, and exudate in a cavity left by a previous illness such as tuberculosis. Characteristically, aspergilloma either causes no symptoms or mimics tuberculosis, causing a productive cough with purulent or blood-tinged sputum, dyspnea, empyema, and lung abscesses.

Allergic aspergillosis causes malaise, weight loss, wheezing, dyspnea, cough with some sputum production, hemoptysis, pleural pain, and fever.

Aspergillosis endophthalmitis usually appears 2 to 3 weeks after an eye injury or surgery and accounts for half of all cases of endophthalmitis. It causes clouded vision, eye pain, and reddened conjunctiva. Eventually, *Aspergillus* infects the anterior and posterior chambers, where it produces purulent exudate.

 ALERT In invasive aspergillosis, *Aspergillus* invades blood vessels and causes thrombosis, infarctions, and the typical signs and symptoms of septicemia (chills, fever, hypotension, delirium). It can also cause azotemia, hematuria, urinary tract obstruction, headaches, seizures, bone pain and tenderness, and soft-tissue swelling. It's rapidly fatal.

DIAGNOSTIC TESTS

▶ Chest radiography or computed tomography can usually reveal an aspergilloma.
▶ Laboratory tests may show leukocytosis, and galactomannan (a molecule from the fungus) can sometimes be found in the blood. An *Aspergillus* antibody test may be positive.
▶ Sputum culture may grow *Aspergillus*.
▶ Stain of sputum or tissue may show fungal elements consistent with *Aspergillus*.
▶ Tissue biopsy may grow *Aspergillus*.

TREATMENT

Aspergillosis doesn't require isolation. Treatment requires local excision of the lesion and supportive therapy, such as chest physiotherapy, to improve pulmonary function. Endocarditis caused by *Aspergillus* is treated by

surgical removal of infected heart valves and long-term amphotericin B therapy. Allergic aspergillosis requires desensitization and, possibly, steroids. Invasive aspergillosis and aspergillosis endophthalmitis require a 2- to 3-week course of I.V. voriconazole (Vfend) as well as prompt cessation of immunosuppressive therapy. Itraconazole (Sporanox) and other antifungal agents such as amphotericin B or caspofungin (Cancidas) can also be used for treatment. However, the invasive form results in an infection that's so virulent that antifungal therapy can't stop the systemic involvement; eventually, death ensues.

 SAFETY Early treatment is necessary to prevent spread of the disease.

NURSING CONSIDERATIONS

▶ Assist with chest physiotherapy, and instruct the patient to cough effectively.
▶ Monitor the patient's vital signs, intake and output, and diagnostic test results.
▶ Provide emotional support for the patient and family.

Patient teaching

▶ Instruct patients with asthma or cystic fibrosis to see the doctor whenever they notice a change in their symptoms.
▶ Patients with weakened immune systems should see the doctor immediately if they develop shortness of breath, a cough productive with bloody sputum, or unexplained fever.
▶ Tell the patient and family that aspergillosis is not contagious.

 PREVENTION *Aspergillus* is so common in the environment, it is probably impossible to completely avoid breathing in some spores. Everyday exposure to *Aspergillus* is rarely a problem for those with healthy immune systems. However, avoiding dusty environments and activities such as gardening and lawn work, as well as improving air quality with HEPA filtration, may help keep those at increased risk from becoming infected.

Contact Precautions

Bartonella quintana infection

Bartonella quintana, a gram-negative rod belonging to the Rickettsiaceae family, restricts itself to human hosts. Typically transmitted by the human body louse (a small, wingless insect), *B. quintana* is associated with poverty, lack of hygiene, crowded and unhygienic conditions, and cold weather.

During World War I, more than 1 million people became infected with what is now known as "trench fever"—the first clinical manifestation of *B. quintana*. Following the war, the incidence of trench fever dropped dramatically, only to rise again during World War II. (See *Trench fever*.)

In the 1980s, *B. quintana* appeared again as an opportunistic pathogen among those infected with human immunodeficiency virus (HIV). More recently, it has reemerged among indigent populations in the United States and Europe.

Causes

B. quintana multiplies in the intestine of the louse and is excreted in its feces, which then infects the human host through breaks in the skin—either by biting or other means. Infected lice excrete infectious feces 5 to 12 days after ingesting infected blood. Recently, *B. quintana* has been found in cat fleas and cat teeth, which is suggestive of bacteremia in cats. Recent research has found *B. quintana* in ticks.

Poor living conditions and a history of alcoholism are the two main predisposing factors for *B. quintana* infection.

Complications

B. quintana is responsible for a long list of complications. Chronic bacteremia has been reported in patients as many as 8 years after initial infection. Other complications include endocarditis, often requiring valve surgery; lymphadenopathy; peliosis; and

Trench fever

Trench fever is known by a variety of names, including Wolhynia fever, shin bone fever, quintan fever, five-day fever, Meuse fever, and His-Werner disease. It was first described in 1915, when more than 1 million people were affected during World War I. However, recent DNA studies have shown that *B. quintana* infected many soldiers in Napoleon's Grand Army at Vilnius in 1812. The infection is characterized by headache and dizziness, shin and joint pain, and fever. Muscle aches, truncal rashes and, later in the course of disease, hepatosplenomegaly are also common.

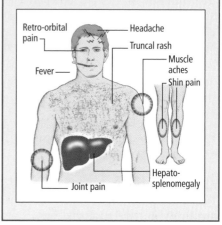

bacillary angiomatosis (more common in those who are HIV positive).

Assessment findings

The initial infection lasts up to 3 days and is marked by a sudden headache, pain behind the eyes, rash, dizziness, shin pain, insomnia, constipation, dyspnea, abdominal pain, and fever. The spleen and liver may also be enlarged. After about 6 weeks, the fever subsides and temperature returns to normal or below normal, only to rise and fall again with relapses occurring about every 6 days (although each successive relapse is less severe). Although it often results in extended disability, no deaths as a result of *B. quintana* have been reported.

ALERT When caring for a patient who has lived on the streets or in shelters, be alert for the presence of parasites such as lice.

DIAGNOSTIC TESTS

▶ Laboratory tests may reveal immunoglobulin G titers of 1:50 or higher, indicating *Bartonella* infection.
▶ Blood cultures may reveal *B. quintana*.
▶ Skin or tissue biopsy may detect *B. quintana*.

TREATMENT

Initial treatment involves ridding the patient of lice. This can be done by treating clothing and bedding with insecticides or by boiling them. Since the lice live on clothing and bedding and only visit the skin to feed, it is usually not necessary to delouse the body.

B. quintana is susceptible to a variety of antibiotics, including penicillins and tetracyclines. For uncomplicated cases, treatment is usually a 4- to 6-week course of oral antibiotics. If the patient is suffering from chronic bacteremia or endocarditis, I.V. antibiotics are required, with gentamicin being the drug of choice. For those who do not require surgery, treatment for 4 to 6 months is recommended. Erythromycin is reported to be more effective in cases of bacillary angiomatosis.

In patients who could not tolerate other therapies, or if other therapies have failed, Lindane (Kwell), which comes in lotion, cream, and shampoo forms, may be prescribed. Lindane is applied to the affected area and washed with soap and water after 8 hours.

NURSING CONSIDERATIONS

◆ Use contact precautions until treatment is complete to prevent spreading the infection.
▶ Have the patient's fingernails cut short to prevent skin breaks and secondary bacterial infection caused by scratching.
▶ Be alert for possible adverse reactions to antiparasitic treatment, including sensitivity reactions and, in some cases, central nervous system (CNS) toxicity.

▶ To prevent self-infestation among health care personnel, avoid direct contact with the patient's hair, clothing, and bedsheets. Use gloves, a gown, and a protective head covering when administering delousing treatment.
▶ After each treatment, inspect the patient for remaining lice and eggs.
▶ Administer antibiotics as ordered.
▶ Be aware of the stigma that is attached to the presence of lice. Provide emotional support to the patient and family.

PREVENTION To prevent reinfestation, everyone in the family or who has had close contact with the patient should be treated with a delousing agent at the same time.

Patient teaching

▶ Instruct the patient to take the antibiotics as prescribed and until completed.
▶ Teach patients the importance of proper hygiene.
▶ Tell the patient and family that blankets, furniture, and carpeting should be sprayed with an insecticide.
▶ All lice must be killed in order to prevent reinfestation. Teach the patient and family how to look for live lice.

PREVENTION The best way to avoid being infested with lice is to not share personal items. Proper personal hygiene as well as environmental cleaning are also important in preventing lice infestation.

Basidiobolomycosis

Basidiobolomycosis, a form of zygomycosis caused by the fungus *Basidiobolus ranarum*, was first isolated in 1955. It is also known as *Entomophthoramycosis basidiobolae*. This fungus is found worldwide in decaying vegetation, food, and soil as well as in the GI tracts of reptiles, amphibians, fish, and insectivorous bats. It is most commonly found in the tropical regions of Africa (it is endemic in Uganda), but cases have also been reported in parts of Asia, India, and South America. It has rarely caused disease in humans in the United States. In recent years, however, its geographical distribution has expanded, as has the variety of manifestations.

CAUSES

The disease is more common in children (80% of cases), especially young boys (3:1), and usually results from traumatic inoculation, such as insect bites, scratches, and minor cuts. Infections are also believed to be the result of lifestyle and dietary behavior. If ingested, *B. ranarum* can cause GI basidiobolomycosis, in which the muscular layer of the GI tract is greatly thickened. Of 15 reported cases of GI basidiobolomycosis worldwide, 5 patients had reptiles or amphibians living in or around their homes, 4 patients did not wash their fruits or vegetables prior to eating, and 3 had camped near a lake or river. Patients diagnosed with basidiobolomycosis usually do not have any underlying disease.

COMPLICATIONS

GI basidiobolomycosis could lead to bowel obstruction and can affect other abdominal organs. If disseminated, *B. ranarum* can lead to severe hypotension, shortness of breath, organ necrosis, septic shock, and death.

ASSESSMENT FINDINGS

Basidiobolomycosis usually manifests as a painless, unilateral, well-circumscribed subcutaneous nodule on the lower extremities and buttocks, accompanied by fever. These nodules tend to grow locally and become ulcerated. (See *Ulcerated nodules of basidiobolomycosis.*)

The presentation of GI basidiobolomycosis is generally nonspecific: abdominal pain, diarrhea, hematochezia, and an elevated white blood cell count. The condition is often misdiagnosed as cancer, peptic ulcer disease, gastroenteritis, diverticulitis, or inflammatory bowel disease.

DIAGNOSTIC TESTS

▶ A complete blood count may reveal leukocytosis as well as an elevated erythrocyte sedimentation rate and C-reactive protein level.
▶ Histopathologic examination of the affected area may show extensive necrotizing inflammation.
▶ Computed tomography of the abdomen can reveal masses that may involve adjacent organs.
▶ Endoscopy can rule out other sources of abdominal pain and diarrhea.
▶ Culture from clinical or surgical specimens may grow *B. ranarum*; surgery may be required to obtain a specimen.

TREATMENT

Initial treatment includes antifungals such as ketoconazole (Extina) and itraconazole (Sporanox), although potassium iodide (Iosat) has been effective as well. If GI basidiobolomycosis is present, surgery may be required to remove the affected parts of the GI tract, followed by antifungal administration. Cutaneous surgery should not progress beyond biopsy because this infection can spread very easily.

The duration of treatment depends on the presentation of the disease as well as the response to treatment. Patients may be required to remain on antifungal therapy for many months or even years.

Ulcerated nodules of basidiobolomycosis

Basidiobolomycosis is usually character-ized by a painless, unilateral, well-circum-scribed subcutaneous nodule on the lower extremities and buttocks, accompa-nied by fever. As these nodules grow in size, they often become ulcerated. Note the extensive swelling and areas of ulcer-ation on the left leg in this patient.

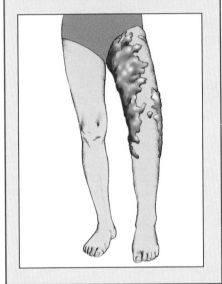

 ALERT Itraconazole capsules and oral solution cannot be used interchangeably. Capsules are to be taken with a full meal, while oral solutions must be taken on an empty stomach.

NURSING CONSIDERATIONS

❯ Ketoconazole and itraconazole are con-traindicated in patients who tend to be hy-persensitive to drugs. Both of these antifun-gals have many drug-drug interactions.
❯ Medical treatments for basidiobolomyco-sis can be toxic to the liver. Be on the lookout for signs and symptoms of hepatotoxicity, and monitor liver function tests carefully.

Patient teaching

❯ Instruct the patient to take medication as prescribed, even if feeling better. Treatment should continue until all tests indicate that the infection has subsided.
❯ Teach the patient about the signs and symptoms of liver disease.
❯ Encourage the patient to keep a list of all medications taken and to share the list with his or her doctor in order to prevent drug-drug interactions.

PREVENTION Because one mode of trans-mission is by ingestion, instruct patients to wash all food prior to eating.

Droplet precautions

Bordetella pertussis infection

The microorganism *B. pertussis* is a gram-negative, pleomorphic bacillus that causes an infection of the respiratory tract. Commonly known as whooping cough or pertussis, this respiratory infection is characterized by a paroxysmal cough. In the United States, the incidence of pertussis has been increasing cyclically, with peaks every 2 to 5 years. Most cases occur from June through September. Pertussis has been reported as a cause of sudden infant death.

Causes

Humans are the only reservoir for *B. pertussis*. It is spread by aerosolized droplets from the coughing of infected people. Once it finds a new host, the microorganism attaches to and damages the ciliated respiratory epithelium.

 SAFETY Pertussis is highly contagious. Transmission can occur following direct contact; sharing confined spaces; or contact with oral, nasal, or respiratory secretions from an infected person.

 PREVENTION Neither previous infection with *B. pertussis* nor vaccination provides lifelong immunity. Protection following vaccination usually decreases after 3 to 5 years and is not measurable after 12 years.

Complications

Premature infants and patients with underlying cardiac, respiratory, or neurologic disease are at higher risk for complications, which include pneumonia, seizures, encephalopathy, and death. More common complications include epistaxis, vomiting, subconjunctival hemorrhages, syncope, insomnia, incontinence, and rib fractures. Compared with older children and adults, infants tend to have more severe symptoms, develop complications, and require hospitalization.

Assessment findings

Typically, pertussis is a 6-week disease that is divided into three stages lasting 1 to 2 weeks each. During the first stage, pertussis mimics common upper respiratory infections, with nasal congestion, rhinorrhea, sneezing, and tearing. The second stage is when the paroxysmal coughing usually starts, with episodes potentially lasting several minutes. In older infants and toddlers, the coughing episodes are followed by a loud "whoop." Younger infants may have apneic episodes and are at risk for exhaustion. Cough-induced vomiting is also common. In the final stage, patients have a chronic cough, which may last for weeks.

 SAFETY Pertussis is most infectious during the initial stage, which usually lasts 1 to 2 weeks, although it may remain communicable for 3 weeks or longer after the onset of a cough.

Diagnostic tests

▶ Sputum or nasopharyngeal culture may be positive for *B. pertussis*.
▶ Antigen detection is the traditional method for diagnosis, and polymerase chain reaction may be positive in the presence of *B. pertussis*.
▶ Chest radiography may reveal infiltrates or edema with atelectasis.

 ALERT Culture results can be negative in previously immunized patients, in people who have received recent antibiotic therapy, or in those who have been coughing for 3 weeks. A negative culture does not necessarily exclude the diagnosis of pertussis.

Treatment

The goals of therapy are to promote rest and ensure proper nutrition. Antibiotic therapy, which is started during the first phase of the disease, does not affect the duration or severity of the disease, but can help prevent its spread. Erythromycin, clarithromycin (Biaxin), and azithromycin (Zithromax) are the drugs of choice.

Cycle of pertussis infection

Infants receive their primary pertussis vaccination before age 6 months, with a booster vaccine given between 16 and 18 months. Because protection following vaccination decreases over time, nonvaccinated or partially vaccinated children are particularly susceptible to contracting pertussis from adults, who frequently serve as reservoirs. For this reason, children should become vaccinated, as should those who handle small children.

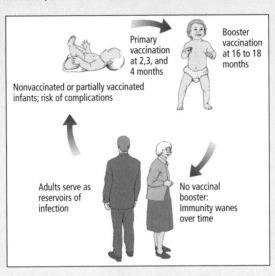

Primary vaccination at 2, 3, and 4 months

Booster vaccination at 16 to 18 months

Nonvaccinated or partially vaccinated infants; risk of complications

Adults serve as reservoirs of infection

No vaccinal booster: Immunity wanes over time

Hospitalization is recommended for those at high risk for severe disease, those with complications, and those who have intractable vomiting.

NURSING CONSIDERATIONS

▶ Obtain a culture specimen either by performing a deep nasopharyngeal aspiration or by holding a Dacron or calcium alginate swab in the patient's posterior nasopharynx for 30 seconds or until the patient coughs.
▶ Keep in mind that *B. pertussis* can grow within 3 to 4 days of infection, but a sample is not considered negative until 10 days.
▶ Report all cases to the state health department or the Centers for Disease Control and Prevention.

 SAFETY Droplet precautions, in addition to standard precautions, are recommended for 5 days after antibiotic therapy is started or, if antibiotics were not given, until 3 weeks after the onset of paroxysmal coughing.

Patient teaching

▶ Encourage parents of young children to have their children vaccinated.

 PREVENTION In 2005, a new combination tetanus, diphtheria, acellular pertussis vaccine (Tdap) was approved for adolescents and adults. Adults under age 65 should receive a single dose of Tdap to replace a single dose of Td (tetanus, diphtheria) vaccine for booster immunization against tetanus, diphtheria, and pertussis.

▶ All members of families with young children should consider getting vaccinated. Research has shown that parents and older siblings are the main source of infection in infants. (See *Cycle of pertussis infection.*)
▶ Instruct patients to cover their mouths when they cough or sneeze and to wash their hands immediately afterward.

Botulism

Caused by the gram-positive, anaerobic bacteria *Clostridium botulinum*, botulism is a rare but severe form of poisoning. *C. botulinum* is found in soil and untreated water worldwide. The bacteria can also be found in undercooked and improperly preserved or canned foods—especially those with a low acid content. *C. botulinum* sometimes occurs normally in the stool of infants. It is one of the most potent bacteria known: If evenly distributed, as little as 1 g can kill more than 1 million people.

There are three main types of botulism, each characterized by the way the disease is transmitted: foodborne botulism, wound botulism, and infant botulism. The number of reported cases worldwide has been decreasing, mostly because of improved canning and food preservation methods. According to the National Institutes of Health, approximately 145 cases of botulism are seen in the United States every year. Of these, almost 65% are infant botulism. However, the incidence of wound botulism, which was once exceedingly rare, is now on the rise, presumably due to increased injectable drug use.

 ALERT All forms of botulism can be fatal and are considered medical emergencies.

Initially used to treat conditions such as cervical dystonia and blepharospasm, two botulinum toxin preparations are licensed in the United States by the Food and Drug Administration. However, on- and off-label use of these preparations has grown. Botulinum toxin A is now available by prescription for therapeutic and cosmetic use. The formulation is normally highly diluted. In 2004, the Centers for Disease Control and Prevention (CDC) confirmed four cases of botulism in adults following cosmetic injection of an unlicensed and highly concentrated botulinum toxin A preparation. All four individuals became severely ill, but they all survived.

 ALERT Botulinum toxin is also considered a major biological weapon. Therefore, with any outbreak of botulism, bioterrorism must be considered.

CAUSES

C. botulinum produces neurotoxin-releasing spores that, when ingested or introduced into a wound, may lead to severe poisoning. The foods most commonly contaminated are home-canned vegetables, cured pork and ham, smoked or raw fish, and honey and corn syrup.

Infant botulism occurs when a child ingests the *C. botulinum* spores that then release the neurotoxin in the intestine.

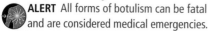 **PREVENTION** Never give honey or corn syrup to an infant younger than 1, not even a small amount on a pacifier.

COMPLICATIONS

Due to the associated weakness, the risk of aspiration is high. Weakness and nervous system problems can become permanent. Death can result if the patient does not receive prompt treatment.

ASSESSMENT FINDINGS

Symptoms often appear 12 to 36 hours after ingestion of the contaminated food, although symptoms can be apparent as early as 6 hours or as late as 10 days after ingestion. Generally, the earlier the symptoms appear, the more critical and severe the illness will be. Severity depends on the amount of toxin ingested and the patient's degree of immunocompromise.

In adults, the most common symptoms include double or blurred vision, droopy eyelids, dry mouth, difficulty swallowing and talking, difficulty breathing, and flaccid paralysis that moves down the body. Deep tendon reflexes are decreased or absent.

In infants, symptoms include weakness and lethargy, constipation, weak cry, poor feeding and sucking, and respiratory distress.

Diagnostic tests

▶ A toxicology screen may identify *C. botulinum.*
▶ Stool culture may identify *C. botulinum.*
▶ The suspected food may also be cultured to isolate *C. botulinum.*
▶ Electromyography will show little response to nerve stimulation in the presence of botulism.
▶ Diagnostic tests should be conducted as needed to rule out diseases that may be confused with botulism, such as myasthenia gravis and Guillain-Barré syndrome.
▶ A mouse-inoculation test will be positive and is the most direct way to confirm a diagnosis of botulism.

Treatment

Botulinus antitoxin, available from the CDC, is administered either I.V. or I.M., although not usually to infants. In infants, the bacteria must be removed by inducing vomiting or by giving an enema. In wound botulism, the toxin is usually removed surgically. For patients with swallowing difficulties, I.V. fluid can be administered, or a nasogastric tube can be inserted until the patient recovers sufficiently. Respiratory distress may require endotracheal intubation. Recovery may take weeks or months as axons on the nerves are regenerated. Fatigue and shortness of breath may continue for years.

 SAFETY Botulism is not contagious and cannot be transmitted from person to person.

Nursing considerations

▶ Obtain a careful history of foods eaten in the past several days. Ask about the health status of other family members with similar food histories.
▶ Monitor respiratory and cardiac function carefully.
▶ Perform frequent neurologic checks.
▶ Purge the GI tract as ordered.

▶ If giving the botulinus antitoxin, check the patient's allergies, especially to horses, because the antitoxin is horse serum. When giving the antitoxin, perform a skin test first, then watch for signs of allergic reaction.
▶ Prevent secondary infection by practicing standard precautions.
▶ Report all cases of botulism to the state health department or the CDC.
▶ Provide emotional support to the patient and family.

Patient teaching

▶ Educate the patient and family about the importance of proper hand hygiene.
▶ Teach the patient and family to cook food thoroughly before ingesting.
▶ Instruct the patient who eats home-canned food to boil the food for 10 minutes before eating to ensure that it is safe to consume. Tell the patient and family to not taste-test any food that is questionable.
▶ Teach patients and families to see their doctors promptly for infected wounds and to avoid injectable street drugs.

 PREVENTION Baked potatoes that were wrapped in aluminum foil should be kept hot until served, or refrigerated. Oils that contain garlic or herbs should be refrigerated.

If doing home canning, follow strict hygiene methods to prevent or kill *C. botulinum*, their spores, and the neurotoxin. Bulging cans or abnormal-smelling preserved foods should not be ingested.

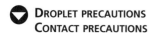

▼ Droplet precautions
  Contact precautions

Bronchiolitis

Bronchiolitis, an inflammation of the lung bronchioles, usually results from a viral infection and can lead to severe illness. This infection usually affects children younger than age 2, although the peak age is 3 to 6 months. Bronchiolitis occurs more frequently in fall and winter months and is a very common cause of hospitalization in infants. Infants who are exposed to cigarette smoke or who live in crowded conditions are at increased risk, as are infants who were born prematurely and those who are not breastfed.

Causes

Respiratory syncytial virus (RSV) is the most common cause of bronchiolitis in children younger than 1. RSV usually only causes mild symptoms in adults, but it can cause severe illness in infants. It is estimated that by the end of their first year, more than half of all infants have been exposed to RSV.

In older children, research has shown that rhinovirus is the most common cause of bronchiolitis. Other viruses that have been implicated include adenovirus, influenza, and parainfluenza. In some cases, bronchiolitis may be caused by multiple infections, such as a combination of RSV and influenza.

Complications

The infant may have severe respiratory distress and become cyanotic. Young infants may become exhausted from the work of breathing and require endotracheal intubation. Secondary infection, such as pneumonia, may also occur. In severe cases of bronchiolitis, and when treatment has been delayed, the infection may be fatal.

Later in life, the patient may develop airway disease, such as asthma.

Assessment findings

Bronchiolitis often starts as a mild upper respiratory infection with symptoms similar to those of a common cold, such as fever, rhinorrhea, and cough. Over the course of 2 or 3 days, however, increased respiratory distress can develop, along with wheezing and a tighter cough. Lung sounds may reveal the presence of crackles and a high-pitched expiratory wheeze. The infant may be tachypneic, hypoxic, and irritable. Nasal flaring, grunting respirations, and use of accessory muscles signal worsening respiratory distress. (See *Observing retractions.*)

The chest may also appear hyperinflated. Affected infants may also be lethargic and dehydrated due to poor feeding.

Diagnostic tests

▶ Blood gases may reveal hypoxemia and hypercarbia.
▶ A complete blood count may reveal leukocytosis.
▶ Chest radiography can rule out pneumonia and other possible causes of the symptoms.
▶ Culture of respiratory secretions may reveal which virus is involved.

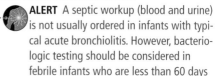 **ALERT** A septic workup (blood and urine) is not usually ordered in infants with typical acute bronchiolitis. However, bacteriologic testing should be considered in febrile infants who are less than 60 days old.

Treatment

In most infants, the disease is self-limiting and can often be treated at home. The goal of treatment is to keep the child well oxygenated. Chest clapping will help loosen secretions, as will humidified air. Suctioning may be required to clear the nasal passages. Clear fluids and rest are recommended. Bronchodilators are often prescribed for infants with bronchiolitis. In extremely ill children, an antiviral medication may be used. However, these medications must be given early in the course of the illness in order to be effective.

Enforce and practice contact and droplet precautions.

▶ Infected patients should be placed in single rooms. If this is not possible, all patients younger than 2 should be grouped based on laboratory confirmation of infection.

 PREVENTION Because many of the viruses that cause bronchiolitis are present in the environment, most cases of bronchiolitis are not preventable. There is also no vaccine currently available for bronchiolitis. However, the medication palivizumab (Synagis) can decrease the likelihood of developing a severe form of RSV and reduce the need for hospitalization. Due to its high cost, however, palivizumab is generally limited to infants who are at extremely high risk of RSV infection.

Patient teaching

▶ Instruct the family to cover their mouths when coughing or sneezing.

▶ Teach the infant's family about the importance of proper hand hygiene, especially before handling the infant and after coughing or sneezing.

▶ Family members with upper respiratory infections should be especially careful around infants and should wear masks when handling an infant.

▶ Teach parents to feed the infected infant more often to prevent dehydration. Also teach them how to recognize potential dehydration (for example, decrease in the number wet diapers, tearless crying).

▶ Explain to family members that antibiotics are not effective against viruses and should only be used in the case of a bacterial infection.

▶ Teach the family about the importance of maintaining a smoke-free environment. If family members smoke, ask them to smoke outside of the house or car.

SAFETY Instruct the family members that the child should be kept at home until the infection has passed to avoid spreading it to others.

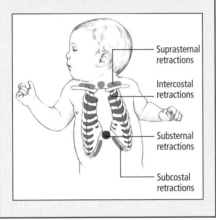

Observing retractions

When you observe retractions in infants and children, be sure to note the exact location of the retractions—an important clue to the cause and severity of respiratory distress. For example, subcostal and substernal retractions usually result from lower respiratory tract disorders; suprasternal retractions, from upper respiratory tract disorders.

Mild intercostal retractions alone may be normal. However, intercostal retractions accompanied by subcostal and substernal retractions may indicate moderate respiratory distress. Deep suprasternal retractions typically indicate severe distress.

- Suprasternal retractions
- Intercostal retractions
- Substernal retractions
- Subcostal retractions

In healthy infants, the disease lasts about a week and then goes away. However, in children with underlying health problems, the infection may be more severe and may require hospitalization.

 PREVENTION RSV is highly contagious and is transmitted by respiratory droplets. It can survive on environmental surfaces for up to 12 hours. Practice proper hand hygiene before and after caring for patients with RSV.

Nursing considerations

▶ Perform frequent respiratory assessments to ensure that the patient's breathing status is not worsening.

▶ Ensure that only humidified oxygen is used.

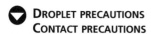

DROPLET PRECAUTIONS
CONTACT PRECAUTIONS

Bronchitis

Bronchitis is inflammation of the lining of the bronchi and may be acute or chronic. Acute bronchitis usually lasts 7 to 10 days, although the patient may have a lingering cough for several weeks or months. Chronic bronchitis is characterized by a productive cough that lasts at least 3 months each year for 2 consecutive years; this form of infection requires early detection and treatment in order to improve the chance for a good outcome. Those with advanced disease have a poor chance for recovery.

CAUSES

Acute bronchitis usually follows a viral respiratory infection, although it can have a bacterial source as well. Those at risk for acute bronchitis include elderly people and young children, people with heart or lung disease, and smokers. Chronic bronchitis is also known as chronic obstructive pulmonary disease and is attributed to a long history of smoking. Tobacco smoke is the cause of chronic bronchitis in almost 80% of cases. (See *Lung changes in bronchitis*.)

Both types of bronchitis are made worse by air pollution, allergies, infections, and certain occupations (such as mining).

COMPLICATIONS

Pneumonia can develop with either acute or chronic bronchitis. Repeated bouts of bronchitis may signal the development of a lung disorder, such as asthma or chronic bronchitis. Patients with chronic bronchitis may develop emphysema, cor pulmonale, or pulmonary hypertension.

ASSESSMENT FINDINGS

Both types of bronchitis have similar symptoms, which include general malaise, headache, chest discomfort, a productive cough, fatigue, a low-grade fever, wheezing,

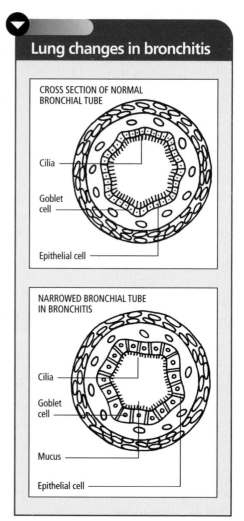

Lung changes in bronchitis

CROSS SECTION OF NORMAL BRONCHIAL TUBE

Cilia

Goblet cell

Epithelial cell

NARROWED BRONCHIAL TUBE IN BRONCHITIS

Cilia

Goblet cell

Mucus

Epithelial cell

and shortness of breath. Lung auscultation may reveal rales. With chronic bronchitis, symptoms may also include swelling of the feet and ankles, blue-tinged lips, and frequent respiratory infections.

DIAGNOSTIC TESTS

▶ Chest radiography can rule out pneumonia and may also show hyperinflation of the lungs.
▶ Lung function tests can rule out other causes of symptoms, such as asthma or emphysema. In chronic bronchitis, tests may reveal increased residual volume, decreased vital capacity and forced expiratory flow, and

normal static compliance and diffusing capacity.

▶ Sputum culture may reveal the virus or bacteria.

▶ In chronic bronchitis, arterial blood gas analysis may show decreased partial pressure of oxygen and normal or increased partial pressure of carbon dioxide.

TREATMENT

Acute bronchitis is usually self-limiting and does not generally require hospitalization. Humidification will help loosen secretions, as will staying well hydrated. Chest physical therapy may help mobilize secretions. Rest is recommended, as is acetaminophen (Tylenol) if a fever is present. If symptoms do not improve within about a week, a bronchodilator, such as albuterol, may be prescribed. If a secondary bacterial infection is present, broad-spectrum antibiotics will be prescribed.

Cough suppressants are not recommended unless the cough interferes with the patient's ability to sleep.

Treatment of chronic bronchitis also includes the use of bronchodilators and may include steroids as well. If an active infection is present, antibiotics are required. It is highly recommended that the patient quit smoking, limit exposure to pollutants and lung irritants, and get the flu vaccine every year as well as a pneumococcal vaccine as recommended. Pulmonary rehabilitation should be considered.

NURSING CONSIDERATIONS

▶ Patients who smoke may need information regarding resources for smoking cessation. Be aware of what is available in your community.

▶ Perform chest physical therapy as indicated.

▶ For patients with chronic bronchitis, encourage daily activity with the use of energy-conservation techniques. Provide frequent rest periods.

◐ Enforce the use of droplet and contact precautions.

Patient teaching

▶ Encourage patients who smoke to take part in a smoking cessation program.

▶ As appropriate, instruct patients to get an annual flu vaccine along with a pneumococcal vaccine.

▶ Explain to patients about air pollution, including second-hand smoke, and how to limit their exposure.

▶ Instruct patients to cover their mouths when they cough.

▶ Teach patients about the importance of proper hand hygiene.

Brucellosis

Brucellosis, which is also known as undulant fever, Malta fever, or Bang's disease, is an acute febrile illness that is transmitted to humans from animals. It's caused by the non-motile, non-spore-forming, gram-negative coccobacilli of the genus *Brucella*, notably *B. suis* (found in swine), *B. melitensis* (found in goats and sheep), *B. abortus* (found in cattle), and *B. canis* (found in dogs). Brucellosis causes fever, profuse sweating, anxiety, general aching, and bone, spleen, liver, kidney, or brain abscesses.

With treatment, brucellosis is seldom fatal, although complications can cause permanent disability.

Causes

Brucellosis is most commonly transmitted via consumption of unpasteurized dairy products or through contact with infected animals or their secretions or excretions. Transmission can also occur if the bacteria enter the body through an open wound. It's most prevalent among farmers, stock handlers, butchers, and veterinarians. Because of such occupational risks, brucellosis infects six times more men than women, especially those between ages 20 and 50; it's less common in children. Hydrochloric acid in gastric juices kills *Brucella* bacteria. As a result, people with achlorhydria are particularly susceptible to this disease.

ALERT *B. canis* is a species of *Brucella* that can infect dogs. Transmission to humans from dogs is rare, as most pet owners do not come into contact with their dog's blood, semen, or placenta. However, immunocompromised people, such as transplant patients or people with human immunodeficiency virus, should not handle dogs known to be infected with *B. canis*.

Although brucellosis occurs throughout the world, it's most prevalent in the Middle East, Africa, the former Soviet Union, India, South America, and Europe; it's seldom found in the United States, with only 100 to 200 cases being reported each year. The incubation period usually lasts from 5 to 60 days, but in some cases it can last for months.

Complications

Brucella can cause a variety of complications, including endocarditis, orchitis, hepatosplenomegaly, arthritis, osteomyelitis, eczematous rashes, petechiae, purpura, pleural effusions, pneumothorax, and abscesses in the testes, ovaries, kidneys, spleen, liver, bone, and brain.

Assessment findings

The onset of brucellosis is usually insidious, but the disease course falls into two distinct phases. Characteristically, the acute phase causes fever, chills, profuse sweating, fatigue, headache, backache, enlarged lymph nodes, hepatosplenomegaly, weight loss, and abscess and granuloma formulation in subcutaneous tissue, lymph nodes, liver, and spleen. Despite this disease's common name—undulant fever—few patients have a truly intermittent (undulant) fever; in fact, fever is commonly insignificant. It may be observed if the patient goes without treatment for a long time.

The chronic phase produces recurrent depression, sleep disturbances, fatigue, headache, sweating, and sexual impotence; hepatosplenomegaly and enlarged lymph nodes persist. In addition, abscesses may form in the testes, ovaries, kidneys, and brain (meningitis and encephalitis). About 10% to 15% of patients with such brain abscesses develop hearing and visual disorders, hemiplegia, and ataxia.

Diagnostic tests

▶ Cultures of blood and bone marrow and biopsies of infected tissue may provide a definitive diagnosis. Culturing is best done during the acute phase.

▶ On blood work, an increased erythrocyte sedimentation rate and normal or reduced white blood cell count may indicate the presence of infection.

▶ Diagnosis must rule out infectious diseases that produce similar symptoms, such as typhoid and malaria.

TREATMENT

Treatment consists of bed rest during the febrile phase. Antibiotic therapy includes a combination of doxycycline (Doryx) and either gentamicin or rifampin (Rifadin). In severe cases, I.V. corticosteroids are given for 3 days, followed by oral corticosteroids. Standard precautions are required until lesions stop draining.

NURSING CONSIDERATIONS

▶ In suspected cases of brucellosis, take a full history. Ask about the patient's occupation and whether he or she has recently traveled or eaten unprocessed food such as dairy products (especially unpasteurized dairy products).

▶ Report all cases of brucellosis to the state health department or the Centers for Disease Control and Prevention.

▶ During the acute phase, monitor and record the patient's temperature every 4 hours. Be sure to use the same route (oral or rectal) every time. Ask the dietary department to provide between-meal milkshakes and other supplemental foods to counter weight loss. Watch for heart murmurs, muscle weakness, vision loss, and joint inflammation, all of which may signal complications.

▶ During the chronic phase, watch for depression and disturbed sleep patterns. Administer sedatives as ordered, and plan your care to allow adequate rest.

▶ Keep suppurative granulomas and abscesses dry. Properly dispose of all secretions and soiled dressings. Reassure the patient that the infection *is* curable.

▶ Before discharge, stress the importance of continuing medication for the prescribed duration. To prevent recurrence, advise the patient to avoid using unpasteurized milk or other dairy products. Warn meat packers and other people at risk of occupational exposure to wear gloves and goggles.

Patient teaching

▶ Tell patients to not consume unpasteurized milk, cheese, or ice cream. If unsure whether something is pasteurized, it is better to avoid consuming it.

▶ Instruct patients who are traveling to high-risk areas to avoid such things as "village cheeses," which are unpasteurized and pose a particular risk.

▶ Teach hunters and animal herders to use rubber gloves when handling the viscera of animals.

California serogroup viral disease

California serogroup viral disease is an acute inflammatory viral infection that commonly affects the brain, spinal cord, and meninges. It is caused by a virus from a group of related viruses called the California serogroup viruses. The group includes the La Crosse, Jamestown Canyon, Morro Bay, and Tahyna viruses. California serogroup viral disease commonly occurs in children ages 6 months to 16 years, with a peak incidence from ages 4 to 10. Adults may contract the virus, but they typically remain asymptomatic; when symptoms occur, adults develop fever or aseptic meningitis. California serogroup viral disease affects males more than females, possibly because males participate more frequently in outdoor activities.

CAUSES

California serogroup viral disease is transmitted to humans through the bite of an infected mosquito. After the mosquito inoculates the skin, the virus replicates, causing primary viremia. Next the virus spreads to the liver, spleen, and lymph nodes. If replication is efficient, the virus may continue spreading to the central nervous system through the cerebral capillary endothelial cells or the choroid plexus, causing viral encephalitis or aseptic meningitis. Most cases occur in the midwestern states during late summer and early fall.

COMPLICATIONS

Most patients with California serogroup viral disease recover completely; however, nearly 20% develop recurrent seizures or behavior problems. The associated mortality rate is less than 1%.

ASSESSMENT FINDINGS

The incubation period for California serogroup viral disease is typically 3 to 7 days. Within 1 to 4 days, the child commonly develops abdominal pain, chills, fever, headache, nausea, photophobia, and vomiting. As encephalitis develops, the child may experience lethargy, somnolence, incoordination, focal motor abnormalities, and seizures. Nearly 10% of children progress to a coma state. The duration of illness is typically 10 to 14 days. Adults are commonly asymptomatic, have a benign febrile illness, or develop aseptic meningitis. If aseptic meningitis develops, signs and symptoms include fever, headache, photophobia, and neck stiffness.

DIAGNOSTIC TESTS

▶ Cerebrospinal fluid analysis reveals normal to mildly elevated pressure, a normal glucose level, a normal or mildly elevated protein level, and leukocytosis.
▶ An elevated antivirus antibody titer indicates the presence of viral infection.
▶ Enzyme-linked immunosorbent assay detects specific immunoglobulin M antibodies to the virus.
▶ Results of a complete blood count are commonly normal or may reveal mild leukocytosis.
▶ Computed tomography or magnetic resonance imaging may rule out other neurologic disorder, such as cerebral hematoma.
▶ Electroencephalography may reveal seizure activity.

TREATMENT

Antiviral agents aren't effective against these viruses. Treatment is supportive: Measures include anticonvulsants, such as fosphenytoin (Cerebyx) or phenytoin (Dilantin) to treat seizures; an antipyretic and analgesic, such as acetaminophen (Tylenol) or ibuprofen (Advil) to relieve headache and fever; and I.V. fluids and electrolyte supplementation to prevent dehydration and electrolyte imbalances.

NURSING CONSIDERATIONS

▶ Monitor intake and output in addition to vital signs.

▶ Monitor the patient's neurologic status. Observe level of consciousness and watch for signs of increased intracranial pressure (increasing restlessness, confusion, vomiting, seizures, and changes in vital signs, behavior, motor function, and pupil size).

▶ Maintain seizure precautions. If a seizure occurs, don't restrain the patient. Place something flat and soft, such as a pillow or hand, under the patient's head. Clear the area of any hard objects and protect the patient from injury. Don't force anything into the patient's mouth if the teeth are clenched—a tongue blade could lacerate the mouth and lips or displace teeth, causing respiratory distress. Turn the patient's head to the side, if possible, to provide an open airway. After the seizure passes, reassure the patient and explain that he or she just had a seizure.

▶ Assess for signs of dehydration, such as tachycardia, dry mucous membranes, and decreased urine output.

▶ Maintain the patient on bed rest.

▶ Monitor serum electrolyte levels.

▶ Administer I.V. fluids and electrolyte replacement therapy as prescribed, and evaluate their effectiveness.

▶ Provide good oral hygiene; phenytoin may cause gingival hyperplasia, especially in children.

▶ Maintain a quiet environment. Darkening the patient's room may decrease photophobia and headache. If the patient naps during the day and is restless at night, plan daytime activities to minimize napping and promote nighttime sleep.

▶ Maintain adequate nutrition. It may be necessary to give the patient small, frequent meals or to supplement meals with enteral feedings.

▶ If behavioral changes occur, reassure the patient and family that the changes are usually temporary and will eventually disappear.

▶ Observe standard precautions.

Patient teaching

▶ Teach the patient and family about the disease process and treatment plan.

▶ Instruct the patient and family about preventive measures, including using insect repellant with a 10% to 30% concentration of N,N-diethyl-meta-toluamide (DEET) on skin and clothing for outdoor activities (avoid use of DEET on the hands of young children and infants younger than 2 months); covering an infant's stroller or playpen with mosquito netting when outside; wearing long sleeves for outdoor activities; repairing holes in screens on doors and windows to prevent mosquitoes from entering the home; and eliminating areas that attract mosquitoes, such as standing water in birdbaths, flower pots, old tires, and unused containers, which are excellent breeding grounds for mosquitoes.

CONTACT PRECAUTIONS

Campylobacteriosis

Campylobacteriosis is an intestinal infection caused by *Campylobacter*, which are spiral-shaped bacteria that invade and destroy the epithelial cells of the jejunum, ileum, and colon. The bacteria may spread to the bloodstream in people with compromised immune systems, causing a life-threatening infection. Most people recover in 2 to 5 days, although recovery may take up to 10 days in some.

CAUSES

Campylobacteriosis is transmitted via consumption of contaminated food, such as raw poultry, fresh produce, water, or unpasteurized milk, and through contact with the stool of an infected person. Transmission can also result from contact with the stool of infected pets and wild animals. Risk factors include recent family history of infection with *C. jejuni* and travel to an area with poor hygiene or sanitation practices.

Campylobacteriosis, which occurs more frequently in the summer months, is the most common bacterial cause of diarrheal illness in the United States. (See *Campylobacteriosis transmission.*)

COMPLICATIONS

Complications associated with campylobacteriosis include bacteremia, severe dehydration and electrolyte disturbances, and Guillain-Barré syndrome. Some patients develop arthritis. Patients with campylobacteriosis who are immunocompromised are more susceptible to sepsis, endocarditis, meningitis, and thrombophlebitis because of the spread of the bacteria into the bloodstream.

ASSESSMENT FINDINGS

Signs and symptoms of campylobacteriosis usually develop 2 to 4 days after ingestion of

Campylobacteriosis transmission

Campylobacteriosis is transmitted by ingesting contaminated food, such as raw poultry, fresh produce, water, or unpasteurized milk, and through contact with infected stool. Only a few organisms are needed to cause illness in humans. One drop of liquid from raw chicken meat can cause infection in a person. An estimated 100 people die from *C. jejuni* infections each year in the United States.

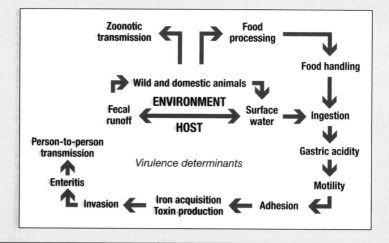

contaminated food or water. The patient's history typically reveals consumption of contaminated food or water, followed by an acute onset of mild or severe diarrhea. There may also be a history of recent close contact with a person experiencing diarrhea.

On examination, the patient may complain of cramping, abdominal pain, nausea, and vomiting. Fever may be present, and there may be traces of blood in the stool.

Diagnostic tests

▶ Stool culture identifying *Campylobacter* confirms the diagnosis of campylobacteriosis.

Treatment

Campylobacteriosis typically resolves on its own and isn't usually treated with antibiotics unless severe signs and symptoms are present. If severe symptoms are present, antibiotics such as ciprofloxacin (Cipro) and erythromycin (Ery-tab) may be ordered. Fluid and electrolyte imbalances are corrected with increased fluid intake or I.V. fluid replacement, as indicated.

Nursing considerations

▶ Monitor the patient's intake and output in addition to vital signs.
▶ Assess for signs of dehydration, such as tachycardia, tachypnea, and decreased urine output.

▶ Encourage the patient to consume extra fluids until diarrhea ceases.
▶ Monitor the patient's electrolyte levels, and assess the effects of replacement electrolyte therapy and I.V. fluids.
▶ Perform good hand hygiene before and after contact with the patient or the patient's environment and when moving from a contaminated area to a clean area during patient care.
◖ Observe standard precautions. Use contact precautions for diapered or incontinent persons for the duration of illness or to control institutional outbreaks.

Patient teaching

▶ Instruct the patient and family about proper hand hygiene.

 PREVENTION Teach the patient and family about preventive measures, including proper food handling and preparation (cooking poultry products thoroughly, using separate cutting boards for meat and other foods, and carefully cleaning cutting boards, countertops, and utensils with soap and hot water) and avoiding consumption of unpasteurized milk and untreated water.

Candidiasis

Candidiasis (also called candidosis or moniliasis) is usually a mild, superficial fungal infection caused by the genus *Candida*. It usually infects the nails (onychomycosis); skin (diaper rash); mucous membranes, especially the oropharynx (thrush); vagina (moniliasis); esophagus; and GI tract. Invasive candidiasis occurs when a *Candida* species enters the bloodstream, causing candidemia and then spreading throughout the body to affect the kidneys, liver, lungs, endocardium, brain, or other structures. Candidemia is the fourth most common bloodstream infection among hospitalized patients in the United States. Such systemic infection is most prevalent among drug abusers, patients who are already hospitalized, patients with a central venous catheter, burn victims, very-low-birth-weight babies, diabetics, or immunosuppressed patients. The prognosis varies, depending on the extent of infection. If the invasive form doesn't respond to treatment, organ failure and death may occur.

CAUSES

Most cases of *Candida* infection result from *C. albicans*. Other infective strains include *C. parapsilosis*, *C. tropicalis*, *C. glabrata*, and *C. guilliermondii*. These fungi are part of the normal flora of the GI tract, mouth, vagina, and skin. They cause infection when some change in the body (such as rising glucose levels from diabetes mellitus or lowered resistance from an immunosuppressive drug, radiation, aging, or a disease such as cancer or human immunodeficiency virus [HIV] infection) permits their sudden proliferation or when they're introduced systemically by central venous or urinary catheters, drug abuse, total parenteral nutrition, or surgery.

COMPLICATIONS

The most common complications include *Candida* dissemination with organ failure of the kidneys, brain, GI tract, eyes, lungs, and heart.

ASSESSMENT FINDINGS

The patient's history may reveal an underlying illness, such as cancer, diabetes, or HIV infection; antineoplastic therapy; or drug abuse. Symptoms of superficial candidiasis correspond to the site of infection:

▶ Skin—Scaly, erythematous, papular rash, sometimes covered with exudate, appearing below the breast, between the fingers, and at the axillae, groin, and umbilicus; in diaper rash, papules appear at the edges of the rash

▶ Nails—Red, swollen, darkened nail bed; occasionally, purulent discharge and the separation of a pruritic nail from the nail bed

▶ Oropharyngeal mucosa (thrush)—Cream-colored or bluish white curdlike patches of exudate on the tongue, mouth, or pharynx that reveal bloody engorgement when scraped; the areas may swell, causing respiratory distress in infants, or they may be painful or cause a burning sensation in the throat and mouth of adults

▶ Esophageal mucosa—Dysphagia, retrosternal pain, regurgitation and, occasionally, scales in the mouth and throat

▶ Vaginal mucosa—White or yellow discharge, with pruritus and local excoriation; white or gray raised patches on vaginal walls, with local inflammation; dyspareunia

Systemic *Candida* infection produces chills; high, spiking fever; hypotension; prostration; myalgia; arthralgia; and a rash. Specific signs and symptoms depend on the site of infection:

▶ Lung—Hemoptysis, cough, fever

▶ Kidney—Fever, flank pain, dysuria, hematuria, pyuria, cloudy urine

▶ Brain—Headache, nuchal rigidity, seizures, focal neurologic deficits

▶ Endocardium—Systolic or diastolic murmur, fever, chest pain, embolic phenomena

▶ Eye—Endophthalmitis, blurred vision, orbital or periorbital pain, scotoma, exudate

DIAGNOSTIC TESTS

▶ Culture of blood, sputum, skin scraping, vaginal scraping, or wound reveals *Candida*.
▶ Echocardiography reveals vegetation on heart valves in a patient with cardiac involvement.
▶ Funduscopy may reveal *Candida* endophthalmitis in a patient with invasive candidiasis.

TREATMENT

Initial treatment is aimed at improving the underlying condition that predisposes the patient to candidiasis, such as controlling diabetes or removing the central venous catheter or indwelling urinary catheter, if possible.

Nystatin is an effective antifungal for superficial candidiasis. Clotrimazole (Mycelex), fluconazole (Diflucan), ketoconazole (Extina), and miconazole (M-Zole 7) are effective in mucous membrane and vaginal candidal infections. Ketoconazole or fluconazole is the treatment of choice for chronic candidiasis of the mucous membranes. Treatment for systemic infection consists of I.V. antifungal drugs, such as fluconazole, caspofungin (Cancidas), micafungin (Mycamine), and anidulafungin (Eraxis). Other drugs that are sometimes used to treat invasive candidiasis include voriconazole (Vfend) and amphotericin B (Abelcet).

NURSING CONSIDERATIONS

▶ Swab nystatin on the oral mucosa of an infant with thrush. Treat the infant after a feeding because feedings will wash the medication away. The infant's mother should also be treated to prevent the infection from being passed back and forth.
▶ Provide the patient with a nonirritating mouthwash to loosen tenacious secretions and a soft toothbrush to avoid irritation.
▶ Relieve the patient's mouth discomfort with a topical anesthetic, such as lidocaine (Xylocaine). Because lidocaine can suppress

the gag reflex and cause aspiration, it should be administered at least 1 hour before meals.
▶ Provide a soft diet for patients with severe dysphagia. Tell patients with mild dysphagia to chew food thoroughly to ensure sure they don't choke.
▶ Place dry padding in the intertriginous areas of obese patients to prevent irritation.

PREVENTION Assess the need for indwelling urinary catheters and central venous catheters daily during multidisciplinary rounds. Make sure catheters that are no longer needed are removed.

▶ Assess the patient for underlying causes of candidiasis such as diabetes mellitus.

ALERT If the patient is receiving amphotericin B for systemic candidiasis, he or she may have severe chills, fever, anorexia, nausea, and vomiting. Premedicate with acetaminophen (Tylenol), antihistamines, or antiemetics to help reduce adverse effects.

▶ Check vital signs frequently in patients with systemic infection. Provide appropriate supportive care. In patients with renal involvement, carefully monitor intake and output as well as urine blood and protein levels.
▶ Perform good hand hygiene before and after contact with the patient or the patient's environment and when moving from a contaminated area to a clean area during patient care.
▶ Make sure patients with candidemia receive an ophthalmic examination.
▶ Observe standard precautions.

Patient teaching

▶ Encourage women in their third trimester of pregnancy to be examined for vaginal candidiasis to protect their neonate from infection at birth.
▶ Instruct patients who are using nystatin to swish it around in the mouth for several minutes before swallowing.

CONTACT PRECAUTIONS

Carbapenem-resistant Enterobacteriaceae infection

Carbapenem-resistant Enterobacteriaceae (CRE) are gram-negative bacteria, such as *Klebsiella pneumoniae* and *Escherichia coli*, that produce the enzyme carbapenemase. The enzyme carbapenemase makes these bacteria resistant to nearly all antibiotics and increases the risk for dissemination. Carbapenem-resistant *K. pneumoniae* is the most common species seen in the United States, followed by carbapenem-resistant *E. coli*. CRE are associated with increased mortality in patients who have prolonged hospitalizations and in critically ill patients with invasive devices, such as central venous catheters, indwelling urinary catheters, and endotracheal tubes.

CAUSES

CRE enter health care facilities through a colonized or infected patient or colonized health care worker. CRE are transmitted mainly through person-to-person contact and from patient to patient through the hands of health care workers. CRE have become prevalent with the overuse of antibiotics, which has given bacteria the chance to develop defenses—such as carbapenemase—against antibiotics.

COMPLICATIONS

Complications associated with CRE infection include sepsis, multisystem organ failure, and death.

ASSESSMENT FINDINGS

Some patients are colonized with CRE; they carry the bacteria but remain asymptomatic. Others become infected and develop signs and symptoms. Systemic infection produces chills, fever, tachycardia, and hypotension. Other signs and symptoms depend on the site of infection:

▶ Lungs—Tachypnea; crackles on auscultation; rusty, viscous sputum (if *K. pneumoniae* is the causative organism); cough; fever; and hypoxemia
▶ Urinary tract—Fever, urgency, frequency, dysuria, and suprapubic tenderness
▶ Wound—Purulent drainage, erythema, swelling, warmth, fever, and malaise

DIAGNOSTIC TESTS

▶ Culture and sensitivity of blood, sputum, urine, or wound reveals specific CRE.
▶ Complete blood count reveals leukocytosis.
▶ Chest radiography shows infiltrate or consolidation if pneumonia is present.

TREATMENT

CRE infection is treated with antibiotics, such as cefepime (Maxipime). Susceptibility testing helps determine antibiotic treatment options, which are limited. Incision and drainage may be necessary for treatment of an infected wound. Antipyretics such as acetaminophen (Tylenol) are given for fever. I.V. fluids are given to prevent dehydration. Vasopressors such as phenylephrine (Neo-Synephrine) may be necessary to reverse hypotension in patients with septic shock.

NURSING CONSIDERATIONS

▶ All acute care facilities should implement contact precautions for patients colonized or infected with CRE or carbapenemase-producing Enterobacteriaceae.
▶ Monitor vital signs as well as intake and output.
▶ Administer antibiotics as prescribed.
▶ Provide wound care if a wound infection is present.
▶ Administer antibiotics and I.V. fluids as prescribed.
▶ Perform routine mouth care.
   (See *Infection prevention and control guidance for CRE in acute care facilities.*)

 PREVENTION Assess the need for central venous and indwelling urinary catheters during multidisciplinary rounds. Immediately discontinue those that are no longer needed.

Infection prevention and control guidance for CRE in acute care facilities

The Centers for Disease Control and Prevention (CDC) recommends that all acute care facilities implement contact precautions for patients who are colonized or infected with CRE or *Klebsiella* carbapenemase-producing Enterobacteriaceae. The CDC has not made recommendations regarding when to discontinue contact precautions.

Laboratory guidelines

Clinical microbiology laboratories should:
• Follow Clinical and Laboratory Standards Institute guidelines for susceptibility testing and develop a protocol for carbapenemase production detection.
• Establish systems to ensure that infection prevention staff is promptly notified of all Enterobacteriaceae isolates that are not susceptible to carbapenem or *E. coli* isolates that test positive for a carbapenemase.

Surveillance

Acute care facilities should review the clinical culture results for the preceding 6 to 12 months to determine whether any cases of previously unrecognized CRE have been present in the facility.
• If cases of previously unrecognized CRE are found, a point prevalence survey should be performed to investigate the presence of CRE in high-risk units.
• If no cases of previously unrecognized CRE are found, continued monitoring for clinical infection is recommended.

If CRE or carbapenemase-producing *Klebsiella* or *E. coli* is found in one or more clinical cultures *or* if the point prevalence survey reveals unrecognized colonization, the facility should investigate for possible transmission.
• Conduct active surveillance patient testing in those with epidemiologic links to a patient with a CRE infection.
– Continue periodic testing until no new cases of either colonization or infection suggesting cross-contamination are identified.
– If transmission of CRE is not identified after repeated active surveillance testing, alter the surveillance strategy by performing periodic prevalence surveys in high-risk units.
• In CRE-endemic areas, an increased risk of CRE importation exists, and the procedures outlined may not be sufficient to prevent transmission. Facilities in these areas should monitor clinical cases and consider additional strategies to reduce rates of CRE.

▶ Disinfect reusable patient care equipment with an appropriate disinfectant after use.
◗ Observe contact precautions.
▶ Precautions.
▶ Change gloves when contaminated and when moving from a soiled area of the body to a clean area during patient care.

Patient teaching

▶ Teach the patient and family about proper hand hygiene.
▶ Instruct the patient to take the entire quantity of antibiotics exactly as prescribed, even if feeling better.

Cat scratch disease

Cat scratch disease is a bacterial infection caused by the fastidious gram-negative bacillus *Bartonella henselae*. Most people with cat scratch disease have a history of being scratched or bitten by a cat or kitten. Cat scratch disease is more common in children and young adults. In the United States, approximately 22,000 cases are diagnosed each year. Most cases are seen during the late summer, fall, and winter months.

CAUSES

Fleas, which carry *B. henselae*, inoculate a cat or kitten with the bacteria while biting. The cat, in turn, transmits the bacteria to a person through a bite or scratch. Kittens transmit the disease more often than cats. Nearly 40% of cats carry the bacteria at some point in their lives but show no signs of illness; therefore, it's impossible to detect whether a cat is a carrier. There is no evidence to suggest that fleas can directly transmit the bacteria to humans. Cat scratch disease is not transmitted from person to person.

COMPLICATIONS

Immunocompromised individuals, such as transplant recipients, those undergoing immunosuppressive cancer treatment, and patients with human immunodeficiency virus, are more likely to develop complications. Complications associated with cat scratch disease occur in approximately 14% of diagnosed cases and include bacillary angiomatosis and Parinaud's oculoglandular syndrome. Encephalitis occurs in less than 5% of infected patients. These complications are rare and typically occur in individuals with compromised immune systems.

ASSESSMENT FINDINGS

The incubation period is typically 3 to 14 days. Signs and symptoms include a mild infection with suppurative papules at the site of injury that commonly occurs 3 to 10 days after injury. One to 2 weeks later, lymphadenopathy develops, especially in the lymph nodes around the head, neck, and upper extremities. (See *Lymph node swelling in cat scratch disease*.) Nearly half of those affected also develop a rash, general malaise, fever, headache, fatigue, and anorexia.

Lymph node swelling in cat scratch disease

Cat scratch disease is an infectious disease that develops from cat scratches, bites, or other exposure to cat saliva. The bacteria *B. henselae* causes chronic swelling of the lymph nodes. Cat scratch disease is thought to be the most common cause of chronic lymph node swelling in children.

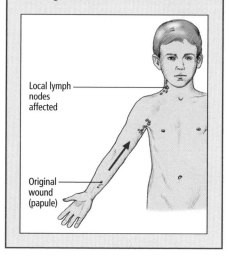

Local lymph nodes affected

Original wound (papule)

DIAGNOSTIC TESTS

❱ Indirect fluorescent antibody testing reveals *B. henselae* antibody.
❱ The skin-test response to cat scratch disease antigen is positive.
❱ A complete blood count may reveal leukocytosis, an elevated erythrocyte sedimentation rate, and elevated C-reactive protein.
❱ Lymph node biopsy can rule out other possible causes of swollen lymph nodes.

TREATMENT

Cat scratch disease typically resolves on its own in about 3 weeks and isn't usually treated with antibiotics unless severe signs and symptoms are present. Swollen lymph nodes may take 2 to 3 months to resolve. If severe symptoms are present, antibiotics such as ciprofloxacin (Cipro) or trimethoprim-sulfamethoxazole (Bactrim) may be prescribed. Acetaminophen (Tylenol) is used to relieve headache and fever. If a lymph node is very large or painful, it may be drained to help relieve the pain.

NURSING CONSIDERATIONS

▶ Perform good hand hygiene before and after contact with the patient or the patient's environment and when moving from a contaminated area to a clean area during patient care.
▶ Clean cat bites or scratches thoroughly with running water and soap.
▶ Administer antibiotics as prescribed.
▶ Apply warm compresses to swollen lymph nodes.
▶ Observe standard precautions.

Patient teaching

▶ Instruct the patient and family about the disease process and the treatment plan.
▶ Tell the patient to take the entire quantity of the drug exactly as prescribed, even if feeling better.

 PREVENTION Teach the patient and family about measures to prevent cat scratch disease, such as keeping pet cats indoors, staying away from strays, avoiding activities that may lead a cat to bite or scratch, controlling fleas on cats, not allowing cats to lick any open wounds, and cleaning bites or scratches immediately with running water and soap.

Cellulitis

Cellulitis is an infection of either the dermis or subcutaneous layer of the skin that commonly follows damage to the skin. Bacteria enter the skin through cracks, peeling, insect bites or stings, animal bites, human bites, injury, trauma, diabetic ulcers, or wounds from recent surgery. Skin disorders, such as eczema, psoriasis, ulcers, and fungal infections, also provide a portal of entry for bacteria. Once inside the dermis, the bacteria cause inflammation and infection.

Cellulitis can occur anywhere on the body, but the lower extremities are the most common site, especially the skin over the tibia and foot. It may also occur on the abdomen or chest following surgery or trauma and on the abdomen of those who are morbidly obese. Orbital cellulitis, an acute infection of the orbital tissue and eyelids, may also occur.

Cellulitis may be more severe in patients with chronic disorders, such as diabetes and human immunodeficiency virus, and in those who are immunosuppressed following chemotherapy or organ transplantation. If treated promptly, the prognosis is usually good. Left untreated, cellulitis can quickly become life-threatening.

Causes

Cellulitis can be caused by a variety of organisms, including bacteria and fungi; however, group A *Streptococcus* and *Staphylococcus aureus* are the most common causes. The most common pathogens in children include *Haemophilus influenzae, Streptococcus pneumoniae*, and *S. aureus*. Methicillin-resistant *S. aureus* (MRSA), once primarily a health care–associated pathogen, has also emerged as a common cause. The community-acquired strain of MRSA has a distinct susceptibility pattern and is more virulent than its nosocomial counterpart. Community-acquired MRSA skin and soft tissue infections were first seen in children, athletes involved in contact sports, and prisoners. In many areas of the country today, community-acquired MRSA has emerged as the primary *S. aureus* organism, even in patients without the previously identified risk factors. Community-acquired MRSA strains continue to be commonly seen in children and young adults, but they occur in all age groups.

Complications

Possible complications include sepsis, local abscess, progression to other tissue areas, tissue necrosis, thrombophlebitis, osteomyelitis, meningitis (if cellulitis involves the face), and lymphangitis. Complications of orbital cellulitis include cavernous sinus thrombosis, hearing loss, septicemia, meningitis, and optic nerve damage.

Assessment findings

Signs and symptoms of cellulitis include warmth and pain at the site of infection, erythema that increases as the infection spreads, skin that appears tight and glossy, lymphadenopathy, myalgia, malaise, chills, nausea, vomiting, and fever. Orbital cellulitis generally produces unilateral eyelid edema, hyperemia of the orbital tissue, reddened eyelids, and matted lashes. Although the eyeball is initially unaffected, proptosis develops later. Other indications of orbital cellulitis include extreme orbital pain, impaired eye movement, chemosis, and purulent discharge from the indurated areas. The severity of associated systemic symptoms (chills, fever, and malaise) in cellulitis varies according to the cause.

Diagnostic tests

▶ Visual inspection reveals cellulitis.
▶ A complete blood count shows leukocytosis, and the erythrocyte sedimentation rate may be elevated.
▶ Culture of fluid from the abscess is positive for the causative organism.
▶ Ophthalmologic examination is indicated in cases of orbital cellulitis to assess whether the eyeball has been affected.

▶ In patients with orbital cellulitis, computed tomography or magnetic resonance imaging of the sinuses and orbital tissue will determine the cause.

TREATMENT

Treatment of cellulitis may include I.V. or oral antibiotics for 7 to 10 days, depending on the infecting organism. Antibiotic ointment or eyedrops may also be prescribed for orbital cellulitis. Surgical incision and drainage may be necessary if an abscess develops. Elevating the affected extremity and applying warm soaks to the site help relieve pain and decrease edema. Warm compresses should be applied every 3 to 4 hours to relieve discomfort in orbital cellulitis. Analgesics may be prescribed to relieve pain. I.V. fluids may be necessary to prevent dehydration.

NURSING CONSIDERATIONS

▶ Monitor vital signs at least every 4 hours.
▶ Elevate the affected extremity to promote comfort and decrease edema.
▶ Encourage fluids and administer I.V. fluids and electrolytes as prescribed to maintain fluid and electrolyte balance.
▶ Apply warm compresses to the site every 3 to 4 hours to relieve pain and decrease edema.
▶ Give good skin care to prevent skin breakdown and further infection.
▶ Provide meticulous wound care after surgery.
▶ Administer antibiotics as prescribed.
▶ Assess pain level, and administer pain medication as needed.
▶ Perform good hand hygiene before and after contact with the patient or the patient's environment and when moving from a contaminated area to a clean area during patient care.
▶ Observe standard precautions; if a resistant organism is isolated, observe contact precautions.

Patient teaching

▶ Instruct the patient and family about proper hand hygiene.
▶ Teach the patient to apply warm compresses every 3 to 4 hours at home.
▶ Stress the importance of completing the prescribed antibiotic therapy, even if feeling better.
▶ Teach the patient with orbital cellulitis how to instill antibiotic eyedrops during the day and ointment at night.
▶ Teach the patient measures to protect the skin and prevent cellulitis, including moisturizing the skin to prevent cracking, wearing properly fitting shoes, carefully trimming nails, and wearing protective athletic equipment while playing sports.
▶ Tell the patient to maintain good hygiene and to carefully clean abrasions and cuts that occur near the eye to prevent orbital cellulitis.
▶ Instruct the patient to properly care for the skin if injury occurs by cleaning the area with soap and water, covering it with a bandage, and changing the bandage daily until healing begins.
▶ Advise the patient to report signs of infection, such as redness, pain, warmth, swelling, and drainage.
▶ Wear appropriate protective equipment when participating in work or sports activities.

Chagas disease

Chagas disease, also known as American trypanosomiasis, is caused by the parasite *Trypanosoma cruzi*, which is transmitted by bugs called triatomines. The disease is common in Central America, Mexico, and South America, where nearly 11 million people are infected. The insect that causes the disease thrives in poor living conditions, such as houses with thatched roofs and mud walls, so people who live in rural areas are at highest risk. Many people in the United States who have Chagas disease were infected in endemic countries. If left untreated, infection is lifelong and can be life-threatening.

CAUSES

Chagas disease is transmitted to humans through contact with the feces of an infected triatomine or "kissing" bug, which survives by sucking the blood of humans and animals. Triatomines are found in houses made from mud, adobe, straw, and palm thatch. During the day, the bugs hide in the walls and roofs. During the night, they emerge from hiding to eat, defecate, and inoculate individuals as they sleep. Chagas disease can also be transmitted through blood transfusion, organ transplantation, laboratory exposure, maternal-fetal transmission, and contaminated food and drink. Chagas disease is not transmitted from person to person.

COMPLICATIONS

Complications associated with Chagas disease include cardiac conduction defects, apical aneurysm, thrombus formation, stroke, and death.

ASSESSMENT FINDINGS

During the acute phase, which lasts 4 to 8 weeks, patients commonly have mild symptoms of febrile illness, such as fatigue, body aches, headache, rash, loss of appetite, diarrhea, and vomiting. A small skin lesion,

Romaña's sign

Unilateral palpebral edema, also known as schizotrypanosomic conjunctivitis or Romaña's sign (after the Argentinian researcher who first reported it in 1935), is a characteristic manifestation of Chagas disease.

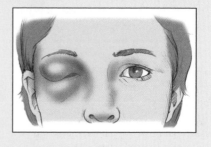

known as a chagoma, may develop at the site where the parasite enters the body. If swelling occurs around the eye, the eyelid may swell as well; this is known as Romaña's sign. (See *Romaña's sign*.)

Several days later, fever develops and lymph nodes become enlarged. This phase is sometimes fatal in children, but typically the patient survives. Rarely, acute myocarditis or meningoencephalitis is detected. Without treatment, the disease progresses into the chronic phase. About 80% of people remain asymptomatic throughout life and are considered to be in the indeterminate phase of chronic illness. It is estimated that over many years about 30% of patients with Chagas disease progress to clinically significant disease mainly affecting the heart. The first sign is typically a conduction defect, most frequently a right bundle branch block. Later in the illness the patient may develop ventricular tachycardia, sinus bradycardia, high-degree heart block, thrombus formation, and dilated cardiomyopathy with heart failure. These abnormalities place the patient at risk for sudden death. Chagas disease can also damage the GI tract, leading to dysphagia, esophageal reflux, weight loss, aspiration, prolonged constipation, and abdominal pain.

DIAGNOSTIC TESTS

▶ A blood smear identifies the parasite during the acute phase.

▶ Blood culture identifies *T. cruzi* during all phases of infection.

▶ A complete blood count shows leukocytosis.

▶ Serology tests will reveal immunoglobulin M antibodies.

▶ Polymerase chain reaction detects *T. cruzi*.

▶ Chest radiography may reveal cardiac enlargement.

▶ A barium enema may identify a dilated and elongated sigmoid colon, with rectal dilation.

▶ Echocardiography may identify cardiac abnormalities, such as cardiomyopathy, decreased ejection fraction, valve dysfunction, and dyskinesias.

TREATMENT

Nifurtimox or benznidazole may be given during the acute phase or to patients with congenital Chagas disease. These drugs may also be given to patients with chronic Chagas disease, but care during this phase is mostly supportive. For cardiac problems, antiarrhythmics or a permanent pacemaker may be needed, as well as diuretics, digitalis or vasoactive drugs. For GI problems, the patient's diet may need to be adjusted to one that is high in fiber with increased fluids, unless fluids are contraindicated by heart failure or renal problems. Laxatives and enemas may be needed. Pneumatic dilation of the lower esophageal sphincter may be performed to facilitate the passage of food. For fecal impaction, manual disimpaction or, in severe cases, surgical decompression may be required. Other surgical interventions that may be needed include a transhiatal subtotal esophagectomy or an abdominal rectosigmoidectomy.

 Prevention Blood treated with gentian violet can prevent the transmission of Chagas disease because it kills the parasite in the blood.

NURSING CONSIDERATIONS

▶ Monitor vital signs, including pulse oximetry. Monitor cardiac rhythm and report abnormalities to the physician.

▶ Administer medications as ordered and observe for adverse effects. If administering antiarrhythmics, note any improvement in cardiac arrhythmia.

▶ Provide a diet high in fiber and encourage fluid intake, if not contraindicated.

▶ Monitor GI status, and record all bowel movements. Administer laxatives or enemas as needed and note effects of treatment.

Patient teaching

▶ Teach the patient and family about the infection, including the cause, diagnosis, and treatment.

▶ Review all prescribed medication, including dosage, administration, and possible adverse effects.

▶ Discuss dietary recommendations. Refer the patient to a nutritionist if necessary.

 PREVENTION Teach patients living in endemic areas to inspect the home for causative insects, disinfect the home with synthetic pyrethroid insecticides, and place screens on windows and doors. The CDC recommends that travelers to Latin America sleep indoors in well-constructed facilities to lower their risk of exposure to triamines, which live in poorer-quality dwellings.

Chancroid

Chancroid, also known as soft chancre, is a highly contagious but treatable sexually transmitted infection characterized by painful genital ulcers and inguinal adenitis. Chancroidal lesions may heal spontaneously and usually respond well to treatment in the absence of secondary infections. The disease is usually found in developing and Third World countries. Only a small number of cases are diagnosed in the United States each year, most of which occur in people who have traveled outside the country to areas where the disease is relatively common. A high rate of human immunodeficiency virus (HIV) infection has been reported among patients with chancroid.

CAUSES

Chancroid results from infection with *Haemophilus ducreyi*, a gram-negative *Streptobacillus*, and is usually transmitted through sexual contact. Nonsexual transmission may occur when pus from the ulcer makes contact with skin in other parts of the body or with another person. Poor hygiene may predispose men—especially those who are uncircumcised—to this disease.

There is no evidence of natural resistance to this infection. A person can be readily reinfected after treatment if preventive measures are not taken. The disease has not been reported in infants born to women with active chancroid at the time of vaginal delivery.

COMPLICATIONS

Complications of chancroid may include phimosis, secondary infections, and urethral fistulas.

ASSESSMENT FINDINGS

After a 3- to 5-day incubation period, a small papule appears at the entry site, usually the groin or inner thigh; in men, it may appear on the penis; in women, on the inner thighs,

Chancroidal lesion

Chancroid produces a soft, painful chancre, similar to that of syphilis. Without treatment, it may progress to inguinal adenitis and the formation of buboes (enlarged, inflamed lymph nodes).

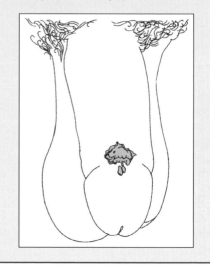

anus, vulva, vagina, or cervix. (See *Chancroidal lesion*.)

Occasionally, this papule may erupt on the tongue, lip, breast, or navel. The papule rapidly ulcerates, becoming painful, soft, and malodorous; it bleeds easily and produces pus. It is gray and shallow, can have sharply defined borders or irregular edges, and can measure up to 2″ (5.1 cm) in diameter. It is estimated that about half of infected men have only a single ulcer, whereas women tend to have four or more ulcers. Women may report pain with urination and intercourse, but they are often unaware of the ulcers due to their typical locations. Within approximately 2 weeks, inguinal adenitis develops, creating suppurated, inflamed nodes that may rupture into large ulcers or buboes. Headache and malaise occur in 50% of patients. During the healing stage, phimosis may develop.

DIAGNOSTIC TESTS

▶ Culture of exudates will reveal the causative organism.

▶ Dark-field examination and serologic testing can rule out other sexually transmitted infection, such as syphilis and genital herpes.

▶ HIV antibody testing can rule out HIV infection.

TREATMENT

The treatment of choice is azithromycin (Zithromax), erythromycin (E-Mycin), ceftriaxone (Rocephin), or ciprofloxacin (Cipro). Antibiotics usually treat the infection quickly with little scarring, although larger ulcers may take longer to heal. The safety of azithromycin for pregnant or lactating women hasn't been established. Aspiration of fluid-filled nodes may also be indicated to prevent the spread of infection.

NURSING CONSIDERATIONS

▶ Make sure the patient isn't allergic to the prescribed drug before administering the first dose.

▶ Observe standard precautions.

Patient teaching

▶ Instruct the patient not to apply lotions, creams, or oils on or near the genitalia or other lesion sites.

▶ Tell the patient to abstain from sexual contact until healing is complete (usually about 2 weeks after treatment begins) because the infection is contagious as long as the patient has any open sores.

▶ Stress the importance of washing the genitalia daily with soap and water. Instruct uncircumcised men to retract the foreskin for thorough cleaning.

▶ Advise the patient to avoid sexual contact with infected people, to use condoms during sexual activity, and to wash the genitalia with soap and water after sexual activity. Explain that abstinence is the only sure way to prevent chancroid.

Chlamydia trachomatis infection

Chlamydial infections—including urethritis in men and urethritis and cervicitis in women—are linked to the organism *C. trachomatis*. Trachoma inclusion conjunctivitis, a chlamydial infection that rarely occurs in the United States, is a leading cause of blindness in Third World countries. Lymphogranuloma venereum, a rare disease in the United States, is also caused by *C. trachomatis*. (See *Lymphogranuloma venereum*.)

CAUSES

Transmission of *C. trachomatis* primarily follows vaginal or rectal intercourse or oral-genital contact with an infected person. Because symptoms of chlamydial infection commonly appear late in the course of disease, sexual transmission of the organism typically occurs unknowingly. Children born to mothers who have chlamydial infections may contract associated conjunctivitis, otitis media, and pneumonia during passage through the birth canal.

Chlamydial infections are the most common sexually transmitted infections in the United States, affecting an estimated 4 million people each year.

COMPLICATIONS

Complications associated with *C. trachomatis* infection include epididymitis, neonatal death, pelvic inflammatory disease, premature rupture of membranes, preterm delivery, salpingitis, spontaneous abortion, and sterility.

ASSESSMENT FINDINGS

Both men and women with chlamydial infection may be asymptomatic or may show signs of infection on physical examination. Individual signs and symptoms vary with the specific type of chlamydial infection and are determined by the organism's route of transmission to susceptible tissue.

A woman with cervicitis may develop cervical erosion, mucopurulent discharge, pelvic pain, and dyspareunia. A woman with endometritis or salpingitis may experience

---

Lymphogranuloma venereum

A rare disease in the United States, lymphogranuloma venereum is caused by serovars L_1, L_2, or L_3 of *C. trachomatis*. The most common clinical manifestation of lymphogranuloma venereum among heterosexuals, especially male patients, is enlarged inguinal lymph nodes (usually unilateral). These nodes may become fluctuant, tender masses. Regional nodes draining the initial lesion may enlarge and appear as a series of bilateral buboes. Untreated buboes may rupture and form sinus tracts that secrete a thick, yellow, granular discharge.

Women and homosexually active men may have proctocolitis or inflammatory involvement of perirectal or perianal lymphatic tissues, resulting in fistulas and strictures.

By the time most patients seek treatment, the self-limited genital ulcer that sometimes occurs at the inoculation site is no longer present. The diagnosis usually is made serologically and by excluding other causes of inguinal lymphadenopathy or genital ulcers.

The treatment of choice is doxycycline. Treatment cures infection and prevents ongoing tissue damage, although the patient may develop a scar or an indurated inguinal mass. Buboes may require aspiration or incision and drainage through intact skin.

signs of pelvic inflammatory disease, such as pain and tenderness in the abdomen, cervix, uterus, and lymph nodes; chills; fever; breakthrough bleeding; bleeding after intercourse; and vaginal discharge. She may also have dysuria. A woman with urethral syndrome may experience dysuria, pyuria, and urinary frequency.

A man with urethritis may experience dysuria, erythema, tenderness of the urethral meatus, urinary frequency, pruritus, and urethral discharge. In urethritis, such discharge may be copious or scant and clear, purulent, or mucoid. A man with epididymitis may experience painful scrotal swelling and urethral discharge. A man with prostatitis may have lower back pain, urinary frequency, dysuria, nocturia, and painful ejaculation.

A patient with proctitis may have diarrhea, tenesmus, pruritus, bloody or mucopurulent discharge, and diffuse or discrete ulceration in the rectosigmoid colon.

DIAGNOSTIC TESTS

▶ Culture of the site of infection will reveal *C. trachomatis*.
▶ Nucleic acid probe will be positive for *C. trachomatis*.

TREATMENT

The recommended first-line treatment for adults and adolescents who have chlamydial infections is drug therapy with tetracycline (Sumycin), erythromycin (E-Mycin), or azithromycin (Zithromax). For pregnant women, erythromycin stearate (Erythrocin Stearate) or azithromycin may be used.

NURSING CONSIDERATIONS

▶ Make sure the patient isn't allergic to any drug before administering the first dose.
▶ Make sure the patient fully understands the dosage requirements of the prescribed medication.
▶ Urge the patient to inform sexual contacts of his or her infection so they can receive appropriate treatment.
▶ If required in your state, report all cases of chlamydial infection to the appropriate public health authorities, who will then conduct follow-up notification of the patient's sexual contacts.
▶ Check the neonate of an infected mother for signs of chlamydial infection. Obtain appropriate specimens for testing.
▶ Observe standard precautions.

Patient teaching

▶ Stress the importance of completing the course of antibiotics even after symptoms subside.
▶ Teach the patient to follow meticulous personal hygiene measures.
▶ Suggest that the patient and his or her sex partners receive testing for human immunodeficiency virus.
▶ Tell the patient to return for follow-up testing.
▶ Instruct the patient to avoid touching any discharge and to wash and dry the hands thoroughly before touching the eyes to prevent eye contamination.
▶ To prevent reinfection during treatment, urge the patient to abstain from sexual intercourse until he or she and his or her partner are free from infection.

CONTACT PRECAUTIONS

Cholera

Cholera, also known as Asiatic or epidemic cholera, is an acute enterotoxin-mediated GI infection caused by the gram-negative bacillus *Vibrio cholerae*. It produces profuse, watery diarrhea that starts suddenly and has a "fishy" odor, vomiting, massive fluid and electrolyte loss and, possibly, hypovolemic shock, metabolic acidosis, and death. Infection confers only transient immunity. A similar bacterium, *Vibrio parahaemolyticus*, causes food poisoning. (See *Vibrio parahaemolyticus food poisoning*.)

CAUSES

Humans are the only hosts and victims of *V. cholerae*, a motile, aerobic organism. It is transmitted through food and water contaminated with fecal material from carriers or people with active infections. Infection also occurs after eating shellfish from recognized environmental reservoirs of cholera.

Cholera occurs during the warmer months and is most prevalent among lower socioeconomic groups. Susceptibility to cholera may be increased by a deficiency or absence of hydrochloric acid.

COMPLICATIONS

Complications associated with cholera include hypoglycemia, severe electrolyte depletion, hypovolemic shock, metabolic acidosis, renal failure, liver failure, bowel ischemia, and bowel infarction.

ASSESSMENT FINDINGS

After an incubation period ranging from several hours to 5 days, cholera produces acute, painless, profuse, watery diarrhea and effortless vomiting (without preceding nausea). As diarrhea worsens, the stools contain white flecks of mucus (rice-water stools).

 ALERT Because of massive fluid and electrolyte losses from diarrhea and vomiting (fluid loss in adults may reach 1 L/hour), cholera causes intense thirst, weakness, loss of skin turgor, wrinkled skin, sunken eyes, pinched facial expression, muscle cramps (especially in the extremities), cyanosis, oliguria, tachycardia, tachypnea, thready or absent peripheral pulses, falling blood pressure, fever, and inaudible, hypoactive bowel sounds.

Vibrio parahaemolyticus food poisoning

Vibrio parahaemolyticus is a common cause of gastroenteritis in Japan. Outbreaks also occur on cruise ships and in the eastern and southeastern coastal areas of the United States, especially during summer.

V. parahaemolyticus, which thrives in a salty environment, is transmitted by ingesting uncooked or undercooked contaminated shellfish, particularly crab and shrimp. After an incubation period of 2 to 48 hours, *V. parahaemolyticus* causes watery diarrhea, moderately severe cramps, nausea, vomiting, headache, weakness, chills, and fever. Food poisoning is usually self-limiting and subsides spontaneously within 2 days. Occasionally, however, it's more severe and may even be fatal in debilitated or elderly persons.

Diagnosis requires bacteriologic examination of vomitus, blood, stool smears, or fecal specimens collected by rectal swab. Diagnosis must rule out other causes of food poisoning and other acute GI disorders.

Treatment is supportive, consisting primarily of bed rest and oral fluid replacement. I.V. replacement therapy is seldom necessary, but oral tetracycline may be prescribed. Thorough cooking of seafood prevents this infection.

Patients usually remain oriented but apathetic, although small children may become stuporous or develop seizures. If complications don't occur, the symptoms subside and the patient recovers within a week. However, if treatment is delayed or inadequate, cholera may lead to metabolic acidosis, uremia and, possibly, coma and death. About 3% who recover continue to carry *V. cholerae* in the gallbladder; however, most are free from the infection after about 2 weeks.

DIAGNOSTIC TESTS

▶ Stool or vomitus culture will reveal *V. cholerae*.
▶ Blood work will reveal elevated blood urea nitrogen and creatinine levels. Increases in serum lactate, protein, and phosphate levels result in a reduced bicarbonate level and an elevated anion gap. The arterial pH is usually low. Calcium and magnesium levels are usually high, and potassium levels are either normal or low.
▶ Dark-field microscopic examination of fresh feces will show rapidly moving bacilli (like shooting stars).
▶ Stool cultures will be negative for *Escherichia coli* infection, salmonellosis, and shigellosis.

TREATMENT

Improved sanitation and the administration of cholera vaccine to travelers in endemic areas can control this disease. The vaccine confers only 60% to 80% immunity and is effective for only 3 to 6 months. Thus, vaccination is impractical in endemic areas.

Treatment requires rapid I.V. infusion of large amounts (50 to 100 ml/minute) of isotonic saline solution, alternating with isotonic sodium bicarbonate or sodium lactate. Potassium replacement may be added to the I.V. solution. Antibiotic therapy can shorten the course of infection and reduce the rehydration requirement.

When I.V. infusions have corrected hypovolemia, fluid infusion decreases to quantities sufficient to maintain normal pulse and skin turgor or to replace fluid loss through diarrhea. An oral glucose-electrolyte solution can be substituted for I.V. infusions. In mild cholera, oral fluid replacement is adequate. If symptoms persist despite fluid and electrolyte replacement, treatment includes tetracycline.

NURSING CONSIDERATIONS

▶ Monitor output (including stool volume) and I.V. infusion accurately. To detect overhydration, carefully observe neck veins, take serial weights, and auscultate the lungs (fluid loss in cholera is massive, and improper replacement may cause potentially fatal renal insufficiency).
▶ Perform good hand hygiene before and after contact with the patient or the patient's environment and when moving from a contaminated area to a clean area during patient care.

 SAFETY Observe standard precautions (wear a gown and gloves when handling feces-contaminated articles or when a danger of contaminating clothing exists); observe contact precautions if the patient is incontinent or diapered, or to control outbreaks in a facility.

Patient teaching

▶ Instruct the patient and family about proper hand hygiene.
▶ Travel precautions to areas where cholera has occurred should include the following:
 - Drink only water that has been boiled or treated with chlorine or iodine. Other safe beverages include tea and coffee made with boiled water and carbonated bottled beverages with no ice.
 - Eat only foods that have been cooked thoroughly and are still hot, or fruit that you have peeled yourself.
 - Avoid undercooked or raw fish or shellfish, including ceviche.
 - Eat only cooked vegetables; avoid salads.
 - Avoid street vendors.
 - Do not bring perishable seafood back to the United States.

Chromomycosis

Chromomycosis is a slowly spreading fungal infection that involves the skin and subcutaneous tissue. It usually affects the upper or lower extremities but may also involve the buttocks, ears, face, shoulders, or trunk. Dissemination is rare. Over a period of years the infection may spread to adjacent tissue, causing large wartlike or cauliflower-like lesions and lymphatic stasis. Chromomycosis commonly occurs among rural barefoot agricultural workers in warm-weather regions. The disease is most common among men ages 30 to 50.

CAUSES

Chromomycosis is caused by dematiaceous fungi: most commonly *Fonsecaea pedrosoi* and *Cladosporidium carrionii*; less commonly, *Phialophora verrucosa*, *Rhinocladiella aquaspersa*, and *Wangiella dermatitidis*. These fungi are found in decaying vegetation, wood, and soil. *F. pedrosoi* is common in the tropical rainforests of Brazil. *C. carrionii* is common in drier climates of Madagascar, Australia, China, Mexico, Cuba, and Africa. Transmission commonly occurs from minor penetrating trauma caused by a splinter of wood or other material. The incubation period is unknown but is thought to be several months. Chromomycosis is not transmitted from person to person.

COMPLICATIONS

Complications of chromomycosis include progression to nearby tissue, abscess, squamous cell cancer, and secondary bacterial infection. Rarely, chromomycosis causes death.

ASSESSMENT FINDINGS

Patients become infected unknowingly. After several years, a small, raised, red papule develops. As the disease advances, the lesion becomes scaly and further progresses to form a wartlike lesion or a cauliflower-like mass that eventually spreads to nearby tissue.

DIAGNOSTIC TESTS

▶ Microscopic examination of scrapings from the lesion will reveal characteristic large, brown, thick-walled cells that divide into two planes.
▶ Punch biopsy and fungal cultures will reveal the causative organism.

TREATMENT

Small lesions are sometimes excised. Cryotherapy with liquid nitrogen may be used alone or in combination with itraconazole (Sporanox). Small lesions may respond to the oral antifungal agents flucytosine (Ancobon), posaconazole (Noxafil), terbinafine (Lamisil), and itraconazole. Larger lesions may require I.V. flucytosine and amphotericin B (Amphocil). If a secondary bacterial infection develops, antibiotics are prescribed according to the causative organism.

NURSING CONSIDERATIONS

▶ Perform good hand hygiene before and after contact with a patient or the patient's environment and when moving from a contaminated area to clean area during patient care.
▶ Clean lesions and provide wound care.
▶ Apply warm compresses every 3 to 4 hours.
▶ Administer antifungal medications as prescribed.
▶ If amphotericin B is prescribed, premedicate with antipyretics, antihistamines, or small doses of corticosteroids to reduce severe adverse effects.
▶ Observe standard precautions.

Patient teaching

▶ Instruct the patient about proper wound care.
▶ Advise the patient to wear shoes when going outdoors to prevent infection.
▶ Teach the patient the importance of proper hand hygiene, particularly before and after wound care.

Clonorchiasis

Clonorchiasis is an infection of the bile ducts caused by the Chinese liver fluke, *Clonorchis sinensis*. This chronic disease sometime lasts 30 years or longer but is rarely fatal. Clonorchiasis is widely found throughout China except in the northwestern region. It also occurs in Japan, Korea, Cambodia, and Vietnam. When found in other parts of Asia, it has typically been brought in from other areas, often via shipments of dried, pickled, or fresh fish imported from endemic areas. In most endemic areas, clonorchiasis commonly occurs in adults over age 30.

Causes

The Chinese liver fluke is found in humans, cats, dogs, swine, rats, and other animals. People are commonly infected by eating raw or undercooked freshwater fish that contain *C. sinensis* larvae housed in cysts. When the person digests the fish, the larvae are released from the cysts and migrate through the common bile duct. Eggs deposited in the bile passages are expelled in human stool. Snails then ingest the fully developed miracidia (ciliated larvae of a parasitic fluke that hatch from an egg). The miracidia produce more larvae, which are deposited into the water. In the water, the *C. sinensis* larvae penetrate a host fish and the cycle begins again. The life cycle from person to snail to fish to person takes at least 3 months to complete. Infection is not directly transmitted from person to person.

Complications

Complications of clonorchiasis include bile duct obstruction and cirrhosis. Clonorchiasis is rarely a direct or contributing cause of death; however, it places the patient at significant risk for cholangiocarcinoma.

Assessment findings

Many patients with clonorchiasis are asymptomatic or develop vague symptoms, which commonly result from bile duct irritation. Signs and symptoms associated with clonorchiasis include loss of appetite, abdominal fullness and pressure, and diarrhea. If bile duct obstruction occurs, the patient may develop jaundice followed by cirrhosis, hepatomegaly, ascites, and edema.

Diagnostic tests

▶ Microscopic examination of stool or duodenal fluid drainage will reveal *C. sinensis* eggs.
▶ Serologic testing with an enzyme-linked immunosorbent assay can be performed but may not be specific for *C. sinensis* infection.
▶ Computed tomography of the abdomen may reveal cholangiocarcinoma.

Treatment

Treatment may include anthelmintics such as albendazole (Albenza) or praziquantel (Biltricide).

Nursing considerations

▶ Perform good hand hygiene before and after contact with the patient or the patient's environment and when moving from a contaminated area to a clean area during patient care.
▶ Administer medications as prescribed.
▶ Observe standard precautions.

Patient teaching

▶ Teach the patient the importance of avoiding raw fish and thoroughly cooking freshwater fish.
▶ Tell the patient that freezing fish for at least 5 days or soaking it in a salt solution for several weeks may also prevent clonorchiasis.
▶ Instruct the patient about proper personal hygiene practices.
▶ Explain to the patient and family the disease process and the importance of breaking the flukes' life cycle.

⬇ **CONTACT PRECAUTIONS**

Clostridium difficile infection

C. difficile is a gram-positive anaerobic bacterium that typically produces two toxins, toxins A and B, and causes antibiotic-associated diarrhea. *C. difficile* infection is most common in elderly people, immunocompromised people, and those who have had a lengthy stay in a health care facility, have undergone GI surgery, or have a serious underlying illness. It's responsible for nearly 25% of all antibiotic-associated cases of diarrhea.

CAUSES

C. difficile colitis can be caused by almost any antibiotic that disrupts the bowel flora, but it's classically associated with clindamycin (Cleocin) use. Symptoms are caused by the exotoxins produced by the organism. Toxin A is an enterotoxin, and toxin B is a cytotoxin.

C. difficile is most often transmitted directly from patient to patient by the contaminated hands of health care workers; it may also be spread indirectly by contaminated equipment such as bedpans, urinals, call bells, rectal thermometers, nasogastric tubes, and contaminated surfaces such as bed rails, floors, and toilet seats.

COMPLICATIONS

Complications of *C. difficile* include electrolyte abnormalities, hypovolemic shock, anasarca, toxic megacolon, colonic perforation, peritonitis, sepsis, hemorrhage, and death.

ASSESSMENT FINDINGS

The patient may have a history of a recent hospitalization or antibiotic therapy. He or she may be asymptomatic or may exhibit any of the following symptoms: soft, unformed, or watery diarrhea (more than three stools in a 24-hour period) that may be foul smelling or grossly bloody; abdominal pain, cramping, or tenderness; nausea and vomiting; and fever. If toxic megacolon develops, the patient may develop increasing abdominal pain and show signs of septic shock (tachycardia, hypotension, oliguria, and tachypnea).

DIAGNOSTIC TESTS

▶ A cell cytotoxin test may show toxins A and B.
▶ Enzyme-linked immunosorbent assay detects toxins A and B.
▶ Stool culture may identify *C. difficile*.
▶ Abdominal radiography may show thumb-printing or colonic distention.
▶ Computed tomography may reveal mucosal wall thickening, colonic wall thickening, or pericolonic inflammation.

TREATMENT

In nearly 20% of people infected with *C. difficile*, withdrawing the causative antibiotic is the only necessary treatment. In the other 80%, oral metronidazole (Flagyl) is required in addition to withdrawing the causative antibiotic. Vancomycin (Vancocin) may be used if metronidazole has been ineffective.

 ALERT About 10% to 20% of patients experience recurrence with the same organism within 14 to 30 days of treatment. Beyond 30 days, a recurrence may be a relapse or reinfection with *C. difficile*. If the previous treatment was metronidazole, low-dose vancomycin may be an effective choice.

If toxic megacolon develops, the treatment is emergency bowel resection to save the patient's life.

NURSING CONSIDERATIONS

▶ Monitor the patient's vital signs, intake and output, and serum electrolyte levels.
▶ Observe the amount and characteristics of the patient's stools.
▶ Encourage fluid intake as indicated, and administer I.V. fluid as prescribed.
▶ Monitor for adverse effects of medication, and evaluate the patient's response to treatment.

SAFETY

Preventing C. *difficile* transmission

For health care workers
- Alcohol-based hand cleansers are less effective against *C. difficile*, so wash your hands well with soap and water.
- Wash your hands before entering and leaving a patient's room.
- Wash your hands before eating and after using the bathroom.

For patients
- Wash your hands before eating and after using the bathroom, bedpan, or urinal.
- Ask health care workers to wash their hands before they provide care.

For visitors
- Wash your hands before entering and leaving the patient's room.

- Wash your hands if you help care for the patient.
- Wash your hands before eating.

For caregivers at home
- Wash your hands well before and after caring for a person with *C. difficile* infection.
- If possible, wear disposable gloves if you must handle stool.
- Clean the bathroom frequently.
- Put disposable waste, such as diapers or other such items, into plastic bags; tie the bags securely; and place them with the regular trash.
- If clothes are heavily soiled with stool, wash them separately in detergent and bleach.

▶ Provide meticulous perianal skin care if the patient is experiencing profuse diarrhea.
▶ Perform good hand hygiene before and after contact with a patient or the patient's environment and when moving from a contaminated area to clean area during patient care.

 SAFETY Thorough cleaning and disinfecting of the immediate environment with 0.5% sodium hypochlorite (bleach) is necessary during hospitalization and after the patient is discharged because the spores of *C. difficile* are resistant to most common facility disinfectants. Make sure reusable equipment is also disinfected with bleach before it's used on another patient.

◯ Institute contact precautions and place these patients in private rooms, if available, or group them with other patients who have *C. difficile*–associated disease.
▶ Dedicate equipment whenever possible.
▶ Keep in mind that patients may remain colonized with *C. difficile* and shed spores even after diarrhea ceases.
▶ See Preventing C. difficile *transmission*.

Patient teaching
▶ Instruct the patient and family about proper hand hygiene practices.

▶ Teach the patient about the infection, including how it is transmitted, a possible cause, and treatment.
▶ Teach the patient about the prescribed medications, including drug, dosage, schedule of administration, and duration of therapy (usually 10 to 14 days).
▶ Caution the patient to avoid alcohol—including over-the-counter medications such as cough syrups that may contain alcohol—while taking metronidazole and for 3 days after cessation of the drug as the combination can cause severe abdominal cramps, nausea, vomiting, and headaches.

 PREVENTION Teach the patient how to disinfect surfaces, contaminated clothing, or household items with a bleach solution to prevent transmission.

▶ Encourage fluid intake; review signs and symptoms of dehydration.
▶ Advise the patient to notify the health care provider if complications or symptoms of relapse develop.

Coccidioidomycosis

Coccidioidomycosis, also called Valley fever or San Joaquin Valley fever, is caused by the fungus *Coccidioides immitis* and occurs primarily as a respiratory infection. Secondary sites of infection include the skin, bones, joints, and meninges. Generalized dissemination is also possible. The primary pulmonary form of coccidioidomycosis is usually self-limiting and seldom fatal. The rare secondary (progressive, disseminated) form produces abscesses throughout the body and carries a mortality rate of up to 60%, even with treatment. Such dissemination is more common in dark-skinned men, pregnant women, and people who are receiving immunosuppressants.

CAUSES

C. immitis lives in the soil in semiarid areas. Coccidioidomycosis is endemic to the southwestern United States, especially between the San Joaquin Valley in California and southwestern Texas; it's also found in Mexico, Guatemala, Honduras, Venezuela, Colombia, Argentina, and Paraguay. It is transmitted by the inhalation of *C. immitis* spores either from the soil in these areas or from the wound dressings or plaster casts of infected people. The infection is most prevalent during warm, dry months.

Because of population distribution and an occupational link (it's common in migrant farm laborers), coccidioidomycosis generally strikes Filipinos, Hispanics, Native Americans, and blacks. Of people who live in endemic regions, it is estimated that 10% to 50% will have evidence of *Coccidioides* exposure. In primary infections, the incubation period is 1 to 4 weeks. Coccidioidomycosis is not transmitted from person to person or from animals to people.

COMPLICATIONS

Patients diagnosed with coccidioidomycosis may develop complications, including bronchiectasis, osteomyelitis, meningitis, hepatosplenomegaly, and liver failure.

ASSESSMENT FINDINGS

About 60% of *C. immitis* infections do not cause any symptoms. However, primary coccidioidomycosis can produce acute or subacute respiratory signs and symptoms (dry cough, pleuritic chest pain, and pleural effusion), fever, sore throat, dyspnea, chills, malaise, headache, and an itchy, macular rash. Chest pain, night sweats, and arthralgias can occur as well. Occasionally, the only sign is a fever that persists for weeks. From 3 days to several weeks after onset, some patients, particularly white women, may develop tender red nodules (erythema nodosum) on their legs, especially the shins, with joint pain in the knees and ankles. Generally, primary disease heals spontaneously within a few weeks.

In rare cases, coccidioidomycosis disseminates to other organs several weeks or months after the primary infection. Disseminated coccidioidomycosis causes fever and abscesses throughout the body, especially in skeletal, central nervous system (CNS), splenic, hepatic, renal, and subcutaneous tissue. Depending on the location of these abscesses, disseminated coccidioidomycosis may cause bone pain and meningitis. Chronic pulmonary cavitation, which can occur in both the primary and the disseminated forms, causes hemoptysis with or without chest pain.

DIAGNOSTIC TESTS

▶ A coccidioidin skin test is positive.
▶ Complement fixation reveals immunoglobulin G antibodies during the first week of illness.
▶ Serum precipitins (immunoglobulins) are positive in the first month of infection.
▶ Immunodiffusion testing of sputum, pus from lesions, and a tissue biopsy may show *C. immitis* spores.
▶ Antibodies in pleural and joint fluid and a rising serum or body fluid antibody titer indicate dissemination.

▶ A complete blood count shows leukocytosis and eosinophilia. The erythrocyte sedimentation rate is increased.

▶ Chest radiography shows bilateral diffuse infiltrates.

▶ If meningitis is present, cerebrospinal fluid shows an increased white blood cell count to more than 500/μl (primarily due to the presence of mononuclear leukocytes), increased protein levels, and decreased glucose levels.

▶ Complement fixation antibodies may be present in ventricular fluid obtained from the brain.

TREATMENT

Mild primary coccidioidomycosis usually requires only bed rest and relief of symptoms. Severe primary disease and dissemination, however, also require long-term I.V. infusion (or, in CNS dissemination, intrathecal administration) of amphotericin B (Amphocin), fluconazole (Diflucan), or itraconazole (Sporanox) and, possibly, excision or drainage of lesions. Severe pulmonary lesions may require lobectomy. Ketoconazole (Nizoral) suppresses *C. immitis* but doesn't eradicate it. Ketoconazole and itraconazole are used for oral treatment of nonmeningeal infection and for long-term therapy.

NURSING CONSIDERATIONS

▶ Perform good hand hygiene before and after contact with a patient or the patient's environment and when moving from a contaminated area to clean area during patient care.

▶ Don't wash off the circle marked on the skin for serial skin tests because the circle aids in reading test results.

▶ In mild primary disease, encourage bed rest and adequate fluid intake. Record the amount and color of sputum. Watch for shortness of breath that may point to pleural effusion. In patients with arthralgia, provide analgesics as ordered.

▶ In CNS dissemination, monitor the patient carefully for a decreased level of consciousness or change in mood or affect.

▶ Before intrathecal administration of amphotericin B, explain the procedure to the patient and reassure the patient that he or she will receive analgesics before a lumbar puncture. If the patient is to receive I.V. amphotericin B, infuse it slowly, as ordered, because rapid infusion may cause circulatory collapse. During infusion, monitor vital signs (temperature may rise but should return to normal within 1 to 2 hours). Watch for decreased urine output, and monitor laboratory results for elevated blood urea nitrogen and creatinine levels and for hypokalemia. Tell the patient to immediately report hearing loss, tinnitus, dizziness, and all signs of toxicity. To ease the adverse effects of amphotericin B, give an antiemetic, antihistamine, and antipyretic as ordered.

▶ Observe standard precautions.

Patient teaching

▶ Instruct the patient and family about proper hand hygiene.

▶ Teach the patient that avoiding dusty environments in endemic regions can help prevent infection. Also, if the patient is at risk for severe disease, tell him or her to avoid activities that will increase exposure to dust (such as digging).

CONTACT PRECAUTIONS

Coxsackievirus infection

Coxsackieviruses, members of the Enterovirus family, are divided into two groups, type A and type B. Type A viruses cause hand, foot, and mouth disease and conjunctivitis; type B viruses cause pleurodynia (fever, abdominal pain, and headache). Both types can cause viral meningitis, myocarditis, and pericarditis. The first coxsackievirus was isolated from human feces in Coxsackie, New York, in 1948. Anyone can become infected by a coxsackievirus, but they are more common in children under age 10. Pregnant women can also transmit the virus to their newborn. In cooler climates, outbreaks commonly occur in the summer and fall in group settings, such as schools, day-care centers, or summer camps; in tropical areas, infection occurs throughout the year.

CAUSES

Coxsackievirus is highly contagious and can be transmitted in a number of ways. It is typically transmitted from person to person through the fecal-oral route, commonly via unwashed hands. Viral transmission can also occur when someone comes in contact with a surface that was contaminated with feces; the virus can survive on most surfaces for several days. Toys, utensils, and diaper changing tables that come in contact with contaminated body fluids can also be vehicles for virus transmission. Moreover, coxsackievirus can be transmitted through respiratory droplets when an infected person sneezes or coughs. The incubation period is typically 3 to 5 days.

COMPLICATIONS

Coxsackievirus can cause serious infections such as viral meningitis, encephalitis, and myocarditis. Newborns that are infected by their mother at or soon after birth can develop symptoms 2 weeks after birth. Affected newborns are prone to developing serious infection, such myocarditis, hepatitis, and meningoencephalitis. Coxsackievirus has been implicated in the development of acute-onset type 1 diabetes, although this relationship continues to be investigated.

ASSESSMENT FINDINGS

Nearly half of the children infected with coxsackievirus are asymptomatic. Others develop headache, fever (lasting about 3 days), muscle aches, sore throat, abdominal discomfort, and nausea. Coxsackieviruses can also cause symptoms that affect specific areas of the body. For example, in hand, foot, and mouth disease, painful red blisters develop in the throat and on the tongue, gums, hard palate, insides of the cheeks, palms of the hands, and soles of the feet. Fever persists for 2 to 3 days, while the associated lesions commonly remain for 7 to 10 days. Hemorrhagic conjunctivitis, also caused by coxsackievirus, affects the conjunctiva of the eye; the child commonly experiences eye pain, photophobia, inflammation, tearing, and blurred vision. Vesicular pharyngitis, also known as herpangina, is characterized by sudden onset of fever, sore throat, and small gray vesicles and ulcers on the tonsils and soft palate. These lesions commonly last for 4 to 6 days.

DIAGNOSTIC TESTS

▶ Diagnosis is typically made based on clinical findings.
▶ Viral testing (although rarely conducted) identifies the coxsackievirus.

TREATMENT

There is no specific treatment for coxsackievirus infection. The infection is typically self-limiting (children usually recover completely within a few days), and treatment is supportive. An antipyretic and analgesic, such as acetaminophen (Tylenol), may be given to control fever and pain. If needed, I.V. fluids may be administered to prevent dehydration. No vaccine currently exists to prevent coxsackievirus infection.

NURSING CONSIDERATIONS

❱ Perform good hand hygiene before and after contact with a patient or the patient's environment and when moving from a contaminated area to clean area during patient care.

❱ Monitor vital signs as well as intake and output.

❱ Monitor cardiovascular status frequently; if myocarditis develops, watch for signs of heart failure (dyspnea, tachycardia, cyanosis, and crackles).

❱ Monitor neurologic status often if the child develops meningitis or encephalitis.

❱ Maintain a quiet environment. Darkening the patient's room may decrease photophobia and headache if the patient develops meningitis or encephalitis. If the patient naps during the day and is restless at night, plan daytime activities to minimize napping and promote nighttime sleep.

❱ Give sponge baths, and administer antipyretics to control fever.

❱ Provide mouth care regularly.

❱ Encourage fluid intake, and administer I.V. fluids as prescribed to prevent dehydration.

❱ Maintain adequate nutrition.

❱ Disinfect reusable patient care equipment with an appropriate disinfectant after use.

❱ Frequently clean items that come in contact with the child's mouth, including toys and pacifiers.

 SAFETY Observe standard precautions; use contact precautions for diapered or incontinent children for the duration of illness to prevent transmission and control facility outbreaks.

Patient teaching

❱ Advise a pregnant woman to notify her health care provider if she experiences symptoms of coxsackievirus infection, especially if she's near her due date.

❱ Instruct the patient to use proper respiratory hygiene (covering the nose and mouth when coughing or sneezing, using a tissue to contain respiratory secretions, disposing of the tissue in the nearest receptacle and then performing hand hygiene), if able.

 PREVENTION Teach the patient and family about the importance of good hand hygiene, especially after using the toilet or changing a diaper and before preparing food or eating. Avoid close contact (kissing, hugging, sharing eating utensils or cups) with infected people.

❱ Advise parents to offer their child plenty of fluids and have the child rest in bed or play quietly indoors until symptoms subside.

 SAFETY Advise parents to keep the infected child out of day care or school until acute symptoms subside to avoid transmitting the infection to other children.

❱ Tell parents to notify the health care provider immediately if a fever higher than 100.4° F (38° C) develops in an infant younger than 6 months or if a fever higher than 102° F (38.8° C) develops in an older child. The health care provider should also be notified immediately if the child experiences anorexia, diarrhea, difficulty breathing, severe sore throat, severe headache, neck stiffness, difficulty feeding, abdominal or chest pain, seizures, vomiting, or testicular pain.

 SAFETY Clean dirty surfaces and soiled items, including toys, with soap and water and then disinfect them with a solution of chlorine bleach (made by adding 1 tbsp of bleach to 4 cups of water).

Creutzfeldt-Jakob disease

Creutzfeldt-Jakob disease (CJD) is a rare, rapidly progressive viral disease that attacks the central nervous system, causing dementia and such neurologic signs and symptoms as myoclonic jerking, ataxia, aphasia, visual disturbances, and paralysis. CJD is always fatal. A new variant of CJD emerged in Europe in 1996. (See *Understanding vCJD*.)

CAUSES

The causative organism in CJD is difficult to identify because no foreign ribonucleic acid or deoxyribonucleic acid has been linked to the disease. CJD is believed to be caused by a specific protein called a prion, which lacks nucleic acids, resists proteolytic digestion, and spontaneously aggregates in the brain. There are three major categories of CJD: It is estimated that up to 85% of cases are sporadic; 5% to 15% are familial, with an autosomal dominant pattern of inheritance; and the remaining cases are categorized as "acquired CJD." Although CJD isn't transmitted by normal casual contact, human-to-human transmission can occur as a result of certain medical procedures, such as corneal and cadaveric dura mater grafts. Isolated cases have resulted from childhood treatment with harvested human growth hormone and from improper decontamination of neurosurgical instruments and brain electrodes.

CJD typically affects adults ages 40 to 65 and occurs in more than 50 countries worldwide. Men and women are affected equally. In people younger than age 30, the incidence is 5 in 1 billion; in all other age groups, the incidence is 1 in 1 million. In the United States, an estimated 200 cases are diagnosed each year.

Understanding vCJD

Like conventional CJD, the variant of the disease (vCJD) is a rare, fatal neurodegenerative disease. Most cases have been reported in the United Kingdom. vCJD is most likely caused by exposure to bovine spongiform encephalopathy (BSE)—a fatal brain disease in cattle also known as mad cow disease—via ingestion of beef products from cattle with BSE.

vCJD affects patients at a much younger age (younger than age 55) than CJD, and the duration of illness is much longer (14 months).

Regulations have been established in Europe to control outbreaks of BSE in cattle and to prevent contaminated meat from entering the food supply. The Centers for Disease Control and Prevention and the World Health Organization are still exploring vCJD and its relationship to BSE.

COMPLICATIONS

Complications associated with CJD include impaired gait, incontinence, akinetic mute state, bronchopneumonia, and death.

ASSESSMENT FINDINGS

Early signs and symptoms of mental impairment may include slowness in thinking, difficulty concentrating, impaired judgment, behavioral changes, and memory loss. Dementia occurs early and is progressive. Involuntary movements (such as muscle twitching, trembling, and peculiar body movements), lack of coordination, and visual disturbances appear with disease progression and advancing mental deterioration. Hallucinations are also common. Coma and death typically occur within 4 months of the onset of symptoms.

Diagnostic tests

▶ Neurologic examination reveals difficulty with rapid alternating movements and point-to-point movements early in the disease.
▶ Electroencephalography shows abnormal brain wave activity.
▶ Cerebrospinal fluid analysis reveals 14-3-3 protein.
▶ Examination of brain tissue at autopsy provides a definitive diagnosis.

Treatment

There's no cure for CJD, and its progress can't be slowed. Palliative care is provided to make the patient comfortable and to ease symptoms. Medications such as sedatives and antipsychotics may be needed to control aggressive behaviors.

The need to provide a safe environment, control aggressive behavior, and meet physiologic needs may require monitoring and assistance in the home or in an institutionalized setting. Family counseling may help in coping with the changes required for home care.

Behavioral modification may be helpful, in some cases, for controlling unacceptable or dangerous behaviors. Reality orientation, with repeated reinforcement of environmental and other cues, may help reduce disorientation.

Nursing considerations

 PREVENTION To prevent disease transmission, use caution when handling body fluids and other materials from patients suspected of having CJD.

 SAFETY Use disposable instruments or special disinfection or sterilization (according to the facility's procedure) for surfaces and objects that are contaminated with neural tissue. No special burial procedures are currently recommended.

▶ Monitor vital signs and neurologic status.
▶ Administer medications as prescribed.
▶ Contact social services and hospice, as appropriate, to assist the family with their needs.
▶ Encourage the patient and family to discuss and complete advance directives.
▶ Offer emotional support to the patient and family.
▶ Refer the patient and family to CJD support groups, and encourage participation.
▶ Observe standard precautions.

Patient teaching

▶ Teach the patient and family about the disease, and assist them through the grieving process.
▶ Teach the patient's family about the importance of proper hand hygiene. Also instruct them to cover cuts and abrasions with waterproof dressings.

CONTACT PRECAUTIONS

Croup

Croup is a severe inflammation and obstruction of the upper airway, occurring as acute laryngotracheobronchitis (most common), laryngitis, and acute spasmodic laryngitis; it must always be distinguished from epiglottiditis. The term *croup* is derived from an old German word for "voice box" and refers to swelling around the larynx or vocal cords. Recovery is usually complete.

CAUSES

Croup usually results from a viral infection but can also be caused by bacteria, allergies, and inhaled irritants. Parainfluenza viruses are the cause in 75% of croup cases; adenoviruses, respiratory syncytial virus (RSV), influenza, and measles viruses account for the rest.

Croup is a childhood disease affecting boys more than girls (typically between ages 3 months and 5 years) and usually occurs during the winter. Up to 15% of patients have a strong family history of croup.

COMPLICATIONS

Children may develop complications, such as respiratory distress, respiratory arrest, epiglottiditis, bacterial tracheitis, atelectasis, and dehydration.

ASSESSMENT FINDINGS

The onset of croup usually follows an upper respiratory tract infection. Clinical features include inspiratory stridor, hoarse or muffled vocal sounds, varying degrees of laryngeal obstruction and respiratory distress, and a characteristic sharp, barking, seal-like cough. These symptoms may last only a few hours or can persist for a day or two. As it progresses, croup causes inflammatory edema and, possibly, spasm, which can obstruct the upper airway and severely compromise ventilation. (See *How croup affects the upper airway.*)

How croup affects the upper airway

In croup, inflammatory swelling and spasms constrict the larynx, thereby reducing airflow. This cross-sectional drawing (from chin to chest) shows the upper airway changes caused by croup. Inflammatory changes almost completely obstruct the larynx (which includes the epiglottis) and significantly narrow the trachea.

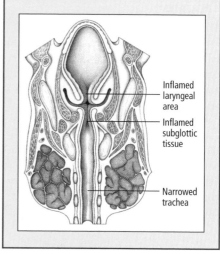

Inflamed laryngeal area

Inflamed subglottic tissue

Narrowed trachea

Each form of croup has additional characteristics. In laryngotracheobronchitis, for example, the symptoms seem to worsen at night. Inflammation causes edema of the bronchi and bronchioles as well as increasingly difficult expiration that frightens the child. Other characteristic features include fever, diffusely decreased breath sounds, expiratory rhonchi, and scattered crackles.

Laryngitis, which results from vocal cord edema, is usually mild and produces no respiratory distress except in infants. Early signs include a sore throat and cough, which rarely may progress to marked hoarseness, suprasternal and intercostal retractions, inspiratory stridor, dyspnea, diminished breath sounds, restlessness and, in later stages, severe dyspnea and exhaustion.

Acute spasmodic laryngitis affects a child between ages 1 and 3, particularly one with allergies and a family history of croup. It typically begins with mild to moderate hoarseness and nasal discharge, followed by the characteristic cough and noisy inspiration (that usually awaken the child at night), labored breathing with retractions, rapid pulse, and clammy skin. The child understandably becomes anxious, which may lead to increasing dyspnea and transient cyanosis. These severe symptoms diminish after several hours but reappear in a milder form over the next one or two nights.

DIAGNOSTIC TESTS

▶ Throat culture may identify the causative organism.
▶ Posteroanterior chest radiography may reveal narrowing of the upper airway.
▶ Laryngoscopy may reveal inflammation and obstruction in epiglottal and laryngeal areas.

TREATMENT

For most children with croup, home care with rest, cool mist humidification during sleep, and antipyretics, such as acetaminophen (Tylenol), relieve symptoms. However, respiratory distress that's severe or interferes with oral hydration requires hospitalization and I.V. fluid replacement to prevent dehydration. If bacterial infection is the cause, antibiotic therapy is necessary. Oxygen therapy may also be required. Increasing obstruction of the airway requires intubation and mechanical ventilation. Inhaled racemic epinephrine and corticosteroids may be used to alleviate respiratory distress.

NURSING CONSIDERATIONS

▶ Monitor and support respirations and control fever.
▶ Provide support and reassurance for the patient and family.
▶ Monitor cough, breath sounds, hoarseness, severity of retractions, inspiratory stridor, cyanosis, respiratory rate and character (especially prolonged and labored respirations), restlessness, fever, and heart rate.
▶ Keep the child as quiet as possible. However, avoid sedation because it may depress respiration. If the patient is an infant, position him or her in an infant seat or prop the baby up with a pillow; place an older child in Fowler's position. If an older child requires a cool mist tent to ease breathing, explain why it's needed.
▶ Control fever with sponge baths and antipyretics. Keep a hypothermia blanket on hand for temperatures above 102° F (38.9° C). Watch for seizures in infants and young children with high fevers. Administer antibiotics as prescribed.
▶ Relieve a sore throat with soothing, water-based ices, such as fruit sherbet and popsicles. Avoid thicker, milk-based fluids if the child is producing heavy mucus or has difficulty swallowing.
▶ Maintain a calm, quiet environment and offer reassurance.
▶ Perform good hand hygiene before and after contact with the patient or the patient's environment and when moving from a contaminated area to a clean area during patient care.

 SAFETY Observe standard precautions; however, if parainfluenza or RSV infection is the cause, observe contact precautions.

Patient teaching

▶ Warn parents that ear infections and pneumonia are complications of croup that may appear about 5 days after recovery. Stress the importance of immediately reporting earache, productive cough, high fever, or increased shortness of breath.
▶ Teach the parents effective home care. Suggest the use of a cool mist humidifier (vaporizer). To relieve croupy spells, tell parents to carry the child into the bathroom, shut the door, and turn on the hot water. Breathing in warm, moist air quickly eases an acute episode of croup.

Cryptococcosis

Cryptococcosis, also called torulosis or European blastomycosis, is caused by a fungus—usually *Cryptococcus neoformans*—that is found in soil and bird droppings. *C. gattii*, another species, less commonly causes symptoms in humans. Typically beginning as an asymptomatic pulmonary infection, cryptococcosis can disseminate to extrapulmonary sites as well, most commonly the central nervous system (CNS) but also the skin, bones, prostate gland, liver, and kidneys.

With appropriate treatment, the prognosis in patients with pulmonary cryptococcosis is generally good. CNS infection can be fatal, but appropriate treatment dramatically reduces mortality.

CAUSES

Cryptococcosis is transmitted through inhalation of the airborne fungus *C. neoformans*, which is contained in particles of soil and bird droppings. Because cryptococcosis can be transmitted through pigeon droppings, it's largely an urban infection. Cryptococcosis isn't transmitted from person to person. It's more prevalent in men than women, usually those between ages 30 and 60, and is rare in children. Cryptococcosis also occurs in dogs, cats, horses, cows, monkeys, and other animals.

Cryptococcosis is especially likely to develop in immunocompromised individuals, such as those with Hodgkin's lymphoma, sarcoidosis, leukemia, or lymphoma, and in those who are receiving immunosuppressive agents. People with acquired immunodeficiency syndrome (AIDS) are by far the most commonly affected group today, accounting for more than 80% of all cases. However, people without compromised immune systems develop cryptococcosis occasionally as well.

COMPLICATIONS

Cryptococcosis may cause ataxia, optic atrophy, hydrocephalus, deafness, paralysis, chronic brain syndrome, and personality changes. Without treatment, meningitis results in death within weeks to months. In immunocompromised patients who develop cryptococcal meningitis, the overall mortality rate following treatment is nearly 30%. Of those who survive, 40% have significant neurologic deficits, including vision loss, decreased mental function, hydrocephalus, and cranial nerve palsies. Relapse occurs in 20% to 25% of patients.

ASSESSMENT FINDINGS

Symptoms commonly begin 2 to 11 months after exposure to *C. gattii*; the incubation period for *C. neoformans* is unknown. Typical signs and symptoms of cryptococcosis include fever, cough with pleuritic pain, shortness of breath, night sweats, weight loss, weakness, and CNS disturbances. CNS involvement occurs gradually (cryptococcal meningitis) and causes progressively severe frontal and temporal headache, fatigue, diplopia, blurred vision, dizziness, ataxia, aphasia, vomiting, tinnitus, memory changes, inappropriate behavior, irritability, psychotic symptoms, seizures, and fever. Left untreated, CNS symptoms will progress to coma and death, usually as a result of cerebral edema or hydrocephalus.

Skin involvement produces red facial papules and other skin abscesses, with or without ulcerations; bone involvement produces painful osseous lesions of the long bones, skull, spine, and joints.

DIAGNOSTIC TESTS

▶ Chest radiography may reveal a pulmonary lesion if pulmonary cryptococcosis is present.
▶ Sputum, urine, blood, prostatic secretion, bone marrow aspirate, or pleural biopsy cultures identify *C. neoformans*.

▶ Culture obtained by bronchoscopy reveals *C. neoformans*.

▶ India ink preparation of cerebrospinal fluid (CSF) and culture reveal *C. neoformans*.

▶ CSF analysis shows increased CSF pressure, white blood cell count, and protein and decreased glucose levels.

▶ Blood cultures are positive for *C. neoformans* in severe infection.

▶ Cryptococcal antigen is positive.

TREATMENT

Patients with pulmonary cryptococcosis require close medical observation for a year after diagnosis. Treatment is unnecessary unless extrapulmonary lesions develop or pulmonary lesions progress, in which case oxygen therapy may be necessary to prevent hypoxia. Treatment of disseminated infection calls for I.V. amphotericin B (AmBisome), flucytosine (Ancobon), or fluconazole (Diflucan). Patients with AIDS will also need long-term therapy, usually with oral fluconazole. Treatment involves a single intensive course of treatment until cultures from the infected site return negative. Patients who experience CNS involvement may require a ventriculoperitoneal shunt if hydrocephalus develops. I.V. fluids and electrolyte replacement may be necessary to prevent dehydration and correct electrolyte imbalances.

NURSING CONSIDERATIONS

▶ Monitor vital signs and respiratory status.

▶ Monitor neurologic status, and note any changes in mental status, orientation, pupillary response, and motor function.

▶ Monitor pulse oximetry, and administer supplemental oxygen as prescribed.

▶ Monitor intake and output as well as electrolyte levels. Administer I.V. fluids and electrolytes as prescribed.

▶ Watch for headache, vomiting, and nuchal rigidity, which indicate neurologic involvement.

▶ If cryptococcal meningitis develops, maintain a calm, quiet environment and offer reassurance.

▶ Before giving I.V. amphotericin B, check for phlebitis. Infuse slowly and dilute as ordered—rapid infusion may cause circulatory collapse.

ALERT Patients receiving amphotericin B for disseminated infection may have severe chills, fever, anorexia, nausea, and vomiting. To help reduce adverse effects, premedicate with acetaminophen (Tylenol), an antihistamine such as diphenhydramine (Benadryl), an antiemetic, and small doses of a corticosteroid.

▶ Before therapy, draw blood for a serum electrolyte analysis to determine baseline renal status.

▶ During drug therapy, watch for decreased urine output, elevated blood urea nitrogen and creatinine levels, and hypokalemia.

▶ Monitor results of complete blood count, urinalysis, magnesium and potassium levels, and hepatic function tests.

▶ Ask the patient to report any hearing loss, tinnitus, or dizziness.

▶ Provide psychological support to help the patient cope with long-term hospitalization.

▶ Observe standard precautions.

Patient teaching

▶ Teach the patient about the disease process and treatment plan.

▶ Advise immunocompromised patients to avoid contact with birds as well as areas contaminated by bird droppings.

▶ Explain the importance of taking antifungal agents exactly as prescribed for as long as prescribed.

CONTACT PRECAUTIONS

Cryptosporidiosis

Cryptosporidiosis, also known as "crypto," is a highly contagious intestinal infection that typically results in acute, self-limiting diarrhea. However, in immunocompromised patients—who contract it more often—cryptosporidiosis causes chronic, severe, life-threatening symptoms. Those at greatest risk for cryptosporidial infection include patients with hypogammaglobulinemia, patients receiving immunosuppressants for cancer therapy or organ transplantation, and malnourished children. Cryptosporidiosis is especially prevalent in patients with acquired immunodeficiency syndrome.

In addition to immunocompromised patients, travelers to foreign countries, medical personnel caring for patients with the disease, and children are at particular risk. Cryptosporidiosis is spread easily in day-care facilities and among household contacts and medical providers. Backpackers, hikers, and campers who drink unfiltered or untreated water are also at increased risk. Contaminated water, such as in a swimming pool or contaminated stream, is a frequent source of infection. This disease occurs worldwide. (See *Preventing cryptosporidiosis*.)

CAUSES

Cryptosporidiosis is caused by the protozoan *Cryptosporidium*. These small spherules inhabit the microvillus border of the intestinal epithelium. There, the protozoa shed infected oocysts into the intestinal lumen, where they pass into the stool. Millions of these parasites can be released in a single bowel movement from an infected human or animal. *Cryptosporidium* oocysts are particularly hardy, resisting destruction by routine water chlorination. This increases the risk of infection through contact with contaminated water. Cryptosporidiosis may also be found in soil or on surfaces that have been

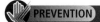 **PREVENTION**

Preventing cryptosporidiosis

At present, there is no vaccine available for cryptosporidiosis. In order to prevent infection, strict food preparation guidelines should be followed. Water should not be swallowed when swimming, and exposure to fecal matter should be avoided. In addition, proper handwashing should be observed. *Cryptosporidium* is poorly treated with chlorine or iodine; therefore, water suspected of contamination should be treated by boiling or filtration with an absolute 1-micron filter prior to ingesting.

contaminated with the feces from infected humans or animals. The disease can also be transmitted via contaminated food and person-to-person contact.

COMPLICATIONS

Complications resulting from cryptosporidiosis include severe fluid and electrolyte depletion, malnutrition, rectal excoriation and breakdown, papillary stenosis, sclerosing cholangitis, and cholecystitis.

ASSESSMENT FINDINGS

Although asymptomatic infections can occur in both healthy and immunocompromised patients, the typical patient with cryptosporidiosis develops symptoms after an incubation period of about 7 days. (The incubation period may be shorter in an immunocompromised patient.) The patient initially complains of watery, nonbloody diarrhea. He or she may also report abdominal pain, anorexia, nausea, fever, and weight loss. In the 10% of patients who develop biliary tract involvement, right upper abdominal pain may be severe. Signs and symptoms usually subside within 2 weeks but may recur sporadically for months to years.

The history of an immunocompromised patient typically reveals a more gradual onset of symptoms. These patients may also develop more severe diarrhea with daily fluid losses as high as 20 L.

For all patients with cryptosporidiosis, auscultation of the abdomen may reveal hyperactive bowel sounds. Palpation may reveal abdominal tenderness.

DIAGNOSTIC TESTS

▶ Microscopic examination of stool reveals the presence of oocysts. Detecting *Cryptosporidium* can be difficult, so patients may be asked to submit several stool samples over several days.

▶ Light and electron microscopy at the apical surfaces of intestinal epithelium obtained through biopsies of the small bowel reveals *Cryptosporidium*.

▶ Alkaline phosphatase levels may be elevated in patients with biliary tract involvement.

TREATMENT

Treatment for cryptosporidiosis consists mainly of supportive measures to control symptoms. Such measures include fluid replacement to prevent dehydration as well as administration of analgesics to relieve pain and antidiarrheal and antiperistaltic agents to control diarrhea. Nitazoxanide (Alinia), an antiprotozoal agent, may be prescribed.

NURSING CONSIDERATIONS

▶ Closely monitor the patient's fluid and electrolyte balance.

▶ Encourage adequate intake of fluids, especially those rich in electrolytes.

▶ Monitor the patient's intake and output, and weigh the patient daily to evaluate the need for fluid replacement. Watch closely for signs of dehydration, and provide fluid replacement as indicated.

▶ Administer analgesics, antidiarrheal and antiperistaltic agents, and antibiotics as indicated. Watch the patient for signs of adverse reactions as well as for therapeutic effects.

▶ Apply perirectal protective cream to prevent excoriation and skin breakdown.

▶ Encourage frequent small meals to help prevent nausea.

▶ Report all cases of cryptosporidiosis to local or state health departments, which will in turn contact the Centers for Disease Control and Prevention.

 SAFETY Observe standard precautions; use contact precautions for diapered or incontinent patients for the duration of illness or to control facility outbreaks.

Patient teaching

▶ Teach the patient about prescribed medications. Make sure he or she understands how to take the drugs and what adverse reactions to watch for. Stress the importance of calling the health care provider immediately if the patient develops an adverse reaction.

▶ Teach the patient and family to recognize the signs and symptoms of dehydration, including weight loss, poor skin turgor, oliguria, irritability, and dry, flushed skin. Instruct the patient to report such findings to the physician.

▶ Teach the patient and family about good personal hygiene, especially proper hand-washing technique. Explain how to safely handle potentially infectious material, such as soiled bed sheets.

▶ Advise the patient's family and close contacts to have their stools tested.

Cyclospora cayetanensis infection

C. cayetanensis is a protozoan parasite from the phylum Apicomplexa, a group of organisms closely related to pathogens that affect birds. These parasites cause a GI infection known as cyclosporiasis. *C. cayetanensis* is a coccidian parasite, which means those who are infected shed oocysts in their feces. Because the oocysts that are shed in the stool must mature outside the host in order to become infective to someone else, direct person-to-person transmission through the fecal-oral route is unlikely. If an infected person contaminates the environment and the oocysts have adequate time to mature, indirect transmission can occur. However, the time required for the oocysts to mature is thought be days to weeks, so indirect transmission is rare.

People of all ages are at risk for *C. cayetanensis* infection. It is seen worldwide but is more common in tropical areas. The infection has been identified in travelers to areas such as Peru, Nepal, Guatemala, Haiti, and Indonesia. Infections in the United States tend to peak during the spring and summer months.

CAUSES

Most cases of *C. cayetanensis* infection have been associated with contaminated food products. Outbreaks in humans have been linked to basil, snow peas, leafy green vegetables, Guatemalan raspberries, and Asian freshwater clams. However, transmission can also occur through drinking or swimming in contaminated water.

 ALERT *C. cayetanensis* is a recently identified microorganism. It was originally mistaken for other microorganisms, including cyanobacteria and other coccidia. Currently, here is little available information about the reservoir animal hosts and environmental survival time. It is thought that the oocysts tend to be resistant to extreme and undesirable conditions and can survive for long periods of time, but only if kept moist.

COMPLICATIONS

Complications associated with *C. cayetanensis* infection include dehydration, electrolyte imbalances, and weight loss.

ASSESSMENT FINDINGS

C. cayetanensis infection affects the small bowel, causing profuse, watery diarrhea 1 to 7 days after contamination. Other associated symptoms include abdominal cramping, bloating, and pain; anorexia; nausea; fatigue; and increased flatus. The patient may also develop body aches, a low-grade fever, and other flu-like symptoms. Some patients, especially those who are immunocompromised, may remain symptomatic for weeks to months and experience significant weight loss. In locations where *C. cayetanensis* infection is endemic, some people remain asymptomatic.

DIAGNOSTIC TESTS

▶ Acid-fast staining of stool specimens identifies *Cyclospora* oocysts. Oocysts may be unstained or stained light pink to dark red; those that are unstained have a wrinkled appearance. Because oocysts may be shed intermittently, a negative stool specimen doesn't rule out the diagnosis. Several stool specimens may be necessary before a diagnosis is made.
▶ Ultraviolet fluorescence microscopy reveals *Cyclospora* oocysts.
▶ Hot modified safranin technique identifies *Cyclospora* oocysts, which stain brilliant reddish orange.

TREATMENT

Trimethoprim-sulfamethoxazole (Bactrim) is the treatment of choice for *C. cayetanensis* infection. Although it is less effective, ciprofloxacin (Cipro) may be used in patients who cannot tolerate trimethoprim-sulfamethoxazole. I.V. fluids may also be necessary to prevent dehydration in some patients. Antipyretics, such as acetaminophen (Tylenol), are administered to control fever. If left untreated, the illness may be prolonged with episodes of remitting and relapsing symptoms.

NURSING CONSIDERATIONS

▶ Report cases of *C. cayetanensis* infection to the local health department so an outbreak investigation can be conducted to identify the contaminated food or water source.
▶ Monitor vital signs as well as intake and output. Assess for signs of dehydration, such as tachycardia, tachypnea, dry mucous membranes, thirst, poor skin turgor, and decreased urine output.
▶ Observe and document the amount and characteristics of the patient's stools.
▶ Encourage fluids, and administer I.V. fluids and electrolytes as prescribed. Remember that dehydration occurs rapidly in infants and children. Ice pops, gelatin, and ice chips may be included in the diet to maintain hydration.
▶ Administer antibiotics as prescribed. Make sure the patient isn't allergic to any drug before administering the first dose. Watch for adverse reactions when administering trimethoprim-sulfamethoxazole, and promptly report rash, sore throat, fever, cough, mouth sores, or iris lesions. These are early signs and symptoms of erythema multiforme, which may progress to life-threatening Stevens-Johnson syndrome or blood dyscrasias.

▶ Administer antipyretics, such as acetaminophen, to control fever.
▶ Perform good hand hygiene before and after contact with the patient or the patient's environment and when moving from a contaminated to clean area during patient care.
▶ To prevent skin breakdown in patients who are experiencing profuse diarrhea, provide meticulous perianal skin care.
▶ Observe standard precautions.

Patient teaching

▶ Instruct the patient and family to clean produce well before eating.
▶ Advise patients traveling to endemic areas to boil drinking water and to avoid consuming uncooked fruits and vegetables; *Cyclospora* is resistant to chlorination.
▶ Teach the patient and family about the importance of practicing good hand hygiene, especially after using the toilet, after changing a diaper, and before preparing food or eating meals.
▶ Encourage the patient to drink plenty of fluids while taking trimethoprim-sulfamethoxazole to prevent crystalluria and kidney stone formation.
▶ Advise the patient to avoid prolonged sun exposure, wear protective clothing, and use sunscreen while taking trimethoprim-sulfamethoxazole.
▶ Explain to the patient the importance of taking the antibiotic exactly as prescribed, for as long as it's prescribed, even if feeling better.

Cytomegalovirus infection

Cytomegalovirus (CMV) infection is caused by the cytomegalovirus, a deoxyribonucleic acid, ether-sensitive virus belonging to the herpes family. Also known as generalized salivary gland disease, CMV infection occurs worldwide and is transmitted by human contact.

CAUSES

CMV has been found in the saliva, urine, semen, breast milk, feces, blood, and vaginal and cervical secretions of infected people. The virus is usually transmitted via contact with these infected secretions, which can harbor the virus for months or even years. It may be transmitted by sexual contact and can travel across the placenta, causing a congenital infection. Immunosuppressed patients, especially those who have received transplanted organs, run a 90% chance of contracting CMV infection. Recipients of blood transfusions from donors with positive CMV antibodies are at some risk.

Between 50% and 80% of adults in the United States are infected with CMV by age 40; infection usually occurs during childhood or early adulthood. Approximately 1 in 150 children is born with congenital CMV infection. In most of these infants, the disease is so mild that it's overlooked.

COMPLICATIONS

CMV infection during pregnancy can be hazardous to the fetus, possibly leading to stillbirth, brain damage, and other birth defects or to severe neonatal illness.

ASSESSMENT FINDINGS

CMV probably spreads through the body in lymphocytes or mononuclear cells to the lungs, liver, GI tract, eyes, and central nervous system, where it commonly produces inflammatory reactions.

Most patients with CMV infection have mild, nonspecific complaints or none at all, even though antibody titers indicate infection. In these patients, the disease usually runs a self-limiting course. However, immunocompromised patients and those receiving immunosuppressants may develop pneumonia or other secondary infections. In patients with acquired immunodeficiency syndrome (AIDS), disseminated CMV infection may cause chorioretinitis (resulting in blindness), colitis, encephalitis, abdominal pain, diarrhea, or weight loss. Infected infants ages 3 to 6 months usually appear asymptomatic but may develop hepatic dysfunction, hepatosplenomegaly, spider angiomas, pneumonitis, and lymphadenopathy. (See *CMV infection in immunosuppressed patients.*)

Congenital CMV infection is seldom apparent at birth, although the neonate's urine contains the virus. CMV can cause brain damage that may not show up for months after birth. It also can produce a rapidly fatal neonatal illness characterized by jaundice, petechial rash, hepatosplenomegaly, thrombocytopenia, hemolytic anemia, microcephaly, psychomotor retardation, mental deficiency, and hearing loss. This form is sometimes rapidly fatal.

In some adults, CMV may cause CMV mononucleosis, with 3 weeks or more of irregular, high fever. Other findings in CMV mononucleosis may include a normal or elevated white blood cell count, lymphocytosis, and increased atypical lymphocytes.

DIAGNOSTIC TESTS

▶ Virus may be isolated in urine, saliva, throat, cervix, or biopsy specimens.

▶ Chest radiography typically shows bilateral, diffuse, white infiltrates.

▶ Complement fixation studies, hemagglutination inhibition antibody tests and, for congenital infections, indirect immunofluorescent tests for CMV immunoglobulin M antibody help confirm the diagnosis.

CMV infection in immunosuppressed patients

The table below lists types of immunosuppressed patients, their risk factors for CMV infection, associated disorders, and prevention tips.

Patient	Risk factors	Associated disorders	Prevention
Fetus	Primary maternal infection in early pregnancy	Cytomegalic inclusion disease	Maternal avoidance of exposure
Organ transplant recipient	Seropositive donor, seronegative recipient; intensive immunosuppression, particularly with anti-lymphocyte globulins or cyclosporine	Febrile leukopenia, pneumonia, GI disease	Donor matching, CMV immunoglobulin, ganciclovir, or high-dose acyclovir
Bone marrow transplant recipient	Graft-versus-host disease, older age, seropositive recipient, viremia	Pneumonia, GI disease	Ganciclovir or high-dose acyclovir
Patient with AIDS	Less than 100 CD4+ cells/μl; CMV seropositivity	Chorioretinitis, GI disease, neurologic disease	Ganciclovir or foscarnet

TREATMENT

Treatment is aimed at relieving symptoms and preventing complications. In the immunosuppressed patient, CMV may be treated with ganciclovir (Cytovene), valganciclovir (Valcyte), cidofovir (Vistide) and, possibly, foscarnet (Foscavir).

NURSING CONSIDERATIONS

▶ Monitor vital signs.
▶ Monitor complete blood count, platelet count, and creatinine levels during treatment.
▶ Provide emotional support to the parents of children with severe congenital CMV infection; brain damage or death may result.
▶ Observe standard precautions.

Patient teaching

▶ Teach the parents of infected children about practicing good personal hygiene, especially handwashing with soap and water after contact with the infected child's diapers or saliva.
▶ Instruct patients about measures to prevent CMV infection, such as giving children under age 6 a hug or kissing them on the head rather than on the mouth and not sharing food, drinks, or utensils with young children.
▶ Tell pregnant day-care workers who have never been infected with CMV to work with children older than age 2½ to reduce the risk for infection.

Dengue fever

Dengue fever, a virus that causes flu-like symptoms, is transmitted by the bite of an infected mosquito. The incubation period is generally 5 to 10 days. Dengue fever occurs in tropical regions, with approximately 100 million cases reported annually. Increased travel to endemic areas, along with overpopulation and inadequate public health systems, may be responsible for the increased spread of the virus. Dengue fever is considered the most important mosquito-borne virus affecting humans.

 PREVENTION The Pan American Health Organization has developed a task force dedicated to the prevention and control of dengue fever. Its goal is to promote behavioral and environmental changes and achieve effective communication between government, community, and health agencies regarding recognition, treatment, and prevention of the illness.

CAUSES

Dengue fever is caused by one of four types of virus (DENV-1, DENV-2, DENV-3, and DENV-4) of the genus *Flavivirus*. It is transmitted by *Aedes aegypti* and *Aedes albopictus* mosquitoes. Infection with one type of dengue virus provides lifelong immunity against that particular strain but may not provide protection from the other three virus strains.

 PREVENTION Several dengue fever vaccines are being investigated, two of which have advanced to human testing. Developing an effective vaccine presents a challenge, however, because the vaccine must be effective against all four types of dengue virus.

COMPLICATIONS

Dengue hemorrhagic fever (DHF) is a more severe form of dengue fever in which fevers may reach 106° F (41° C) and cause seizures.

This complication occurs when a patient infected with one dengue virus serotype becomes infected with a second type of dengue virus. Thrombocytopenia and hemoconcentration occur, causing leakage of intravascular volume from capillaries. This may lead to the development of dengue shock syndrome (DSS), which may be fatal.

Other rare complications include liver failure, encephalopathy, myocarditis, or brain injury resulting from DSS or intracranial hemorrhage.

ASSESSMENT FINDINGS

Dengue fever presents with flu-like symptoms: weakness, malaise, frontal headache, eye pain, and bone, joint, and muscle pain. An acute high fever—up to 103° to 106.5° F (39.5° to 41.4° C)—follows chills, erythematous mottling of the skin, and facial flushing (a specific indicator of dengue). Fever generally lasts for 5 to 7 days. Nausea, vomiting, change in taste, and abdominal pain may occur. A generalized maculopapular rash may develop within 1 to 2 days of the fever, accompanied by a secondary morbilliform, maculopapular rash that spares the palms of the hands and soles of the feet. This rash may last 1 to 5 days and may desquamate. Myalgia of the lower back, arms, and legs may occur, along with arthralgia of the knees and shoulders. Hypotension may result from hypovolemia. Acute symptoms last approximately 1 week, but weakness, anorexia, and malaise may linger for several more weeks. Some infections may produce few or no symptoms, especially in children.

DHF findings include a positive tourniquet test (10 or more petechiae developing after a blood pressure cuff is inflated midway between the patient's systolic and diastolic pressure for 5 minutes), ecchymosis or purpura, and bleeding from injection sites, mucosa, or other sites. Melena may also occur. DSS includes all the signs of DHF in addition to a rapid, weak pulse; narrow pulse pressure; hypotension; cold, clammy skin; and restlessness.

DIAGNOSTIC TESTS

▶ Blood cultures can isolate the specific virus.

▶ An enzyme-linked immunosorbent assay will detect immunoglobulins IgM and IgG (more than 6 days after onset of symptoms). With DHF:

▶ Blood work may show a rise in hematocrit of 20%, with an even larger increase after treatment with fluids. Thrombocytopenia may also be present.

▶ Chest radiography may identify pleural effusion.

TREATMENT

There is no specific treatment for dengue fever. Supportive care should be provided, such as hydration with oral fluids and normal saline I.V. Administration of acetaminophen will help with fever as well as muscle and joint pain. Nonsteroidal anti-inflammatory drugs and aspirin should be avoided due to bleeding complications that may occur with DHF. If DHF or DSS develops, additional supportive care may be needed. In most cases, the patient will be treated at home, with hospitalization necessary only if DHF or DSS develops or if the patient becomes severely dehydrated. With DHF and DSS, blood products may be administered.

NURSING CONSIDERATIONS

▶ Encourage oral fluid intake, and administer I.V. fluids as ordered.

▶ Administer prescribed medications, such as acetaminophen, and evaluate for effects.

▶ Monitor vital signs as well as intake and output.

▶ Provide comfort measures, such as tepid baths to reduce fever and massage and position changes to relieve muscle and joint pain.

▶ Monitor for signs of complications, such as hypotension, restlessness, change in mental status, petechiae, epistaxis, microscopic hematuria, and melena.

▶ Monitor laboratory results of complete blood count, especially hematocrit and platelet levels.

▶ If seizures occur, institute seizure precautions.

Patient teaching

▶ Teach the patient about the infection, including how it is transmitted, possible causes, and treatment.

▶ Discuss the signs and symptoms of possible complications, and outline any complications that should be reported to the practitioner immediately. Stress that complications may occur after the fever has abated.

▶ To prevent the complication of Reye syndrome, advise parents of children with dengue fever to avoid giving aspirin.

 PREVENTION People who reside in a tropical environment should be advised to remove any potential settings for mosquito breeding, such as water storage devices (for example, discarded tires). Use of insecticides may also be required in areas of outbreak. To prevent mosquito bites when traveling to a tropical region, advise the patient and family to utilize insect repellent and mosquito netting and to wear protective clothing.

Dermatophytosis

Dermatophytosis (tinea) is a group of superficial fungal infections usually classified according to their anatomic location. Dermatophytosis may affect the scalp (tinea capitis), the bearded skin of the face (tinea barbae), the body (tinea corporis, occurring mainly in children), the groin (tinea cruris, or jock itch), the nails (tinea unguium, also called onychomycosis), or the feet (tinea pedis, or athlete's foot). These disorders vary from mild inflammations to acute vesicular reactions.

CAUSES

Tinea infections are caused by dermatophytes (fungi) of the genera *Trichophyton*, *Microsporum*, and *Epidermophyton*. Transmission can occur directly (through contact with infected lesions) or indirectly (through contact with contaminated articles or surfaces, such as shoes, towels, or shower stalls). Some cases result from contact with contaminated animals or soil. Warm weather, humidity, and tight clothing encourage fungus growth.

COMPLICATIONS

Hair or nail loss and secondary bacterial or candidal infections, resulting in inflammation, itching, tenderness, and maceration, are common complications of tinea infection. About 20% of infected people develop chronic conditions.

ASSESSMENT FINDINGS

Tinea lesions vary in appearance and duration. Inspection of a patient with tinea capitis may expose small, spreading papules on the scalp that may progress to inflamed, pus-filled lesions (kerions). Patchy hair loss with scaling may be visible. Tinea barbae appears as pustular folliculitis in the bearded area.

In patients with tinea corporis, inspection and palpation reveal flat skin lesions at any site except the scalp, bearded skin, or feet. These lesions may be dry and scaly or moist and crusty; as they enlarge, their centers heal, producing the classic ring-shaped appearance.

In patients with tinea cruris, inspection and palpation reveal raised, sharply defined, itchy red lesions in the groin that may extend to the buttocks, inner thighs, and external genitalia.

Tinea unguium starts at the tip of one or more toenails (fingernail infection is less common). Inspection reveals gradual thickening, discoloration, and crumbling of the nail, with accumulation of subungual debris. Eventually, the nail may be completely destroyed.

A patient with severe tinea pedis may complain of extreme itching and pain on walking. Inspection findings include scaling and blisters between the toes and, possibly, a dry, squamous inflammation that affects the entire sole.

DIAGNOSTIC TESTS

▶ A potassium hydroxide test coupled with microscopic examination of lesion scrapings usually help confirm tinea infection.
▶ Wood's light examination may help confirm some types of tinea capitis.
▶ Culture of the affected area may help to identify the infecting organism.

TREATMENT

Local tinea infections usually respond to topical antifungal agents, such as imidazole cream or oral griseofulvin (Griseofulvin) for infections of the skin and hair. Oral terbinafine (Lamisil) or itraconazole is helpful for nail infections. However, topical therapy is ineffective for tinea capitis; oral griseofulvin for 1 to 3 months is the treatment of choice. In addition to imidazole, other antifungals include naftifine (Naftin), ciclopirox (Loprox), terbinafine (Lamisil), and tolnaftate. Topical treatment should continue for 2 weeks after lesions resolve.

Supportive measures include application of open wet dressings, removal of scabs and scales, and administration of a keratolytic, such as salicylic acid, to soften and remove hyperkeratotic lesions of the heels or soles.

Nursing considerations

▶ Be alert for possible adverse reactions to griseofulvin therapy, including sensitivity reactions, GI disturbances, headaches, photosensitivity and, possibly, liver damage.
▶ Monitor liver function in patients taking griseofulvin.
▶ Patients with tinea capitis should discontinue medications and notify the physician if the condition worsens.
▶ Use careful handwashing technique.
▶ For patients with tinea corporis who have excessive abdominal girth, place abdominal pads between skinfolds and change the pads frequently. Check the patient daily for excoriated, newly denuded skin areas. Apply open wet dressings two or three times daily to decrease inflammation and help remove scales.
▶ For tinea unguium, keep the patient's nails short and straight, and gently remove debris under the nails. Prepare the patient for prolonged therapy, and outline possible adverse reactions to griseofulvin, which is contraindicated in patients with porphyria and may require an increase in dosage during anticoagulant (warfarin) therapy.
▶ For patients with tinea cruris, provide sitz baths, as ordered, to relieve itching.
▶ Observe standard precautions.

Patient teaching
▶ Teach the patient and family about transmission and recurrence of the infection.

Teach the patient and family to identify environmental conditions that encourage fungal growth or aggravate the disorder.
▶ Instruct the patient to wear loose-fitting, cotton clothing, which should be changed frequently and laundered in hot water to avoid aggravating the condition.
▶ Teach the patient and family about prescribed medications and preparations. Stress the importance of completing the entire treatment regimen, even after the lesions appear to have healed. Instruct patients to notify the physician if adverse reactions occur.
▶ Advise the patient to avoid scratching because scarring and secondary infection may occur.
▶ Instruct patients with tinea cruris to dry the affected area thoroughly after bathing and to dust evenly with antifungal powder. Suggest sitz baths to relieve itching.
▶ Encourage patients with tinea pedis to expose the feet to air whenever possible and to wear sandals or leather shoes and clean cotton socks. Tell them to wash the feet twice daily and, after drying them thoroughly, dust the feet evenly with an antifungal powder to absorb perspiration and prevent excoriation.

PREVENTION Advise patients not to share clothing, hats, towels, bed linens, pillows, combs, brushes, or nail clippers with others and to keep the lesions covered. Stress the importance of good handwashing technique and diligent personal hygiene in preventing the spread of infection.

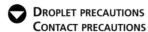

DROPLET PRECAUTIONS
CONTACT PRECAUTIONS

Diphtheria

Diphtheria is an acute, highly contagious, toxin-mediated infection caused by *Corynebacterium diphtheriae*, a gram-positive rod that usually infects the respiratory tract, primarily the tonsils, nasopharynx, and larynx. The GI and urinary tracts, conjunctivae, and ears are rarely involved.

CAUSES

Transmission usually occurs through intimate contact or by airborne respiratory droplets from asymptomatic carriers or convalescing patients. Many more people are asymptomatic carriers than contract active infection. Diphtheria is more prevalent during the colder months because of closer person-to-person indoor contact; however, infection may occur at any time during the year.

Thanks to effective immunization, diphtheria is rare in many parts of the world, including the United States. Since 1972, however, the incidence of cutaneous diphtheria has been increasing in the United States, especially in areas of the Pacific Northwest and the Southwest where crowding and poor hygienic conditions prevail. Most victims are children younger than age 15; about 10% of patients die as a result of the infection.

COMPLICATIONS

The extensive pseudomembrane formation and swelling that occur during the first few days of infection can cause respiratory obstruction. Other complications of diphtheria include myocarditis, polyneuritis (primarily affecting motor fibers but possibly also sensory neurons), encephalitis, cerebral infarction, bacteremia, renal failure, pulmonary emboli, and bronchopneumonia; these complications are caused by *C. diphtheriae* or other super-infecting organisms. Serum sickness may result from antitoxin therapy.

ASSESSMENT FINDINGS

Most diphtheria infections go unrecognized, especially in partially immunized individuals. After an incubation period of less than a week, clinical cases of diphtheria characteristically show a thick, patchy, grayish green membrane over the mucous membranes of the pharynx, larynx, tonsils, soft palate, and nose as well as fever, sore throat, and crouplike symptoms such as a rasping cough, hoarseness, and the like. Attempts to remove the membrane usually cause bleeding, which is highly characteristic of diphtheria and distinguishes it from mononucleosis. If this membrane causes airway obstruction (particularly likely in laryngeal diphtheria), symptoms include tachypnea, stridor, possibly cyanosis, suprasternal retractions, and suffocation, if untreated. Adenopathy and cervical swelling can occur. In cutaneous diphtheria, skin lesions resemble impetigo. Symptoms of streptococcal pharyngitis and bacterial epiglottiditis are similar to those of diphtheria but are more acute in onset. With epiglottiditis, no membrane is evident on indirect laryngoscopy.

DIAGNOSTIC TESTS

▶ Physical examination shows the characteristic membrane.
▶ Throat culture, or culture of other suspect lesions growing *C. diphtheriae*, confirms the diagnosis.

TREATMENT

Treatment must not wait for confirmation by culture. Standard treatment includes diphtheria antitoxin administered I.M. or I.V.; antibiotics, such as penicillin or erythromycin, to eliminate the organisms from the upper respiratory tract and other sites and to terminate the carrier state; measures to prevent complications; and possible tracheotomy if airway obstruction occurs.

NURSING CONSIDERATIONS

⬤ Maintain droplet precautions for pharyngeal diphtheria and contact precautions for cutaneous diphtheria until at least 1 week after antibiotic therapy has ended and two consecutive negative nasopharyngeal cultures are obtained at least 24 hours apart.

▶ Give drugs as ordered. Diphtheria antitoxin, which is made from horse serum, is the only specific treatment available, so obtain eye and skin tests to determine sensitivity to the antitoxin. Although time-consuming and risky, desensitization should be attempted if sensitivity tests are positive. If sensitivity tests are negative, give the antitoxin before laboratory confirmation because mortality increases directly with any delay in antitoxin administration. After giving antitoxin or penicillin, be alert for anaphylaxis; keep epinephrine 1:1,000 and resuscitation equipment handy. In patients who receive erythromycin, watch for thrombophlebitis.

▶ Monitor respirations carefully, especially in laryngeal diphtheria (usually, such patients are in a high-humidity environment). Watch for signs of airway obstruction, and be ready to give immediate life support, including intubation and tracheotomy.

▶ Watch for signs of shock, which can develop suddenly as a result of systemic vascular collapse, airway obstruction, or anaphylaxis.

▶ Obtain cultures as ordered.

▶ If neuritis develops, tell the patient it's usually transient. Be aware that peripheral neuritis may not develop until 2 to 3 months after the onset of illness.

▶ Report all cases of diphtheria to local public health authorities.

▶ Provide psychological support to the patient and family.

 ALERT Be alert for signs of myocarditis, such as a sudden decrease in pulse rate, irregular heartbeat, pallor, or the development of heart murmurs. Monitor for electrocardiogram changes. Ventricular fibrillation is a common cause of sudden death in patients with diphtheria. Be prepared to intervene immediately.

Patient teaching

▶ Teach the patient and family about the disease, diagnosis, and treatment, including medications and possible adverse effects.

▶ Explain how to properly dispose of nasopharyngeal secretions, and teach proper infection precautions.

▶ Explain the need for follow-up testing. Advise the patient to expect a prolonged convalescence period.

▶ Discuss the signs and symptoms of possible complications, including any complications that should be reported to the practitioner immediately.

▶ Treatment of exposed individuals with antitoxin remains controversial. Suggest that the patient's family receive diphtheria toxoid (given as combination diphtheria and tetanus toxoid or as a combination including pertussis vaccine for children younger than age 6) if they haven't been immunized.

 PREVENTION Stress to all parents the need for childhood immunizations. Protective immunity doesn't last longer than 10 years after the last vaccination, so it's important to get tetanus-diphtheria boosters every 10 years.

Diphyllobothriasis

Diphyllobothriasis is a cestode, or tapeworm, infection. Tapeworms are capable of self-fertilization; however, *Diphyllobothrium* eggs complete their development in an aquatic environment and then become infective.

Humans are the primary host, with adult worms surviving in the intestinal tract. Ranging in size from 3' to 49' (1 to 15 m), *Diphyllobothrium* is the longest tapeworm species that infects humans. Infection can be long term, lasting decades. Infestation is seen worldwide but is rare in the United States, occurring only in Alaska or the western part of the country.

CAUSES

Diphyllobothriasis is caused by infection with the *Diphyllobothrium latum* organism, which is present in raw or undercooked fish. Infection occurs when the primary host (humans) ingests the cysts in the flesh of the intermediate host (fish). Cestodes are worms without an intestinal tract. They survive by attaching their head to the intestinal mucosa of the host and absorbing nutrients there. The body of the cestode contains segments called proglottids (male and female gonads) that produce up to one million eggs per day, per worm. These eggs are passed in the feces of the host. (See "Life cycle of *D. latum*.")

COMPLICATIONS

Intestinal obstruction may occur as a result of massive infection. Other complications include cholecystitis or cholangitis, which result from migration of proglottids, and megaloblastic anemia, which is indistinguishable from pernicious anemia.

ASSESSMENT FINDINGS

Diphyllobothriasis is frequently asymptomatic. Rarely, eggs may be discovered in feces. There has been some documentation of a patient vomiting a ball of fish tapeworms. When signs and symptoms do occur, they may include abdominal pain, diarrhea, malaise, anorexia, and weight loss. Less common signs include fatigue, dizziness, numbness of the extremities, hunger, and pruritus ani. Vitamin B_{12} deficiency results from absorption of the vitamin by the tapeworm, which leads to pernicious anemia. Signs and symptoms of pernicious anemia include a smooth, beefy red, painful tongue; enlarged liver and spleen; dyspnea; weak extremities and disturbed coordination; irritability; depression; delirium; and ataxia. Signs of intestinal obstruction include abdominal distention and pain.

DIAGNOSTIC TESTS

▶ Stool culture reveals eggs and parasite particles. It may take two to three specimens for positive identification due to the irregular release of eggs by the tapeworm. Eggs appear 5 to 6 weeks after infestation.
▶ The vitamin B_{12} level may be decreased.
▶ Abdominal radiography can identify intestinal obstruction, if present.
▶ Blood work may reveal slightly decreased hemoglobin and hematocrit levels and eosinophilia.

TREATMENT

Most patients with diphyllobothriasis are treated as outpatients. Anthelmintic drugs are used to treat parasites; praziquantel (Biltricide) is the drug of choice for diphyllobothriasis, but its use in this disorder is investigational. Niclosamide is used as an alternative treatment. Both medications are effective after only one dose. Gastrografin has been found to cause detachment and passing of whole worms in the stool. Vitamin B_{12} is given if a deficiency is identified. Surgical intervention may be required in cases of intestinal obstruction.

NURSING CONSIDERATIONS

▶ Collect stool specimens as ordered, and send them to the laboratory promptly.
▶ Monitor for signs and symptoms of pernicious anemia.

Life cycle of *D. latum*

Diphyllobothriasis is caused by the fish tapeworm *D. latum*. Infection occurs following ingestion of raw or undercooked fish containing the tapeworm. The larvae grow in the intestine. An adult worm is segmented (the segments are also known as proglottids), with eggs forming in each segment. The eggs are then passed in the stool. Sometimes, a string of proglottids is passed in the stool with the eggs.

Tapeworm infection can result in vitamin B_{12} deficiency and megaloblastic anemia.

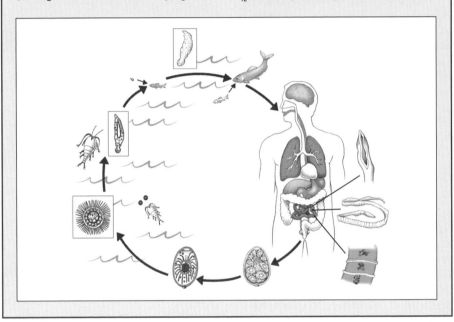

▶ Administer medications as ordered, and evaluate for adverse effects.

▶ Maintain standard precautions.

Patient teaching

▶ Teach the patient about the infection, including how it is acquired and how it is spread.

▶ Discuss diagnostic tests and treatment, including medications and possible adverse effects.

▶ Advise patients taking praziquantel to take it with liquid during a meal; the tablet should not be crushed. Explain that this medication may cause dizziness.

▶ Discuss the signs and symptoms of possible complications of diphyllobothriasis, and indicate any complications that should be reported to the practitioner immediately.

▶ Discuss the need for follow-up stool cultures on the seventh day posttreatment. If the culture is positive for *Diphyllobothrium*, a second course of treatment may be prescribed.

▶ Review proper handwashing technique to prevent fecal-oral contamination.

PREVENTION To prevent diphyllobothriasis, teach patients to avoid eating raw freshwater fish. Recommend that they cook fish to a temperature of 132° F (56 °C) or higher for longer than 5 minutes and to not sample the fish until it is cooked. If not cooking the fish immediately, freeze it for 24 hours. Pickling the fish in brine may also help prevent diphyllobothriasis.

Dysentery

Dysentery is an inflammatory disorder of the lower digestive tract that involves frequent passage of severe diarrhea-type stool. The stool may contain mucus and blood, depending on the causative organism. If left untreated, dysentery can be fatal. In the past, dysentery has also been called flux or bloody flux. There are two types of dysentery—amebic and bacillary. With either type, illness usually lasts 3 to 7 days.

CAUSES

Amebic dysentery is caused by *Entamoeba histolytica* and is common in the tropics or areas that use human excrement as fertilizer. Bacillary dysentery is caused by a bacterial organism, such as *Shigella*, *Salmonella*, or *Campylobacter*, and is usually seen in temperate zones. Bacterial dysentery is usually more severe than amebic dysentery.

Dysentery is transmitted through food and water contaminated with feces. It is spread by improper hand sanitation after defecation and occurs more frequently in overcrowded areas with poor sanitation.

 PREVENTION Although there is no vaccine currently available for dysentery, there are several in the evaluation stages.

COMPLICATIONS

Amebic dysentery may result in abscesses that affect the liver, lungs, or brain. It may also result in nonintestinal infections, such as amebic hepatitis. With either type of dysentery, GI ulceration with bleeding may occur, as well as appendicitis or inflammation of the colon. Bacillary dysentery may move to other organs and cause meningitis, encephalitis, or hemolytic-uremic syndrome and kidney failure. Seizures may also occur secondary to fever. Dysentery caused by *Shigella* may also cause Reiter syndrome, or reactive arthritis.

ASSESSMENT FINDINGS

Both amebic and bacterial dysentery cause watery diarrhea, although the diarrhea is more severe with bacterial dysentery. Diarrhea may have a foul odor, appear bloody, and contain yellowish white mucus. Tenesmus, or the feeling of incomplete emptying of the bowel, may occur. The patient may also experience abdominal cramping and vomiting, which may be bloody. Fever may occur 1 to 3 days after exposure. Palpation of the abdomen may elicit tenderness, and bowel sounds may be hyperactive.

DIAGNOSTIC TESTS

▶ Stool culture for ova and parasites will identify the cause of diarrhea. Several stool specimens may be needed for proper identification.
▶ Stool sampling for occult blood is positive when blood is present.
▶ Serologic tests identify antibodies.

TREATMENT

Metronidazole (Flagyl) is used to treat acute amebic dysentery, along with or followed by a second luminal amebicide, such as paromomycin. Bacterial dysentery may subside on its own or may be treated with an antibiotic. Use of antibiotics, such as ceftriaxone (Rocephin) or ciprofloxacin (Cipro), generally reduces the length of the illness by approximately 2 days. Antibiotics are recommended for older patients, malnourished children and children in day care, anyone infected with human immunodeficiency virus, food handlers, and health care workers. Drug susceptibility tests identify which drug would be most effective against the offending organism. Hydration with oral and I.V. fluids is essential. Electrolyte replacement is also important for patients with dysentery due to the loss of fluid and nutrients through diarrhea. Antidiarrheal medications should be avoided. Fever should be treated with acetaminophen products, and aspirin should be avoided. GI bleeding may require intervention as well as the administration of blood products. A clear liquid diet using electrolyte-rich products should be followed, with I.V. fluids administered if severe dehydration develops. Lactose-containing products should be avoided until symptoms resolve.

Nursing considerations

▶ Follow standard precautions.
▶ Obtain stool cultures as ordered. Multiple specimens may be needed until the organism is identified.
▶ Encourage oral fluid intake, and administer I.V. fluids as ordered.
▶ Administer prescribed medications, and monitor for adverse effects.
▶ Monitor vital signs as well as intake and output. Note the amount and appearance of stool. Watch for passage of blood or bloody vomitus.
▶ Assess for signs and symptoms of dehydration, such as dry mucous membranes, hypotension, tenting of the skin, thirst, and decreased urine output.
▶ Monitor laboratory test results for electrolyte imbalances and replace appropriately as ordered. If bleeding is present, monitor hemoglobin and hematocrit levels and administer blood products, if needed.

Patient teaching

▶ Teach the patient about the infection, including how it is transmitted, possible causes, and treatment.
▶ Discuss the signs and symptoms of possible complications, and indicate any complications that should be reported to the practitioner immediately.
▶ Teach the patient and visitors how to wash hands properly using soap and water, and encourage handwashing before preparing and eating food and after using the bathroom.
▶ Advise the patient to avoid products that contain lactose, due to temporary lactose intolerance, and explain that lactose intolerance may last for years.
▶ Teach the patient about medications that are prescribed, including administration and

possible adverse effects. Stress that the patient should complete the entire dose of medication that is prescribed.
▶ Discuss any follow-up cultures that are needed.

 SAFETY To prevent the transmission of dysentery, teach the patient to wash hands before eating and after using the bathroom, bedpan, or urinal. The nurse and family members should sanitize their hands before entering and when leaving the patient's room using an alcohol-based hand cleanser or soap and water. Soiled diapers should be put into a plastic bag and placed in the regular trash. Stress teaching children at day care and school to wash their hands. Food handlers should not return to work until stool cultures are negative.

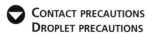

CONTACT PRECAUTIONS
DROPLET PRECAUTIONS

Ebola virus infection

One of the most frightening viruses to come out of the African subcontinent, the Ebola virus first appeared in 1976. More than 400 people in the Democratic Republic of Congo (formerly known as Zaire) and the neighboring Sudan were killed by the hemorrhagic fever that it caused. Ebola virus has been responsible for several outbreaks in the intervening years, including one in Zaire in the summer of 1995.

An unclassified ribonucleic acid (RNA) virus, Ebola is morphologically similar to Marburg virus. Both can cause headache, malaise, myalgia, and high fever, progressing to severe diarrhea, vomiting, and internal and external hemorrhage.

Four strains of the Ebola virus are known to exist: Ebola Zaire, Ebola Sudan, Ebola Tai, and Ebola Reston. All four types are structurally similar, although they have different antigenic properties. However, Ebola Reston causes illness only in monkeys, whereas the other three forms cause disease in humans.

The prognosis for Ebola virus infection is extremely poor, with mortality as high as 90%. The incubation period ranges from 2 to 21 days.

CAUSES

Ebola virus infection is caused by an unclassified RNA virus that is passed from person to person by direct contact with infected blood, body secretions, or organs. Contaminated needles can also cause the infection. Nosocomial and community-acquired transmission can occur. Transmission through semen may occur up to 7 weeks after clinical recovery. The virus can be transmitted even after the patient has died. (See *Preventing the spread of Ebola virus.*)

COMPLICATIONS

As the infection progresses, severe complications, including kidney and liver dysfunction, dehydration, and hemorrhage, may develop. In pregnant females, Ebola virus leads to spontaneous abortion, disseminated intravascular coagulation, azotemia, and massive hemorrhage.

ASSESSMENT FINDINGS

The patient's health history usually reveals contact with an infected person. However, no clear line of infection may be apparent at the beginning of an Ebola virus outbreak. The patient usually complains of flu-like signs and symptoms (such as headache, malaise, myalgia, fever, cough, and sore throat).

As the virus spreads through the body, inspection reveals bruising as capillaries

SAFETY

Preventing the spread of Ebola virus

The CDC recommends the following guidelines to help prevent the spread of this deadly infection:
• Keep the patient on contact and droplet precautions throughout the course of the infection.
• If possible, place the patient in a negative-pressure room at the beginning of hospitalization to avoid the need for transfer as the infection progresses.
• Keep frequently used items (such as a thermometer and stethoscope) in the pa-

tient's room. Thoroughly disinfect this equipment or discard it upon the patient's discharge or death.
• Restrict nonessential staff members from entering the patient's room.
• Make sure that anyone who enters the patient's room wears gloves, mask, eye protection, and a gown to prevent contact with any surface in the room that may have been soiled.

rupture and dead blood cells infiltrate the skin. A maculopapular eruption appears after the fifth day of infection. The patient may also display melena, hematemesis, epistaxis, and bleeding gums. In the final stages of infection, the skin blisters and sloughs off, blood seeps from all body orifices, and the patient begins vomiting his or her liquefied internal organs. Death usually results during the second week of illness from organ failure or hemorrhage.

DIAGNOSTIC TESTS

▶ Specialized laboratory tests—such as an enzyme-linked immunosorbent assay (ELISA) using EBO-2 viral antigens and immunoglobulin G ELISA—reveal specific antigens or antibodies and may show the isolated virus.
▶ Laboratory tests reveal neutrophil leukocytosis, hypofibrinogenemia, thrombocytopenia, and microangiopathic hemolytic anemia.

TREATMENT

No cure exists for Ebola virus infection; treatment is intensive supportive care. Administration of I.V. fluids helps offset the effects of severe dehydration. The patient may receive replacement of plasma heparin before the onset of clinical shock.

Throughout treatment, the patient should remain on contact and droplet precautions. If diagnostic tests indicate that the patient is free from the virus—which typically occurs 21 days after onset in those few who survive—the patient can be released.

NURSING CONSIDERATIONS

◗ Follow the CDC guidelines for contact and droplet precautions when caring for a patient who has Ebola virus.
▶ Check the results of complete blood count and coagulation studies for signs of blood loss and coagulopathy.
▶ Assess the patient daily for petechiae, ecchymoses, and oozing blood. Note and document the size of ecchymoses at least every 24 hours.
▶ Protect all areas of petechiae and ecchymoses from further injury.
▶ Test stools, urine, and vomitus for occult blood.
▶ Watch for frank bleeding, including GI bleeding and, in women, menorrhagia. Note and document the amount of bleeding every 24 hours or more often.
▶ Monitor the patient's family and other close contacts for fever and other signs of infection.
▶ Provide emotional support for the patient and family during the course of this devastating disease. Encourage them to ask questions and discuss any concerns they have about the disease and its treatment.

Patient teaching

▶ Teach the patient about the infection, including how it is transmitted, possible causes, and treatment.
▶ Discuss the signs and symptoms of possible complications, and specify any complications that should be reported to the practitioner immediately.

CONTACT PRECAUTIONS

Ecthyma

Ecthyma is a bacterial infection of the skin that results in an ulcerative pyoderma involving the lower epidermis and dermis. It is considered a deeper form of impetigo, which is a contagious superficial skin infection that occurs in nonbullous and bullous forms. The characteristic ulcer of ecthyma causes deep penetration of the lower epidermis and dermis by the infecting organism and usually results in scarring. The infection often starts in a preexisting break in the skin, such as from a scratch or insect bite. The infection seems to occur more often in children and older adults.

CAUSES

Group A beta-hemolytic streptococci cause ecthyma. Risk factors include crowded living conditions, high temperature and humidity, and poor hygiene. Those with existing impetigo are at especially high risk. Preexisting tissue damage from dermatitis or insect bites, anemia, malnutrition, and a compromised immune system (diabetes, neutropenia, acquired immunodeficiency syndrome) may contribute to the development of this infection. A warm climate favors outbreaks of this infection, which usually occurs in late summer and early fall. The most common transmitters appear to be biting insects, such as mosquitoes and flies, with autoinoculation occurring through scratching.

COMPLICATIONS

A rare but serious complication of ecthyma is glomerulonephritis, caused by a nephritogenic strain of beta-hemolytic streptococci. Other complications of ecthyma include cellulitis, erysipelas, gangrene, lymphangitis, suppurative lymphadenitis, and bacteremia (rare). Scarlet fever may also occur. Permanent skin damage resulting from ecthyma is common. More extensive complications include staphylococcal scalded skin syndrome and toxic shock syndrome.

ASSESSMENT FINDINGS

Ecthyma begins with a red-bordered vesicle or pustule that deepens into ulceration with a gray-yellow crust that is thicker than the crust seen in impetigo. Lesions may enlarge to 1¼ inches (3 cm) in diameter and may be painful. These lesions are usually found on the legs after a scratch or bug bite. Once the crust is gone, a shallow ulceration remains, with a raised and indurated margin. Autoinoculation can transmit ecthyma to other parts of the body, especially to sites that have been scratched open. Lymphadenopathy may occur.

DIAGNOSTIC TESTS

▶ Physical examination may be sufficient for diagnosis.
▶ Gram stain of vesicular fluid and visualization under a microscope usually confirm gram-positive cocci that represent group A streptococci. *Staphylococcus aureus* may also be present.
▶ Culture and sensitivity testing of fluid or denuded skin may indicate the most appropriate antibiotic.
▶ The white blood cell count may be elevated.

TREATMENT

Therapy is basically the same as for impetigo, but response may be slower. Oral broad-spectrum antibiotics, such as penicillin, are prescribed for ecthyma and may need to be continued for several weeks until the condition is resolved. The topical antibiotics mupirocin (Bactroban) and retapamulin (Altabax) may be used for localized lesions. I.V. antibiotics may be used for systemic involvement. Therapy may also include removal of the exudates by washing the lesions two or three times a day with soap and water (or antibacterial soap) or, for stubborn crusts, with warm soaks or compresses of normal saline or a diluted soap solution. Frequent cleaning of linens, towels, and clothing is encouraged. An antihistamine to alleviate itching may be helpful.

NURSING CONSIDERATIONS

▶ Urge the patient not to scratch, as this may cause spread of the infection.

▶ Give medications as indicated. Remember to check for medication allergy, and monitor for adverse drug reactions.

◆ Use meticulous handwashing technique and follow standard and contact precautions to prevent the infection from spreading. Encourage frequent bathing with an antibacterial soap.

▶ Remove crusts by gently washing with bactericidal soap and water. Soften stubborn crusts with cool compresses.

▶ Change bed linens and bedclothes frequently.

▶ Comply with local public health standards and guidelines.

▶ Check family members for ecthyma and impetigo. If ecthyma is present in a school-age child, notify the child's school.

▶ In hospitalized patients, contact precautions should be maintained until 24 hours after effective treatment has been initiated.

Patient teaching

▶ Be sure to discuss the disorder, diagnosis, and treatment with the patient and family. Stress the need to continue prescribed medications as ordered, even after lesions have healed.

▶ Provide written instructions for the care of lesions, including crust removal, application of topical medication, and dressing change technique.

▶ Teach the family how to identify characteristic lesions. Encourage regular inspections, especially of children, to identify new lesions.

▶ Teach the patient proper handwashing technique.

▶ Advise parents to cut their child's fingernails and cover his or her hands with socks or mittens to prevent scratching.

▶ Teach the patient and family about signs and symptoms of complications, such as blood in the urine, increased blood pressure, fever, or increasingly painful lesions. If these occur, urge the patient to seek medical attention.

▶ Encourage use of insect repellents when outdoors to prevent insect bites.

 PREVENTION To prevent further spread of this highly contagious infection, encourage frequent bathing using a bactericidal soap, Tell the patient not to share towels, washcloths, or bed linens with family members. Emphasize the importance of following proper handwashing techniques and maintaining proper hygiene.

CONTACT PRECAUTIONS

Eczema herpeticum

Eczema herpeticum, also known as Kaposi varicelliform eruption, is a rare disseminated herpes infection that occurs at the site of pre-existing skin damage, most commonly atopic dermatitis. This condition may affect multiple organs, such as the lungs, liver, and/or brain. It is potentially life-threatening, although mortality has decreased from 50% to less than 10% since the use of acyclovir and other antibiotics was instituted. Originally thought to only affect children, eczema herpeticum can affect people of any age or gender.

CAUSES

Eczema herpeticum is caused by herpes simplex virus (HSV) type 1 or 2. It may also be caused by coxsackievirus A16 or vaccinia virus. Disorders of the skin, such as eczema, pemphigus, burns, or other dermatoses, can become infected with HSV. Infection is thought to occur by autoinoculation from a latent infection or from contact with someone with an infection. The virus enters the skin when the skin barrier is impaired due to dermatitis or eczema. Skin-to-skin contact with a person who has cold sores or genital herpes usually triggers the infection. Patients with eczema herpeticum have been found to have a decreased amount of natural killer cell activity in atopic dermatitis, which in turn decreases their defense against HSV.

COMPLICATIONS

Complications of eczema herpeticum include systemic involvement affecting the lungs, liver, brain, GI tract, eyes, or adrenal glands. When it affects the eyes, conjunctivitis, blepharitis, keratitis, and uveitis can occur. Blindness can result from herpetic keratitis. These complications are more likely to occur when eczema herpeticum affects the face. Septicemia from secondary bacterial infections may lead to death. The most common secondary infections are caused by

Staphylococcus aureus, Pseudomonas aeruginosa, and *Peptostreptococcus.*

ASSESSMENT FINDINGS

Flu-like symptoms of fever, chills, and malaise may occur in a patient with preexisting dermatitis. Symptoms appear approximately 5 to 12 days after exposure. The skin may initially have clusters of umbilicated vesiculopustules that spread over 7 to 10 days. The vesicles then progress to painful, hemorrhagic, crusted, punched-out erosions that may coalesce to become large, bleeding, denuded, and infected with secondary bacteria. Affected areas include the area of dermatitis, especially in the upper body (particularly the head and neck). The patient may also have lymphadenopathy. There may be a history of contact with someone else with HSV, or the patient may have a history of primary or recurrent herpes. The illness lasts approximately 16 days, with healing occurring in 2 to 6 weeks.

DIAGNOSTIC TESTS

▶ Viral culture swabs and direct fluorescent antibody stain from the infected lesions identify the virus.
▶ Tzanck smear of an erosion or open vesicle shows characteristic epithelial multinucleated giant cells and acantholysis but is not sensitive for HSV infection.
▶ Polymerase chain reaction can detect minute amounts of viral DNA in tissue.
▶ Tissue biopsy identifies changes characteristic of HSV infection but is not done routinely.

TREATMENT

Treatment of eczema herpeticum includes antiviral medication, such as acyclovir (Zovirax) or valacyclovir. For patients who have acyclovir-resistant HSV infection and who are immunocompromised, foscarnet (Foscavir) may be used. Systemic and topical antibiotics should also be used to treat any secondary bacterial infection. If a bacterial infection is not present, it may be prevented through use of a topical cream, such as silver sulfadiazine. Analgesics may be needed for very painful lesions. If the eye is affected, an ophthalmologist should be consulted, although this is a rare occurrence.

NURSING CONSIDERATIONS

● Follow contact precautions while active lesions are present and standard precautions after lesions crust.

▶ When obtaining a culture from the infected lesions, be sure to swab vigorously because extracellular particles may be present.

▶ After checking for allergies, administer medications as ordered and monitor for adverse reactions.

▶ Administer analgesics as ordered, and evaluate the effect after 30 minutes.

▶ Apply cool, moist compresses to help remove any crustation covering the lesions. Be sure to use personal protective equipment when performing skin or wound care.

Provide emotional support to the patient and family, as lesions may be disfiguring.

Patient teaching

▶ Teach the patient about all medication, including dosage, administration, and potential adverse effects. Stress the need to complete the prescription as ordered.

 SAFETY Stress the need for proper hand-washing technique to prevent spread of the infection.

▶ Tell the patient to be sure to wear disposable gloves when applying any topical lotions to the lesions or when cleaning the lesions, and to wash his or her hands afterward.

▶ Review possible complications, such as increased pain, redness, or drainage from the vesicles, which may indicate a secondary infection. Stress the need to seek medical attention if this occurs.

▶ If lesions occur on the face, tell the patient that an ophthalmologist may need to be consulted if the eyes become involved.

▶ Teach the patient proper skin care and how to prevent spread of the infection. Encourage frequent changing of bed linens.

▶ Recommend that patients wear loose, lightweight clothing to prevent irritation to lesions.

▶ Tell the patient to avoid strenuous exercise that may cause sweating until the lesions are healed.

▶ Encourage follow-up care 2 weeks after therapy is initiated to evaluate the patient's response to treatment.

Ehrlichiosis

Human ehrlichiosis, an infectious disease that's transmitted by the bite of an infected tick, was first diagnosed in 1986. The genus *Ehrlichia* contains a number of emerging species that can transmit potentially life-threatening infections; however, most cases are mild to moderate in severity, with the more severe cases affecting immunocompromised patients. Males are affected more than females, possibly due to outdoor exposure, and most cases occur in people over age 50, according to the CDC. Ehrlichiosis may be misdiagnosed as Rocky Mountain spotted fever, as both are transmitted by tick bite and present with similar signs and symptoms.

CAUSES

Ehrlichiosis is caused by *Ehrlichia* organisms, specifically *E. chaffeensis*, which causes human monocytic ehrlichiosis, or *E. ewingii*. These tiny gram-negative organisms multiply within white blood cell (WBC) cytoplasm. Clusters multiply to form large mulberry-shaped aggregates called morulae. Known vectors include the lone star tick (*Amblyomma americanum*), the American dog tick (*Dermacentor variabilis*), and the deer tick (*Ixodes dammini* and *Ixodes scapularis*).

Ehrlichiosis occurs worldwide, with prevalence related to the distribution of tick vectors. In the United States, most cases of ehrlichiosis are reported in the south-central and southern Atlantic areas of the country, but it has also been reported in the upper Midwest. Persons at highest risk include those who live in endemic and highly wooded areas, engage in activities in high grassy areas, and own a pet that may introduce a tick into the home. Because ehrlichiosis is not reportable to the health department, the exact incidence is unknown; however the CDC notes that reports of cases have increased from about 100 per year in 1999 to 600 per year in 2006.

It is unknown whether re-infection can occur or if infection confers immunity. More studies are being done to investigate this topic.

COMPLICATIONS

Complications of ehrlichiosis can be severe, especially if it is left untreated or occurs in immunocompromised patients. It can produce such complications as acute respiratory distress syndrome, disseminated intravascular coagulation (DIC), seizures, and coma. An estimated 1% to 5% of patients die as a result of the infection.

ASSESSMENT FINDINGS

The incubation period for ehrlichiosis is 9 days from the time of the tick bite. Although ehrlichiosis can produce mild flu-like symptoms, some affected individuals may experience more severe symptoms. Early symptoms include fever, chills, severe headache, muscle pain (myalgia), and nausea that develop within 5 to 14 days of the tick bite. A maculopapular or petechial rash appears in about half of the cases, although not necessarily at the site of the tick bite. Hepatomegaly and lymphadenopathy may occur. Most people infected with ehrlichiosis don't seek medical help, but the infection can be fatal without appropriate treatment.

DIAGNOSTIC TESTS

▶ Diagnosis of ehrlichiosis is based on evaluation of signs and symptoms in addition to supporting laboratory data.
▶ A fluorescent antibody test may be positive for *E. chaffeensis* or granulocytic *Ehrlichia*.
▶ Immunofluorescent antibody Ehrlichia titer shows elevated immunoglobulin G.
▶ A complete blood count shows decreased WBCs, indicative of leukopenia, and a low platelet count, indicative of thrombocytopenia. The erythrocyte sedimentation rate may be elevated. Granulocyte staining shows characteristic clusters of organisms inside the cytoplasm of WBCs. Liver enzymes show elevated levels of transaminase.

TREATMENT

Ehrlichiosis is treated with tetracycline or doxycycline (Doryx), producing rapid improvement when used early in the course of disease. Doxycycline shouldn't be used in pregnant or nursing women; rifampin or chloramphenicol may be used in these patients. Seizures, kidney failure, respiratory failure, coma, or death can occur if treatment is delayed. Supportive therapy is provided to help relieve signs and symptoms. Analgesics are provided for headache and body aches, and antipyretics are given for fever.

NURSING CONSIDERATIONS

▶ Monitor the patient for signs and symptoms of respiratory involvement. Monitor pulse oximetry and chest radiography results if the patient demonstrates signs of respiratory distress.
▶ Note any allergies before administering medication. Administer antibiotics as ordered, and observe for signs of adverse effects. Evaluate the effects of analgesics and antipyretics 30 minutes after administration.
▶ Monitor laboratory values for signs of complications, such as DIC.
▶ Assess the patient's skin for signs of rash.
▶ Provide frequent rest periods if the illness is severe.
▶ Report all cases of ehrlichiosis to the state health department or the CDC.

Patient teaching

▶ Teach the patient about the infection and how it is spread. Review signs and symptoms of complications and when to notify the practitioner.
▶ Review prescribed medication, including administration and possible adverse effects.
▶ Teach the patient and family how to remove ticks properly.

 PREVENTION Review with the patient measures to prevent tick bites when outdoors, such as wearing light-colored clothing (to visualize ticks) and long-sleeve shirts and pants. Advise tucking pants inside socks or boots to prevent ticks from crawling up the leg. Tell them to apply insect repellent to clothing and any exposed skin. Repellent with DEET (n, n-diethyl-m-toluamide) is effective but only lasts a few hours before it needs to needs to be reapplied. Advise the patient to stick to trails and avoid dense brush when hiking. Also tell the patient to avoid standing under overhanging foliage.

 SAFETY Tell patients to examine themselves for ticks after being outdoors and to remove any ticks found on the body; studies suggest that a tick must be attached for at least 24 hours in order to cause ehrlichiosis. Tell patients to use a handheld mirror to check all areas of the body. Stress to parents to check children for ticks and to use proper technique to remove any that are found. Clothes can be run through a 20- to 30-minute cycle in a hot dryer to kill ticks.

Elephantiasis

Elephantiasis is a syndrome that results in swelling or thickening of the tissue of the legs, genitals, or female breasts. There are two types of elephantiasis: One is caused by lymphatic filariasis, a parasitic disease, and the other is a nonparasitic form—nonfilarial elephantiasis, or pod coniosis.

The disfigurement caused by elephantiasis is a leading cause of disability worldwide: 10% of women in endemic communities may have swollen limbs, and 50% of men may have genital effects. More than 120 million people are now or have been affected, 40 million of whom are seriously incapacitated and disfigured by the disease. The areas most commonly affected by the disease are India and Africa.

CAUSES

Lymphatic filariasis is caused by threadlike worms that live in and cause damage to the lymphatic system. The disease is transmitted by mosquitoes that pick up the microfilariae when they bite infected humans; the microfilariae develop into the infective larval stage and then are injected into another person during a bite. The most common filarial species is *Wuchereria bancrofti*, but *Brugia malayi* and *Brugia timri* cause the infection in Asia. It takes several mosquito bites over many months to cause the infection. People living in tropical and subtropical settings are at the greatest risk for the infection.

Nonfilarial elephantiasis is thought to be caused by contact with irritant soils associated with volcanic activity. Chemicals from the soil are transmitted through the soles of the feet and then travel to the lymphatic system, blocking proper drainage. Other causes of nonfilarial elephantiasis include certain sexually transmitted infections (e.g., lymphogranuloma venereum), tuberculosis, leishmaniasis, recurring streptococcal infections, and leprosy. In some cases, no cause can be identified (idiopathic).

COMPLICATIONS

Complications of elephantiasis include secondary skin infection. The disease may take years to manifest, and many people never acquire outward clinical manifestations. However, studies have now disclosed that such victims, who appear healthy, actually have hidden lymphatic pathology and kidney damage as well. The debilitating consequences of elephantiasis may cause personal and socioeconomic hardships. Obstruction of blood vessels in the affected extremity may lead to gangrene.

ASSESSMENT FINDINGS

Patients with elephantiasis present with painful, hardened, edematous skin of the lower extremities (most common), genitalia, arms, and breasts. The scrotum may be increased in size, even up to the size of a basketball. The skin is pebbly in appearance and may be darker than skin elsewhere on the body. Ulcerations may be present, and the skin may be warm or hot to touch. Other signs may include fever, chills, and malaise. Hydrocele may also occur.

DIAGNOSTIC TESTS

▶ Microscopic examination may identify the microfilariae in the blood, skin, chylous urine, or hydrocele fluid. Blood collection should be done at night because microfilariae circulate in the blood at night.
▶ Patients with active filarial infection typically have elevated levels of antifilarial immunoglobulin G_4 in the blood, and these can be detected using routine assays.
▶ Slitlamp examination may identify microfilariae in the cornea or anterior chamber of the eye.
▶ Filarial antigens and serologic antibodies are detected in the blood; however, because lymphedema may develop many years after infection, laboratory tests are often negative.
▶ Laboratory tests may show marked eosinophilia.

▶ Ultrasound may identify lymphatic obstruction of the inguinal and scrotal lymphatics.

TREATMENT

Treatment of lymphatic filariasis is ivermectin (Stromectol), an anthelminthic; however, diethylcarbamazine (DEC) has also been used for treatment. With DEC, antihistamines and corticosteroids may also be required to decrease allergic reactions of disintegrating microfilariae resulting from treatment. Other medications that may be used include doxycycline (Doryx) and albendazole (Albenza). For chronic conditions, medication may not be effective and surgery may be required, such as for hydrocele. Surgery for elephantiasis of the limbs is generally ineffective. Additional measures include meticulous skin care and exercise to promote lymphatic drainage.

 PREVENTION The World Health Organization is attempting to eliminate filarial infections by providing mass drug administration to areas of the world where people are at risk for lymphatic filariasis. Recommended antifilarial drug combinations of either DEC or ivermectin plus albendazole, in addition to regular use of DEC-fortified salt, may prevent occurrence of new infection and disease.

NURSING CONSIDERATIONS

▶ Provide emotional support to patients to help them deal with debilitating features if lymphatic complications or elephantiasis develops.
▶ Provide meticulous skin care, and monitor for complications such as bacterial infection. Provide wound care as indicated, and assess for any worsening or improvement of the wound.
▶ Administer medications as ordered, and monitor for effect as well as adverse reactions.
▶ Assist with exercises of any limbs affected by lymphedema. Due to constricted movement, the patient may also need assistance with activities of daily living.
▶ Refer the patient to a lymphedema specialist to assist with exercises and hygiene that may improve the condition and prevent complications.

Patient teaching

▶ Teach the patient about the specific type of infection present, how it was acquired, and the recommended treatment plan.
▶ Review all prescribed medication, including dosage, administration, and possible adverse effects.
▶ Teach the patient about wound care, if appropriate. Stress the need for good skin care and hygiene to prevent infection.
▶ Teach appropriate exercises to help reduce lymphedema and maintain limb function. Obtain assistance from a physical therapist, as available.
▶ Review with the patient the signs and symptoms of complications and when to notify the physician.
▶ Review follow-up care, usually 1 year after treatment.

 PREVENTION Teach patients in areas endemic to lymphatic filariasis to avoid mosquito bites through the use of mosquito repellent on any exposed areas, especially between dusk and dawn; to utilize mosquito netting while sleeping; and to wear long sleeves and long pants when outdoors.

Encephalitis

Encephalitis is a severe inflammation of the brain characterized by intense lymphocytic infiltration of brain tissue and the leptomeninges. This process causes cerebral edema, degeneration of the brain's ganglion cells, and diffuse nerve cell destruction.

Encephalitis is usually caused by a mosquito-borne or, in some areas, a tickborne virus. Transmission by means other than arthropod bites may occur through ingestion of infected goat's milk and accidental injection or inhalation of the virus.

CAUSES

Encephalitis usually results from infection with arboviruses that are specific to rural areas. In urban areas, encephalitis is most frequently caused by enteroviruses (coxsackievirus, poliovirus, and echovirus). Other causes include herpesvirus, mumps virus, adenoviruses, and demyelinating diseases after measles, varicella, rubella, or vaccination. (See *Types of encephalitis*.)

COMPLICATIONS

Potential complications associated with viral encephalitis include bronchial pneumonia, urine retention, urinary tract infection, pressure ulcers, and coma. Epilepsy, parkinsonism, and mental deterioration may also occur.

ASSESSMENT FINDINGS

Depending on the severity of the infection, all forms of viral encephalitis have similar clinical features. The severity of arbovirus encephalitis may range from subclinical to rapidly fatal necrotizing disease. Herpes encephalitis also produces signs and symptoms that vary from subclinical to acute and often fatal fulminating disease.

If encephalitis is the primary illness, the patient may be acutely ill when he or she seeks treatment because the nonspecific symptoms that occur before the onset of acute neurologic symptoms aren't recognized as signs of encephalitis. Thus, the patient history may include reports of systemic symptoms, such as headache, muscle stiffness, malaise, sore throat, and upper respiratory tract symptoms that existed for several days before the onset of neurologic symptoms.

Signs and symptoms include an altered level of consciousness, from lethargy or drowsiness to stupor, seizures, confusion, hallucinations, tremors, cranial nerve palsies, exaggerated deep tendon reflexes, absent superficial reflexes, and paresis or paralysis of the extremities. The patient may complain of a stiff neck when the head is bent forward.

Other signs include fever, nausea, and vomiting. If the cerebral hemispheres are involved, assessment findings may include aphasia, involuntary movements identified on inspection, ataxia, sensory defects such as disturbances of taste and smell, and poor memory retention.

DIAGNOSTIC TESTS

▶ Serologic assays, such as immunoglobulin (Ig) M antibody-capture enzyme-linked immunosorbent assay (MAC-ELISA) and IgG ELISA may be diagnostic. Early in the infection, IgM antibody is more specific, whereas later IgG is more reactive.
▶ Blood analysis or, rarely, cerebrospinal fluid (CSF) analysis identifies the virus and confirms the diagnosis.
▶ Serologic studies in herpes encephalitis may show rising titers of complement-fixing antibodies. In some types of encephalitis, serologic blood tests may be diagnostic.
▶ Lumbar puncture detects elevated CSF pressure in all forms of encephalitis. Despite inflammation, CSF analysis findings often reveal clear fluid. White blood cell count and protein levels in CSF are slightly elevated, but the glucose level remains normal.
▶ Electroencephalography reveals abnormalities such as generalized slowing of waveforms.

Types of encephalitis

Four main virus agents cause most cases of encephalitis in the United States: eastern equine encephalitis (EEE), western equine encephalitis (WEE), St. Louis encephalitis, and La Crosse encephalitis, all of which are transmitted by mosquitoes. Since 1999, encephalitis due to West Nile virus (WNV) has also been seen in the United States. Most cases of arboviral encephalitis occur from June through September, when the weather is wet and arthropods are most active. In milder parts of the country, where arthropods are active late into the year, cases are seen into the winter months. No vaccines are available for these U.S.-based diseases. However, a Japanese encephalitis vaccine is available for those who will be traveling to Japan, a tickborne encephalitis vaccine is available for those who will be traveling to Europe, and an equine vaccine is available for EEE, WEE, and Venezuelan equine encephalitis (VEE). Public health measures often require spraying of insecticides to kill larvae and adult mosquitoes as well as controlling standing water that can be used as breeding sites for mosquitoes.

EEE

EEE is caused by an alphavirus transmitted to humans and horses by the bite of an infected mosquito. The incubation period is 4 to 10 days. Symptoms begin with a sudden onset of fever, general muscle pains, and headache of increasing severity and can progress to seizures and coma. Overall mortality is 25%; of those who recover, many suffer irreversible brain damage.

WEE

The alphavirus WEE is the causative agent. The enzootic cycle of WEE involves passerine birds, in which the infection is inapparent, and culicine mosquitoes, principally *Culex tarsalis*, a species associated with irrigated agriculture and stream drainages. Most WEE infections are asymptomatic or present as mild, nonspecific illness. Patients with clinically apparent illness usually have a sudden onset with fever, headache, nausea, vomiting, anorexia, and malaise, followed by altered mental status, weakness, and signs of meningeal irritation.

St. Louis encephalitis

The leading cause of St. Louis encephalitis—the most common mosquito-transmitted human pathogen in the United States—is a flavivirus. Mosquitoes become infected by feeding on birds that are infected with the St. Louis encephalitis virus. Mild infections present with fever and headache. More severe infection is marked by intense headache, high fever, neck stiffness, stupor, disorientation, coma, tremors, occasional seizures (especially in infants), and spastic (but rarely flaccid) paralysis.

Tickborne encephalitis

Tickborne encephalitis is caused by two closely related flaviviruses. The eastern subtype causes Russian spring-summer encephalitis and is transmitted by *Ixodes persulcatus*, whereas the western subtype is transmitted by *Ixodes ricinus* and causes central European encephalitis. Infection usually presents as a mild, influenza-type illness or as benign, aseptic meningitis, which may lead to fatal meningoencephalitis. Fever is often biphasic, and there may be severe headache and neck rigidity, with transient paralysis of the limbs, the shoulders or, less commonly, the respiratory musculature. A few patients are left with residual paralysis. Although the great majority of tickborne encephalitis infections follow exposure to ticks, infection has occurred through the ingestion of infected cows' or goats' milk. An inactivated tickborne encephalitis vaccine is currently available in Europe and Russia.

WNV encephalitis

WNV is a flavivirus that is transmitted principally by *Culex* species mosquitoes, but it also can be transmitted by *Aedes*, *Anopheles*, and other species. The mild form of WNV encephalitis infection presents as a febrile illness of sudden onset often accompanied by malaise, anorexia, nausea, vomiting, eye pain, headache, myalgia, rash, and lymphadenopathy. A minority of patients with severe disease develop a maculopapular or morbilliform rash involving the neck, trunk,

(continued)

Types of encephalitis *(continued)*

arms, or legs. Some patients experience severe muscle weakness and flaccid paralysis. Neurologic presentations include ataxia, cranial nerve abnormalities, myelitis, optic neuritis, polyradiculitis, and seizures.

La Crosse encephalitis
The La Crosse encephalitis virus, a bunyavirus, is a zoonotic pathogen cycled between the daytime-biting treehole mosquito, *Aedes triseriatus*, and the vertebrate amplifier hosts (chipmunks, tree squirrels) in deciduous forest habitats. It usually presents as a nonspecific summertime illness with fever, headache, nausea, vomiting, and lethargy. Severe disease is characterized by seizures, coma, paralysis, and a variety of neurologic sequelae after recovery.

Japanese encephalitis
Japanese encephalitis is a flavivirus transmitted to humans by *Culex* mosquitoes, primarily *C. tritaeniorhynchus*, which breed in rice fields. Mild infections occur without apparent symptoms other than fever and

headache. More severe infection is marked by quick onset, headache, high fever, neck stiffness, stupor, disorientation, coma, tremors, occasional seizures (especially in infants), and spastic (but rarely flaccid) paralysis.

Murray Valley encephalitis
Murray Valley encephalitis is endemic in New Guinea and in parts of Australia. It is estimated that 1 in 1,000 affected people develop symptoms, which include fever, headache, rash, myalgia, nausea and vomiting. More severe symptoms include seizures, lethargy, confusion, and loss of consciousness. Murray Valley encephalitis infections are common, and the small number of fatalities has mostly been in children.

VEE
VEE is an alphavirus that causes encephalitis in horses and humans. Adults usually develop only an influenza-like illness; overt encephalitis is usually confined to children. VEE is a significant veterinary and public health problem in Central and South America.

TREATMENT

The antiviral agent acyclovir (Zovirax) is effective only against herpes encephalitis. Antibiotics may be prescribed if the infection is caused by bacteria. Treatment for all other forms of encephalitis is supportive. Drug therapy includes reduction of intracranial pressure with I.V. mannitol and corticosteroids; phenytoin (Dilantin) or another anticonvulsant; sedatives for restlessness; and aspirin or acetaminophen (Tylenol) to relieve headache and reduce fever. Ribavirin (Copegus) and interferon alpha-2b were found to have some effect against West Nile virus encephalitis.

Other supportive measures include adequate fluid and electrolyte intake to prevent dehydration and appropriate antibiotics for associated infections, such as pneumonia or

sinusitis; maintenance of the patient's airway; administration of oxygen to maintain arterial blood gas levels; and maintenance of nutrition, especially during periods of coma. Isolation is unnecessary.

NURSING CONSIDERATIONS

▶ Assess neurologic function often. Observe level of consciousness and signs of increased intracranial pressure (increasing restlessness, vomiting, seizures, and changes in pupil size, motor function, and vital signs). Also watch for cranial nerve involvement (ptosis, strabismus, and diplopia), abnormal sleep patterns, and behavior changes.

▶ Administer fluids as ordered, but avoid fluid overload, which may increase cerebral edema. Measure and record intake and output accurately.

▶ Maintain adequate nutrition. Give the patient small, frequent meals, or provide nasogastric tube or parenteral feedings.

▶ Maintain a quiet environment. Darkening the room may decrease headache.

▶ If the patient has seizures, initiate seizure precautions.

Patient teaching

▶ Teach the patient and family about the disease and its effects. Explain the diagnostic tests and treatment measures.

▶ Explain to the patient and family that behavior changes caused by encephalitis usually disappear, but permanent problems sometimes occur.

 PREVENTION Help patients prevent mosquito-borne encephalitis by urging them to wear long-sleeved shirts and long pants if going outside between dusk and dawn. Encourage the use of mosquito repellant and mosquito netting. Tell patients to eliminate areas that attract mosquitoes, such as standing water in birdbaths or old tires, and to repair holes in screens on doors and windows to prevent mosquitoes from entering the home.

Endometritis

Endometritis, which occurs in women of childbearing age, is inflammation of the endometrium, the inner lining of the uterus. Inflammation extends into the myometrium, the middle layer of the uterine wall, and the parametrial tissue. Endometritis may be classified as obstetric or nonobstetric, acute or chronic, and is the most common cause of postpartum fever. It may follow the occurrence of pelvic inflammatory disease. Infection following vaginal delivery is estimated at 1% to 3%; the incidence following cesarean section is higher, at over 13% depending on risk factors and whether perioperative prophylactic antibiotics were given.

CAUSES

Chlamydia, gonorrhea, acute salpingitis, acute cervicitis, or tuberculosis may cause endometritis. Predisposing conditions may include prolonged rupture of membranes during pregnancy, pelvic inflammatory disease, childbirth, or miscarriage. Risk factors include any sexually transmitted infection; multiple sex partners; and conditions or procedures, such as conization or cauterization of the cervix, that alter or destroy cervical mucus, allowing bacteria to ascend into the cervical cavity. Additionally, any procedure that risks transfer of contaminated cervical mucus into the endometrial cavity by an instrument, such as a biopsy curette or an irrigation catheter, or by tubal insufflation, abortion, or recent intrauterine device insertion, increases the risk of endometritis. Chronic endometritis may be caused by retained products of conception after delivery or elective abortion.

Endometritis is generally caused by more than one microorganism. A polymicrobial mixture of aerobic and anaerobic organisms is usually found and may include gram-positive cocci such as *Streptococcus agalactiae, Streptococcus viridans, Streptococcus faecalis, Staphylococcus aureus,* and *Staphylococcus epidermidis*; gram-negative organisms such as *Escherichia coli, Klebsiella pneumoniae, Proteus mirabilis, Enterobacter aerogenes, Gardnerella vaginalis,* and *Neisseria gonorrhoeae; Chlamydia trachomatis* and mycoplasmas such as *Ureaplasma urealyticum;* and *Bacteroides* species (*B. bivius* is most common), *Peptococcus* species, *Peptostreptococcus* species, and *Fusobacterium* species.

COMPLICATIONS

Possible complications of endometritis include septicemia, septic shock, wound infection, pelvic or uterine abscess, pelvic hematoma, peritonitis, or septic pelvic thrombophlebitis. Infertility may also result from endometritis.

ASSESSMENT FINDINGS

Patients with acute endometritis may have mucopurulent or purulent vaginal discharge oozing from the cervix; edematous, hyperemic endometrium, possibly leading to ulceration and necrosis (with virulent organisms); lower abdominal pain and tenderness; fever; rebound pain; abdominal muscle spasms; and thrombophlebitis of uterine and pelvic vessels (with severe forms). In patients with severe infection, abdominal palpation may reveal a boggy uterus. Patients with chronic endometritis may have recurring episodes, which is increasingly common because of widespread use of intrauterine devices. The patient may also complain of vaginal odor, fever ranging from 100° to 104° F (37.8° to 40° C), malaise, dyspareunia, and dysuria.

DIAGNOSTIC TESTS

▶ Pelvic examination reveals tenderness of the uterus and cervix; cervical discharge may be present.
▶ Urine cultures rule out or identify urinary tract infection.
▶ A white blood cell count may reveal leukocytosis. The sedimentation rate is elevated.
▶ Endocervical cultures may identify gonorrhea or chlamydia.

▶ Blood cultures may identify organisms related to septicemia.

▶ Computed tomography may exclude other potential causes of abdominal pain.

▶ Ultrasonography may identify retained products of conception or intrauterine hematoma.

TREATMENT

Most patients with endometritis should be treated as inpatients with administration of I.V. antibiotics, such as gentamicin and/or clindamycin (Cleocin). Improvement is usually evident after 48 to 72 hours of treatment. In mild cases, oral antibiotics may be used on an outpatient basis. Doxycycline (Doryx) may be ordered if chlamydia is the cause of endometritis. A second- or third-generation cephalosporin combined with metronidazole (Flagyl) is also a frequent treatment choice.

If endometritis is caused by retained products of conception, dilation and curettage may be performed. If the cause of endometritis is chlamydia or gonorrhea, treatment of sexual partners is necessary.

 PREVENTION Prophylactic antibiotics for patients undergoing cesarean delivery may help prevent endometritis. Use of condoms helps prevent sexually transmitted infections that may cause endometritis. Avoidance of intrauterine devices may also prevent endometritis.

NURSING CONSIDERATIONS

▶ Assist with pelvic examination and obtaining cervical cultures.

▶ After establishing the patient's drug allergies, administer analgesics and antibiotics as ordered. Note the effects of pain medication 30 minutes after administration.

▶ Check for fever. Administer antipyretics as ordered. Provide tepid baths for comfort.

▶ Monitor intake and output for dehydration, and encourage oral fluids. With severe infection, I.V. fluids may be administered.

▶ Perform abdominal assessments every shift and as needed. Watch for abdominal rigidity and distention, which are possible signs of peritonitis.

▶ Provide frequent perineal care if vaginal drainage occurs. Note any abnormal vaginal bleeding.

▶ Encourage the patient to discuss her feelings, and offer emotional support as needed. If the patient has fertility problems, refer her to a fertility specialist.

▶ Monitor for signs of septicemia, such as fever and hypotension. Notify the physician immediately if signs are noted.

Patient teaching

▶ Explain the disorder to the patient, including the cause, diagnosis, and treatment.

▶ Teach the patient about all medications, including dosage, administration, and possible adverse effects.

▶ Stress the need for the patient's sexual partner to be examined, if appropriate. Discuss the use of condoms to prevent the spread of sexually transmitted infection.

▶ Tell the patient to immediately report signs and symptoms of complications, such as fever, severe abdominal pain, abdominal rigidity or distention, or unusual vaginal discharge or bleeding.

Enterobiasis

Enterobiasis (also called pinworm, seatworm, or threadworm infection, or oxyuriasis) is a benign intestinal disease caused by a thin, small, white roundworm that is about the length of a staple. Found worldwide, this disease is common even in temperate regions that have good sanitation. Enterobiasis is the most prevalent helminthic infection in the United States and is especially prominent among school-age children. More than 40 million Americans are estimated to be infected. (See *Pinworm infection.*)

CAUSES

Enterobiasis is caused by the nematode *Enterobius vermicularis*. Adult pinworms live in the intestine; female worms migrate to the perianal region to deposit their ova. Direct transmission occurs when a person's hands transfer infective eggs from the anus to the mouth. Indirect transmission occurs when an indi-

vidual comes in contact with contaminated articles, such as linens and clothing. Rarely, a pinworm ova is ingested while breathing; this is possible if the ova is airborne, such as may occur when shaking out linens.

Enterobiasis infection and re-infection occur most commonly in children between ages 5 and 14 and in certain institutionalized groups because of poor hygiene and frequent hand-to-mouth activity. Crowded living conditions increase the likelihood of the infection spreading to several members of a family.

COMPLICATIONS

Complications are uncommon but may include vulvovaginitis, salpingitis, appendicitis, bowel ulceration, and pelvic and liver granuloma.

ASSESSMENT FINDINGS

The patient's history may reveal contact with an infected person or infected articles. Asymptomatic enterobiasis is commonly overlooked. In symptomatic infection, intense perianal pruritus may occur, especially at night, when the female worm exits the anus to deposit ova. Occasionally, worms or ova may be found on underclothing, pajamas, or sheets 2 to 3 hours after the patient falls asleep. Worms or ova may also be found under the fingernails as a result of scratching the infected area.

Pruritus causes irritability, scratching, skin irritation and, sometimes, vaginitis. Inspection may reveal perianal erythema and irritation. Heavy infections can result in abdominal pain and weight loss.

DIAGNOSTIC TESTS

▶ A history of anal pruritus suggests enterobiasis.
▶ Diagnosis results from identification of *Enterobius* ova recovered from the perianal area.
▶ A stool sample is usually free of ova and worms because the worms deposit their ova outside the intestine and die after returning to the anus.

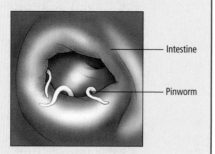

Pinworm infection

Enterobiasis is caused by a small, thin, white worm that lives in the intestine. It is the most common worm infection in the United States. Although anyone may be infected, it occurs most commonly in children, institutionalized persons, and household members of those who are infected.

Intestine

Pinworm

▶ Microscopic inspection of a perianal sample will be diagnostic.

TREATMENT

Drug therapy with pyrantel, mebendazole, or albendazole (Albenza) destroys the causative parasites. Effective eradication requires simultaneous treatment of the patient's family members and, in institutions, other patients. The medication should be given in two doses—the first when the infection is discovered and the second 2 weeks later. Household linens and bedclothes should be washed. The patient should shower first thing in the morning to remove eggs. The patient and family members should all follow strict handwashing technique, including cleaning under the fingernails.

NURSING CONSIDERATIONS

▶ Obtain a specimen for evaluation by placing cellophane tape—sticky side out—on the base end of a test tube and rolling the tube around the perianal region. Make sure you collect the sample in the morning before the patient bathes or defecates. Then send the tape for examination under a microscope.
▶ Administer drugs, as ordered, to combat infection and relieve distressing symptoms.
▶ Before giving the tablet form of pyrantel, make sure the patient isn't sensitive to aspirin, since the pyrantel tablet has an aspirin coating.
▶ Follow up as needed with others who have come in contact with the patient.
▶ Report all outbreaks of enterobiasis to school authorities.

Patient teaching

▶ If pyrantel is prescribed, tell the patient and family that this drug colors the stool bright red and may cause vomiting (emesis will also be red).
▶ Tell parents to adhere strictly to the prescribed drug dosage as directed by a physician.

 SAFETY To help prevent the spread of enterobiasis, tell parents to bathe children daily (showers are preferable to tub baths) and to change underwear and bed linens daily and wash them in hot water. Teach proper handwashing technique.

▶ To avoid aerosolization of eggs that may be on linens, tell the patient's family not to shake bed linens.
▶ Educate children about appropriate personal hygiene, and stress the need for proper handwashing after defecation and before handling food. Discourage nail biting. If the child can't stop, suggest that he or she wear gloves until the infection clears.

Droplet Precautions

Epiglottitis

Epiglottitis, also known as supraglottitis, is an acute inflammation of the epiglottis and surrounding area. It is a life-threatening emergency that rapidly causes edema and induration of the epiglottis and may result in airway obstruction. If left untreated, epiglottitis can result in complete airway obstruction. Epiglottitis can occur from infancy to adulthood in any season, but it is seen more often in children. The illness is fatal in 8% to 12% of patients, typically children between ages 2 and 8, and affects males more frequently than females.

Causes

Epiglottitis usually results from infection with the bacteria *Haemophilus influenzae* type b (Hib); occasionally, pneumococci or group A streptococci is the culprit. Since the introduction of the Hib conjugate vaccine in 1990, the incidence of epiglottitis has decreased significantly.

Complications

Airway obstruction and death may occur within 2 hours of onset.

Assessment findings

The patient or his or her parents may report a previous upper respiratory tract infection. Additional complaints include sore throat, dysphagia, and the sudden onset of a high fever.

On inspection, the patient may be febrile, drooling, pale or cyanotic, restless, apprehensive, and irritable. Nasal flaring and chest and neck muscle retraction may also be observed. Inspiratory stridor will be present. The patient may sit in a tripod position: upright, leaning forward with the chin thrust out, mouth open, and tongue protruding. This position helps relieve severe respiratory distress. The patient's voice usually sounds thick and muffled.

Manipulation may trigger sudden airway obstruction, so do not attempt throat inspection until immediately prior to intubation. The patient's throat appears red and inflamed.

 ALERT Epiglottitis can progress to complete airway obstruction within minutes. To prepare for this medical emergency, keep the following in mind:

❱ Watch for increasing restlessness, tachycardia, fever, dyspnea, and intercostal and substernal retractions. These are warning signs of total airway obstruction and the need for an emergency tracheotomy.

❱ Keep the following equipment available at the patient's bedside in case of sudden, complete airway obstruction: a tracheotomy tray, endotracheal tubes, manual resuscitation bag, oxygen equipment, and a laryngoscope with blades of various sizes.

❱ Remember that using a tongue blade or throat culture swab can initiate sudden, complete airway obstruction.

❱ Before examining the patient's throat, arrange for trained personnel (such as an anesthesiologist) to be present in case the patient requires insertion of an emergency airway.

Diagnostic tests

❱ Lateral neck radiographs show an enlarged epiglottis and distended hypopharynx.

❱ Direct laryngoscopy reveals the hallmark of acute epiglottitis: a swollen, beefy-red epiglottis. The throat examination should follow radiography studies and, in most cases, shouldn't be performed if significant obstruction is suspected or if immediate intubation isn't possible.

❱ Additional radiographs of the chest and cervical trachea help to confirm the diagnosis.

❱ Arterial blood gases will reveal respiratory acidosis.

❱ Blood cultures can be used to find the causative organism.

Treatment

A patient with acute epiglottitis and airway obstruction requires emergency hospitalization. He or she should be placed in a cool-mist tent with supplemental oxygen. If complete or near-complete airway obstruction occurs, the patient may also need emergency endotracheal intubation or a tracheotomy. Arterial blood gas monitoring or pulse oximetry may be used to assess progress.

Treatment may also include parenteral fluids to prevent dehydration when the disease interferes with swallowing as well as a 10-day course of parenteral antibiotics— usually ampicillin. If the patient is allergic to penicillin or could have ampicillin-resistant endemic *H. influenzae,* chloramphenicol or another antibiotic may be prescribed. Corticosteroids may be prescribed to reduce edema during early treatment. Oxygen therapy may also be used.

 PREVENTION The American Academy of Pediatrics recommends that all children receive the Hib vaccine. Hib immunization should begin at age 2 months and continue for three or four doses depending on the product used. Since the introduction of the Hib vaccine, the incidence of epiglottitis has decreased dramatically.

Nursing considerations

▶ Place the patient in a sitting position to ease respiratory difficulty unless he or she finds another position to be more comfortable.
▶ Place the patient in a cool-mist tent. Change the sheets frequently because they become saturated quickly.
▶ Encourage the parents to remain with their child. Offer reassurance and support to relieve family members' anxiety and fear.
▶ Monitor the patient's temperature, vital signs, and respiration rate and pattern frequently. Also monitor arterial blood gas levels (to detect hypoxia and hypercapnia) and pulse oximetry values (to detect decreasing oxygen saturation). Report changes.
◗ Observe droplet precautions to prevent the infection from spreading.
▶ Observe the patient continuously for signs of impending airway closure, which may develop at any time.
▶ Minimize external stimuli.
▶ Start an I.V. line for antibiotic therapy and fluid replacement if the patient can't maintain adequate fluid intake. Draw blood for laboratory analysis as ordered.
▶ Record intake and output precisely to monitor and prevent dehydration.
▶ Because patients who have a tracheostomy are unable to cry or call out, anticipate the needs of these patients as much as possible. Provide emotional support. Reassure the patient and family that a tracheostomy is a short-term intervention (usually 4 to 7 days). Monitor the patient for signs of secondary infection, such as increasing temperature, increasing pulse rate, and hypotension.

Patient teaching

▶ Inform the patient and family that epiglottal swelling usually subsides after 24 hours of antibiotic therapy. The epiglottis usually returns to normal size within 72 hours.
▶ If the patient's home care regimen includes oral antibiotic therapy, emphasize the need to complete the entire prescription. Discuss drug storage, dosage, adverse effects, and whether the medication can be taken with food or milk.
▶ If the patient requires the Hib vaccine, discuss the rationale for immunization and help the family obtain the vaccine.
▶ The need for prophylaxis of household contacts of someone with *H. influenzae* should be discussed with the physician in order to avoid producing a carrier state.

Epstein-Barr virus

A member of the herpes group, Epstein-Barr virus (EBV) is one of the most common viral infections and affects most people at some point during their life. The illness is mostly asymptomatic, or symptoms are mild and brief. EBV commonly affects adolescents and causes infectious mononucleosis in up to 50% of cases. Infectious mononucleosis is an acute infection that causes fever, sore throat, and cervical lymphadenopathy, the hallmarks of the infection. It also causes hepatic dysfunction, increased lymphocytes and monocytes, and development and persistence of heterophil antibodies. Mononucleosis primarily affects young adults and children, although in children it's usually so mild that it's commonly overlooked.

EBV has been associated with several neoplasms, the most common of which are nasopharyngeal carcinoma and lymphoma. It has also been associated with Hodgkin disease and non-Hodgkin's lymphoma in AIDS. Chronic EBV can cause oral hairy leukoplakia, which presents as a white lesion on the tongue or oral mucosa and is treatable with antiviral agents.

EBV is not a reportable condition, so its exact incidence is not known. The prognosis is excellent, and major complications are uncommon.

CAUSES

Apparently, humans are the only reservoir of EBV. It is probably contagious starting before symptoms develop until the fever subsides and oropharyngeal lesions disappear. EBV is spread by contact with oral secretions and is frequently transmitted from adults to infants and among young adults by kissing. It has also been transmitted during bone marrow transplantation and blood transfusion.

COMPLICATIONS

Although major complications are rare, mononucleosis may cause splenic rupture, aseptic meningitis, encephalitis, hemolytic anemia, pericarditis, and Guillain-Barré syndrome.

ASSESSMENT FINDINGS

The patient's history may reveal contact with a person who has infectious mononucleosis.

After an incubation period of about 4 to 6 weeks, the young adult patient may experience prodromal symptoms, such as headache, malaise, profound fatigue, anorexia, myalgia and, possibly, abdominal discomfort. After 3 to 5 days, the patient develops a sore throat, which may be described as the worst he or she has ever had, and dysphagia related to adenopathy. A fever is usually present, typically with a late afternoon or evening peak of 101° to 102° F (38.3° to 38.9° C).

Inspection commonly reveals exudative tonsillitis, pharyngitis and, sometimes, palatal petechiae, periorbital edema, a maculopapular rash that resembles rubella, and jaundice.

Palpation reveals nodes that are mildly tender with symmetrical enlargement. Cervical adenopathy with slight tenderness may be present, but the patient may also have inguinal and axillary adenopathy. The patient may also have splenomegaly and, less commonly, hepatomegaly. Auscultation of the chest is usually normal. A faint maculopapular rash occurs occasionally, mostly related to treatment with ampicillin, which is prescribed for a misdiagnosis of strep throat.

DIAGNOSTIC TESTS

The following abnormal laboratory test results confirm infectious mononucleosis:
▶ The monospot (heterophil) test is positive for infectious mononucleosis.
▶ Laboratory tests may reveal an increase in white blood cell count during the second and third weeks of illness. Liver function studies are abnormal.
▶ There is a fourfold increase in heterophil antibodies (agglutinins for sheep red blood cells) in serum drawn during the acute phase; these antibodies remain elevated for 3 to 4 weeks.

❱ Antibodies to EBV and cellular antigens are shown on indirect immunofluorescence. Such testing is usually more definitive than testing for heterophil antibodies but may not be necessary because the vast majority of patients are heterophil positive.

TREATMENT

Infectious mononucleosis isn't easily prevented and is resistant to standard antimicrobial treatment. Therefore, therapy is essentially supportive: relief of symptoms, bed rest during the acute febrile period, and acetaminophen or ibuprofen for headache and sore throat. If severe throat inflammation causes airway obstruction, steroids can relieve swelling and prevent the need for a tracheotomy. Splenic rupture, marked by sudden abdominal pain, requires emergent splenectomy. Patients with infectious mononucleosis who have throat cultures positive for group A streptococcal infection should not be treated as this represents colonization of the bacteria. If tonsillar or lymph node hypertrophy causes upper airway obstruction, steroids may be prescribed. Use of interferon alpha and the infusion of donor T cells or EBV-specific cytotoxic T cells are currently under investigation. Although EBV is inhibited in vitro by several antiviral agents, only EBV-associated oral hairy leukoplakia responds effectively to acyclovir.

NURSING CONSIDERATIONS

❱ Administer medications to treat symptoms as needed.

 SAFETY Maintain standard precautions. EBV is not readily transmitted, so further isolation is not required.

❱ Provide warm saline gargles for symptomatic relief of sore throat.

❱ Be cautious when performing abdominal palpation because the spleen can rupture easily.

❱ Provide adequate fluids and nutrition.
❱ Plan care to provide frequent rest periods.

Patient teaching

❱ Explain that convalescence may take several weeks, usually until the patient's white blood cell count returns to normal.

❱ Because transmission can occur through saliva, advise patients to avoid kissing until they are recovered. Parents should be cautious with drooling babies or children with hand-to-mouth behaviors.

❱ Stress the need for bed rest during the acute illness. Warn the patient to avoid excessive activity, which could lead to splenic rupture.

❱ Advise patients who are students that they can continue less demanding school assignments and see friends but that they should avoid lengthy or difficult projects until after recovery.

❱ To minimize throat discomfort, encourage the patient to drink milkshakes, fruit juices, and broths and to eat cool, bland foods. Instruct the patient to use warm saline gargles, analgesics, and antipyretics as needed for sore throat and fever.

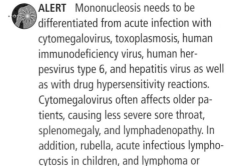 **ALERT** Mononucleosis needs to be differentiated from acute infection with cytomegalovirus, toxoplasmosis, human immunodeficiency virus, human herpesvirus type 6, and hepatitis virus as well as with drug hypersensitivity reactions. Cytomegalovirus often affects older patients, causing less severe sore throat, splenomegaly, and lymphadenopathy. In addition, rubella, acute infectious lymphocytosis in children, and lymphoma or leukemia share some of the same features as infectious mononucleosis.

CONTACT PRECAUTIONS

Erysipelas

Erysipelas, also known as "St. Anthony's fire," is a skin infection caused by bacterial inoculation into an area of skin trauma, most commonly on the face or legs. The infection characteristically extends into the lymphatic system, causing lymph node tenderness and swelling. The incidence of erysipelas has been increasing since 1980. It affects children and adults, although peak incidence is reported in patients ages 60 to 80. If bacteremia develops, it can be fatal; however, the overall mortality rate is less than 1%.

CAUSES

Streptococcus pyogenes (beta-hemolytic group A streptococci) is the most common causative organism. Other bacteria less commonly associated with erysipelas are non–group A streptococci (groups G, C, and B) and, rarely, staphylococci. The infection enters a break in the skin barrier, such as with a surgical incision, psoriatic lesions, trauma, stasis ulcer, insect bites, or eczema. Risk factors include an impaired immune system or lymphatic system, diabetes, alcoholism, nephritic syndrome, recent streptococcal pharyngitis, and arteriovenous insufficiency.

COMPLICATIONS

Infection may spread to other areas of the body via the lymphatic system within the dermis, causing septic arthritis, endocarditis, and septic shock. Recurrence may cause disfigurement, and lymphatic destruction may cause elephantiasis. Other complications include abscess, thrombophlebitis, and gangrene. Acute glomerulonephritis, endocarditis, and toxic shock syndrome may also occur, but these are rare. Untreated lesions on the trunk, arms, or legs may involve large body areas and lead to death.

Rash of erysipelas

Erysipelas is characterized by a quick-growing rash that has the texture of an orange peel and a sharply demarcated, raised border. The face has traditionally been the most commonly affected area, but the legs now account for up to 80% of cases.

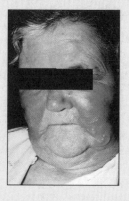

ASSESSMENT FINDINGS

Initial infection may cause fever, chills, fatigue, malaise, and vomiting. A red, warm, painful rash appears 1 to 2 days later. Other characteristics of the rash include a rapidly enlarging lesion with a sharply demarcated, raised edge, a typical finding in this type of infection. Streaking of the skin leading to the lymph nodes may be evident, and lymphadenopathy may be present. The patient may also complain of pruritus, burning, and tenderness from the rash and may report muscle aches and joint pain. Headache and sore throat may also be present. (See *Rash of erysipelas*.)

After treatment, the affected area may show pigment changes that may or may not resolve with time.

DIAGNOSTIC TESTS

▶ Physical examination helps to differentiate erysipelas from cellulitis because of the sharply demarcated, raised, advancing edges of the rash along with lymphatic involvement.

▶ Blood cultures may identify sepsis.

▶ Antistreptolysin O titers are elevated after 10 days.

▶ The white blood cell count may be elevated.

TREATMENT

Because of rapid progression of the infection, treatment should be prompt. Oral or I.V. antibiotics, such as penicillin, clindamycin, or erythromycin, are used to treat erysipelas. I.V. antibiotics may be required for infant, elderly, and immune-compromised patients, and long-term therapy may be needed for patients with recurrent infection. The antibiotics roxithromycin and pristinamycin are used in Europe and have proven to be more effective in treating erysipelas, but they are not approved by the Food and Drug Administration for use in the United States.

The affected limb should be elevated, and the patient should rest the limb as much as possible. Wet dressings should be applied to the lesions and changed at least twice per day, depending on the severity of the infection and whether drainage is present. Debridement may be necessary in cases of necrosis or gangrene. Cold packs, analgesics (aspirin and codeine for local discomfort), and topical anesthetics may be used to increase comfort. Antipyretics may be used to decrease fever.

 PREVENTION Prevention of erysipelas includes prompt treatment of streptococcal infections as well as drainage and secretion precautions.

NURSING CONSIDERATIONS

◑ Maintain contact precautions for drainage not adequately contained and standard pre-cautions if drainage is light or absent. Encourage proper handwashing for all visitors.

▶ Monitor vital signs. Administer antipyretics, such as acetaminophen, to reduce fever.

▶ Apply dressings as ordered. Note wound drainage and appearance. Report any increase in rash size and any areas of necrosis.

▶ Apply cold packs to increase comfort. Administer analgesics for pain, and evaluate their effects after 30 minutes.

▶ After checking for allergies, administer antibiotics ordered. Monitor for adverse effects.

▶ Monitor for signs and symptoms of complications, such as increased pain and drainage from the rash. Also look for signs of bacteremia or shock, such as hypotension and altered mental status.

▶ Provide emotional support. Recurrent erysipelas can cause disfigurement and disability.

Patient teaching

▶ Teach the patient about the infection, including diagnosis and treatment.

▶ Discuss any medication that is prescribed, including dosage, administration, and possible adverse effects. Stress that the patient should complete all the medication as ordered.

▶ Review signs and symptoms of complications and when to seek medical attention.

▶ Teach the patient about wound care as necessary as well as how to assess the wound for complications. Tell the patient that the skin may not return to normal for a few weeks and to expect some peeling.

Erythrasma

Erythrasma is a superficial, chronic skin condition that causes pink patches that develop into brown patches. These patches are commonly found in skin folds, such as under the breast and in the groin, axillae, and toe webs (especially between the fourth and fifth toes). The condition worsens when occlusive clothing is worn and is more prevalent in obese patients and patients with diabetes. Erythrasma is found worldwide but is more prevalent in subtropical and tropical climates. It has a higher incidence in dark-skinned people. Men develop this condition more often in the groin area. (See *Rash of erythrasma.*)

CAUSES

Erythrasma is caused by *Corynebacterium minutissimum*, which is normally present on the skin. These bacteria invade the stratum corneum, the outermost layer of the epidermis. Risk factors for erythrasma include an immune-compromised state, excessive sweating, obesity, diabetes mellitus, poor hygiene, and advanced age. The condition occurs more often in warm weather.

COMPLICATIONS

Complications of erythrasma include wound infection, infective endocarditis and, possibly, septicemia, which may cause death in immune-compromised patients. Other infections that have been related to erythrasma include cellulitis, arteriovenous fistula, intravascular catheter–related infection, primary bacteremia, and meningitis. Recurrence of the condition may be considered a complication.

ASSESSMENT FINDINGS

Patients with erythrasma present with brown-red macular patches that may cause itching. These patches are located in skin folds that are moist and generally occluded, although widespread involvement of the

Rash of erythrasma

Erythrasma is a long-term skin infection that usually occurs in areas where skin overlaps (such as under the breasts and in the groin, axillae, and toe webs). The rash starts as pink patches and progresses to brown patches. The condition is more prevalent in obese patients and patients with diabetes, and it worsens when occlusive clothing is worn.

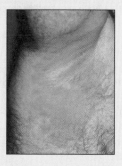

trunk and limbs may occur. The patches may be scaly, and the skin may appear macerated if toe webs are involved. These patches may remain on the skin for years. Patients are otherwise asymptomatic.

DIAGNOSTIC TESTS

▶ Wood's light examination identifies coral-red fluorescence of lesions (the patient should not bathe prior to examination because bathing may cause negative results).
▶ Gram stain identifies gram-positive filamentous rods.
▶ Methylene blue stain may highlight club-shaped rods of *C. minutissimum.*

TREATMENT

Initially, the patient may attempt to treat this condition with the use of antibacterial soap and an over-the-counter topical cream that contains tolnaftate or miconazole. Erythromycin (E-mycin) is the drug of choice to treat erythrasma. Other effective antibiotics include penicillin, tetracycline, and vancomycin. Topical antibiotic therapy may be used, such as fusidic acid (Zeta) or clindamycin (Cleocin). The use of photodynamic therapy improves or clears the condition and should be considered. Additional measures include keeping the affected area clean and dry and avoiding occlusive clothing when possible. Any concomitant infections should be treated. Patients with diabetes should strive for good glycemic control, and patients who are obese should attempt to decrease body mass index in order to prevent complications and recurrence of the condition.

Nursing considerations

▶ Assist the patient in cleaning skin folds and maintaining dryness.
▶ After checking for allergies, administer or apply medication as ordered and evaluate for any adverse reactions.
▶ Monitor affected sites for response to treatment.
▶ Refer the patient to a social worker if he or she is unable to perform grooming tasks independently.

Patient teaching

▶ Maintain standard precautions. Encourage proper handwashing technique for the patient and any caregiver who will be performing personal care for the patient.
▶ Teach the patient about the disorder, including its cause, diagnosis, and treatment.

▶ Review any medication that is ordered, including dosage and administration as well as possible adverse reactions.
▶ Teach the patient about signs and symptoms of possible complications, such as worsening skin condition, fever, chest pain, difficulty breathing, or altered mental status. Tell patients to seek medical care if any of these occur.
▶ Encourage the patient to bathe with antibacterial soap. Recommend the use of deodorant with aluminum chloride if the patient has excessive sweating.

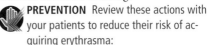 **PREVENTION** Review these actions with your patients to reduce their risk of acquiring erythrasma:
- Strive for and maintain a healthy body weight.
- Maintain good hygiene and keep the skin dry, especially any skin folds.
- Avoid excessive heat.
- Wear absorbent clothing when possible.
- For diabetic patients, review the diet to help establish and maintain adequate glycemic control.

CONTACT PRECAUTIONS

Escherichia coli infection

The Enterobacteriaceae—a group of mostly aerobic, gram-negative bacilli—cause local and systemic infections, including an invasive diarrhea that resembles shigellosis and, more commonly, a noninvasive, toxin-mediated diarrhea that resembles cholera. *E. coli* and other Enterobacteriaceae are the cause of most nosocomial infections. Noninvasive, enterotoxin-producing *E. coli* infections may be a major cause of diarrheal illness in children in the United States.

The prognosis for patients with mild to moderate infection is good. Severe infection requires immediate fluid and electrolyte replacement to avoid fatal dehydration, especially among children, in whom mortality may be quite high.

CAUSES

Although most strains of *E. coli* are harmless and exist as part of the normal GI flora, infection usually results from certain nonindigenous strains. For example, noninvasive diarrhea results from two toxins produced by strains called enterotoxic or enteropathogenic *E. coli*. Enteropathogenic *E. coli* serotype O157:H7 is the most well-known strain in the United States. Strains that produce Shiga toxins, known as Shiga toxin–producing *E. coli*, can result in hemorrhagic colitis (a form of renal failure) and hemolytic-uremic syndrome (HUS). HUS is a serious condition that affects approximately 10% of people who are infected with *E. coli* O157:H7 or other Shiga toxin–producing *E. coli*; of those who are infected, 50% will require dialysis and 5% will die. These toxins interact with intestinal juices and promote excessive loss of chloride and water. In the invasive form, *E. coli* directly invades the intestinal mucosa without producing enterotoxins, thereby causing local irritation, inflammation, and diarrhea. Normal

strains can cause infection in immunocompromised patients.

Transmission can occur directly from an infected person or indirectly by ingestion of contaminated food or water or contact with contaminated utensils. Cattle and other ruminants are an important reservoir in the United States, with the mode of transmission being the ingestion of food or water contaminated with the infected animal's feces. The incubation period can be as short as 12 hours or as long as 4 days.

The incidence of *E. coli* infection is highest among travelers returning from other countries, particularly Mexico, Southeast Asia, and South America. *E. coli* infection also induces other diseases, especially in people whose resistance is low. Outbreaks of *E. coli* O157:H7 have been associated with undercooked hamburger, raw cookie dough, unpasteurized milk, and produce such as onions, melons, and spinach. Waterborne transmission can occur from contaminated drinking water and recreational waters. The infection can also be transmitted following contact with animals at petting zoos.

COMPLICATIONS

Bacteremia, severe dehydration, life-threatening electrolyte disturbances, acidosis, HUS, and shock can develop in patients with *E. coli* infection.

ASSESSMENT FINDINGS

The effects of noninvasive diarrhea depend on the causative toxin but may include the abrupt onset of watery diarrhea with cramping abdominal pain and, in severe illness, acidosis. Invasive infection produces chills, abdominal cramps, and diarrheal stools that contain blood and pus. Diarrhea may range from mild and nonbloody stools to stools that are virtually all blood.

Infantile diarrhea resulting from an *E. coli* infection is usually noninvasive; it begins with loose, watery stools that change from yellow to green and contain little mucus or blood. Vomiting, listlessness, irritability, and anorexia commonly precede diarrhea. This condition can progress to fever, severe dehydration, acidosis, and shock. Bloody diarrhea may occur from infection with *E. coli* O157:H7, which has also been associated with HUS in children.

DIAGNOSTIC TESTS

▶ Clinical observation may be the key to diagnosis. However, if *E. coli* O157:H7 is suspected, notify the laboratory so that appropriate testing of stool specimens can be conducted.

▶ A firm diagnosis requires sophisticated identification procedures, such as bioassays, which are expensive, time-consuming and, consequently, not widely available. Specimens may need to be forwarded to state health labs.

▶ Diagnosis must rule out salmonellosis and shigellosis, other common infections that produce similar signs and symptoms.

TREATMENT

Treatment of *E. coli* infection consists of correcting fluid and electrolyte imbalances. Infants or immunocompromised patients with *E. coli* infection should be given I.V. antibiotics based on the organism's drug sensitivity. Salicylates or opium tincture should be administered for cramping and diarrhea.

NURSING CONSIDERATIONS

▶ Keep accurate intake and output records. Measure stool volume, and note the presence of blood or pus. Replace fluids and electrolytes as needed, monitoring for decreased serum sodium and chloride levels and signs of gram-negative shock. Watch for signs of dehydration, such as poor skin turgor and dry mouth.

◑ Use contact precautions when there is wound drainage, or when there is infection with an antibiotic-resistant strain.

▶ For infants, use contact precautions, give nothing by mouth, administer antibiotics as ordered, and maintain body warmth.

▶ *E. coli* O157:H7 is a reportable disease. Report cases to local public health authorities.

 PREVENTION To prevent spread of this infection, avoid direct patient contact during epidemics. Use proper handwashing technique, and follow standard precautions. Provide the patient with a private room, wear protective clothing as necessary (such as when handling feces or soiled linens), and perform scrupulous handwashing before entering and after leaving the patient's room.

Patient teaching

▶ Teach the patient and family proper handwashing technique.

▶ Advise travelers to foreign countries and those with well water at home to use bottled water and avoid uncooked fruits and vegetables.

▶ Teach the patient about the infection, including how it is transmitted, possible causes, and treatment.

▶ Discuss the signs and symptoms of possible complications, highlighting any that should immediately be reported to the practitioner.

▶ Patients and close contacts may need to be cultured, particularly those who are employed as food handlers or day-care providers. Symptomatic contacts should be restricted from handling food or providing care to patients or other susceptible populations until diarrhea ceases and two cultures are negative.

DROPLET PRECAUTIONS

Fifth disease

Fifth disease, also called erythema infectiosum, is an illness that mostly affects children ages 3 to 15 years but can also affect adults. Fifth disease causes a red rash on the cheeks and a lacy red rash on the trunk and limbs. It is usually a mild illness and, once infected, lasting immunity occurs. Approximately 60% of adults have immunity to fifth disease. No vaccine exists to prevent this infection.

Fifth disease got its name from being considered among the five classic rash-associated infections of childhood. The other classic infections are measles, scarlet fever, rubella (German measles), and another rash infection called fourth disease. Fifth disease is sometimes referred to as "slap face" disease due to the rash that presents on the cheeks in children.

CAUSES

Human parvovirus B19, an erythrovirus, causes fifth disease. It is transmitted from person to person either by respiratory secretions or droplets or through blood products; it is also transmitted from mother to fetus during pregnancy. Fifth disease is contagious in the early stages, before the rash appears. It has an incubation period of 4 to 14 days. Epidemics of fifth disease occur in the late winter or early spring; during school outbreaks, 10% to 60% of students may be infected.

Veterinarians are concerned about a type of parvovirus that affects pets. This is not the same virus, and fifth disease cannot be transmitted from pets to humans or from humans to pets.

COMPLICATIONS

Fifth disease can cause aplastic crisis in patients with a history of sickle cell anemia, thalassemia, autoimmune hemolytic anemia, or pyruvate kinase deficiency. Chronic bone marrow failure may occur in patients with a history of human immunodeficiency virus infection, acute lymphocytic leukemia, and congenital immunodeficiency syndromes. If a woman is infected during pregnancy (usually during the first half of pregnancy), fifth disease may lead to severe anemia or congestive heart failure in the mother and hydrops fetalis (fetal anemia) or intrauterine death of the fetus, although intrauterine death occurs in less than 5% of cases. Other complications that may be triggered by fifth disease include rheumatoid arthritis, idiopathic thrombocytopenic purpura, myocarditis, hepatitis, uveitis, glomerulonephritis, and seizures.

ASSESSMENT FINDINGS

Approximately 20% of patients with fifth disease are asymptomatic. Fifth disease mostly affects the skin and joints. A few days before the rash appears, the patient may complain of coldlike symptoms (fever, sore throat, muscle aches, and nasal congestion). Patients will present with a classic "slapped-cheek" redness on the cheeks that resembles sunburn. This rash may fade within 2 to 4 days. Another macular rash appears on the extremities 1 to 4 days after the initial cheek redness but does not usually affect the palms of the hands or soles of the feet. This rash fades into a lacy pattern that may last up to 3 weeks. It is usually not itchy, but some itching may occur. (See *Fifth disease rashes*.)

Until the rash is entirely gone, other stimuli—such as heat, sunlight, exercise, or stress—may exacerbate it. The patient with fifth disease may not feel ill at all or may feel ill for up to 20 days.

In adults, the rash is often atypical or absent, but 50% of adults with fifth disease suffer symmetrical arthralgia or arthritis, particularly of the hands, wrists, ankles, and knees. This joint pain may last up to several months but usually resolves within 2 weeks. Joint swelling may also occur. Arthropathy is unusual in children.

DIAGNOSTIC TESTS

▶ Physical presentation with the typical rash usually leads to diagnosis.

Fifth disease rashes

One of the first signs of fifth disease is bilateral cheek redness. This is followed by a rash that appears on the extremities and torso. The palms of the hands and soles of the feet are seldom affected. The rash usually begins to fade from the center of the body outward, resembling lace as it fades. Typically, the rash fades completely within 3 weeks.

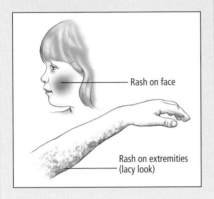

Rash on face

Rash on extremities (lacy look)

▶ Blood antibody screening is revealing. If immunoglobulin M (IgM) antibodies are present, current or recent disease is confirmed. If immunoglobulin G (IgG) antibodies are present, the patient has had the virus in the past. Pregnant women exposed to fifth disease may be monitored for seroconversion.

TREATMENT

Treatment of fifth disease is symptomatic. Acetaminophen (Tylenol) or nonsteroidal anti-inflammatory medications such as ibuprofen may be administered for fever, joint pain, or malaise. Antihistamines and topical antipruritics may be administered if itching occurs. Increased fluids and rest are recommended. Patients with severe anemia or those who are immune-suppressed may need more specific treatment, such as blood transfusions or immune globulin.

Pregnant women who contract fifth disease should have an initial fetal ultrasound to identify any abnormalities; this should be followed by weekly ultrasounds for 8 to 10 weeks after the infection has cleared. If fetal anemia is identified, treatment may involve intrauterine transfusions.

NURSING CONSIDERATIONS

▶ Provide comfort measures as needed, such as tepid baths, position changes, and massage. Evaluate the effects of interventions.
▶ Administer medications as ordered, and evaluate their effects.
▶ Monitor the complete blood count, especially hemoglobin and hematocrit levels, in patients with a history of sickle cell or chronic anemia. Administer blood products as indicated.
● Follow droplet precautions to prevent the infection from spreading.

Patient teaching

▶ Teach patients and families about the illness and how it is transmitted. Review any prescribed medications, including dosage, administration, and possible adverse effects.
▶ Explain that the patient is contagious only in the early stages of the disease; once the rash appears, children may return to school or day care, and adults may return to work and activities.
▶ Encourage parents to teach children not to share utensils or cups, as this is a mode of transmission.
▶ Stress proper and frequent handwashing and proper disposal of soiled tissues to decrease spread of the virus.
▶ Stress that immunocompromised patients should avoid anyone who has cold- or flu-like symptoms.

 SAFETY Teach parents of children with fifth disease to avoid administration of aspirin due to the risk of developing Reye syndrome.

Filariasis

Filariasis is a parasitic infection that is classified according to the body cavity inhabited by the parasite. The areas most commonly affected are cutaneous and lymphatic, but other body cavities can also be affected, such as the lungs. Currently, no form of filarial infection exists in the United States. Internationally, however, lymphatic filariasis affects 120 million people. In 2000, the World Health Organization (WHO) initiated the Global Alliance to Eliminate Lymphatic Filariasis, the goal of which is to eliminate this parasitic infection as a public health problem by 2020.

Causes

Lymphatic filariasis is caused by threadlike worms (nematodes) that live in the lymphatic system; it is transmitted by the bite of a mosquito carrying infective larvae. The larvae develop into adult worms in the lymphatic vessels, causing severe damage and swelling (lymphedema). The most common filarial species is *Wuchereria bancrofti*, but *Brugia malayi* and *Brugia timri* cause the infection in Asia. It takes several mosquito bites over many months to cause the infection. People living in tropical and subtropical settings are at the greatest risk for infection. Cutaneous filariasis caused by *Loa loa* is transmitted by the mango fly or deer fly; *Onchocerca volvulus* transmits microfilariae via the black fly; and *Mansonella streptocerca* transmits infection via a midge. *Dirofilaria immitis* may cause lesions in the lung periphery. Depending on the species, incubation may be 3 to 12 months.

Complications

Filarial infection can cause personal and socioeconomic hardships due to its debilitating consequences. Meningoencephalopathy and localized necrotizing granulomas are severe complications of *L. loa* infection. *D. immitis* may cause pulmonary infarction if the larvae lodge in the branches of the pulmonary arteries. Lymphatic filariasis may result in hydrocele or elephantiasis of the extremities or genitals. A secondary bacterial infection may cause elephantiasis, blindness, and infection of the skin and lymphatic system.

Assessment findings

Assessment findings are based on the type of infection present and the body site affected. Signs and symptoms may be acute or chronic. Patients with lymphatic filariasis may be asymptomatic or may complain of fever and edema of the lymph system, commonly affecting the legs but also seen in the arms, breasts, and genitals. Thickening and hardening of the skin (elephantiasis) as well as skin exfoliation may occur. Filariasis affecting the pulmonary system causes a dry cough, dyspnea, wheezing, and anorexia. Cutaneous filariasis causes itching, subcutaneous lumps, localized pain, and lymphadenitis and may lead to ocular lesions and eye disorders such as glaucoma, optic atrophy, and corneal fibrosis.

Diagnostic tests

▶ Microscopic examination may identify the microfilariae in the blood, skin, chylous urine, or hydrocele fluid. Blood collection should be done at night because microfilariae circulate in the blood at night.

▶ Slitlamp examination may identify microfilariae in the cornea or anterior chamber of the eye.

▶ Filarial antigens and antibodies are detected in the blood.

▶ A complete blood count shows marked eosinophilia.

▶ Serum immunoglobulin (Ig) testing reveals elevated IgE and IgG_4.

▶ Chest radiography may reveal pulmonary infiltrates if the lungs are involved.

▶ Ultrasonography may identify lymphatic obstruction of the inguinal and scrotal lymphatics or vitreous changes in the eye.

▶ Lymph or skin biopsy identifies *L. loa* and *O. volvulus* infection.

TREATMENT

Treatment is based on the type of infection. The anthelminthic ivermectin (Stromectol) is the drug of choice for most infections, although diethylcarbamazine (DEC) has also been used for treatment. With DEC, antihistamines and corticosteroids may also be required to decrease allergic reactions caused by disintegrating microfilariae resulting from treatment. DEC should not be used to treat infections caused by *O. volvulus* because DEC may cause blindness, and use with heavy *L. loa* infection may cause encephalitis. Other medications that may be used include doxycycline (Doryx) and albendazole (Albenza). For chronic conditions such as hydrocele, medication may not be effective and surgery may be required. Additional measures include meticulous skin care and exercise to promote lymphatic drainage. Supportive care should be provided for infection with pulmonary involvement.

 PREVENTION The WHO is attempting to eliminate filarial infections worldwide by providing mass drug administration to areas of the world where people are at risk for lymphatic filariasis. Recommended antifilarial drug combinations of either DEC or ivermectin plus albendazole, in addition to regular use of DEC-fortified salt, may prevent the occurrence of new infection and disease.

NURSING CONSIDERATIONS

▶ Provide emotional support to patients to help decrease fear regarding infection and to help deal with debilitating features if lymphatic complications or elephantiasis develops.
▶ Provide meticulous skin care, and monitor for complications such as bacterial infection.
▶ Administer medications as ordered.
▶ Assist with exercises of any limbs affected by lymphedema.
▶ Monitor for complications based on the type of infection, such as signs of encephalitis or blindness.
▶ Monitor respiratory status in patients infected with *D. immitis*. Monitor pulse oximetry and arterial blood gas results. Provide oxygen and ventilator support as indicated.

Patient teaching

▶ Teach the patient about the specific infection they have, including how it was acquired and the recommended treatment plan.
▶ Review all medication, including dosage, administration, and possible adverse effects.
▶ Review follow-up care, usually 1 year after treatment is complete.

 PREVENTION Teach patients in areas endemic to lymphatic filariasis to avoid mosquito bites through the use of mosquito repellent on any exposed areas, especially between dusk and dawn; utilize mosquito netting while sleeping; and wear long sleeves and long pants when outdoors.

CONTACT PRECAUTIONS

Folliculitis

Folliculitis—a bacterial infection originating in the hair follicle—causes the formation of pustules. The infection can be superficial (follicular impetigo or Bockhart's impetigo) or deep (sycosis barbae). Folliculitis may also lead to the development of furuncles (furunculosis), commonly known as boils, or carbuncles (carbunculosis). These disorders may be recurrent and are particularly troublesome to healthy young adults. The prognosis depends on the severity of the infection and on the patient's physical condition.

CAUSES

The most common cause of folliculitis is coagulase-positive *Staphylococcus aureus*, which is a common and normal skin organism in many people (20% to 30% of adults carry *S. aureus* in their nose). Predisposing factors for folliculitis include an infected wound elsewhere on the body, poor personal hygiene, debilitation, diabetes mellitus, occlusive cosmetics, tight clothes, friction, incorrect shaving technique, exposure to chemicals (cutting oils), and management of skin lesions with tar or with barrier therapy using a steroid. Folliculitis may be caused by bacteria other than *S. aureus*, such as *Propionibacterium*, which causes acne.

COMPLICATIONS

Untreated furunculosis may lead to cellulitis, which in turn may progress to septicemia if the infection reaches the dermal vascular plexus. Skin lesions are usually uncomplicated, but seeding of the bloodstream can lead to pneumonia, lung abscess, osteomyelitis, sepsis, endocarditis, arthritis, or meningitis. In severe cases, residual permanent scarring may result.

ASSESSMENT FINDINGS

The patient history recounts predisposing factors. The patient may complain of pain, erythema, and edema of several days' duration.

In patients with folliculitis, inspection usually reveals pustules on the scalp, arms, and legs in children; on the face in bearded men (sycosis barbae); and on the eyelids (styes) in patients of any age.

The degree of hair follicle involvement in patients with bacterial skin infection ranges from superficial folliculitis (erythema and a pustule in a single follicle) to deep folliculitis (extensive follicle involvement) to furunculosis (red, tender nodules that surround follicles with a single draining point) and, finally, to carbunculosis (deep abscesses that involve several follicles with multiple draining points).

Folliculitis may progress to furunculosis, in which the patient complains of hard, painful nodules, usually on the neck, face, axillae, and buttocks. If nodules enlarge and rupture, inspection will reveal discharged pus and necrotic material on the skin surface. Erythema may persist for days or weeks after nodule rupture.

In severe cases of systemic infection and in carbunculosis, vital sign assessment may reveal fever, and the patient may complain of malaise. Inspection reveals lesions that range from tiny, white-topped pustules to large, yellow, pus-filled lesions. The patient with carbunculosis will complain of extremely painful, deep abscesses that drain through multiple openings onto the skin surface, usually around several hair follicles. Palpation is used to detect pain, tenderness, and edema around the pustule sites; in both furunculosis and carbunculosis, palpation also reveals hard nodules under the skin surface.

A systemic response to the infection may include localized lymphadenopathy.

DIAGNOSTIC TESTS

▶ Wound culture usually shows *S. aureus*, which may be a resistant strain (methicillin-resistant *S. aureus*, or MRSA).

▶ Laboratory tests may reveal leukocytosis.

TREATMENT

Treatment, which emphasizes site care and drug therapy, includes cleaning the infected area thoroughly with antibacterial soap (such as chlorhexidine) and water; applying warm, wet compresses to promote vasodilation and drainage from the lesions; administering a topical antibiotic, such as mupirocin ointment (Bactroban), clindamycin (Cleocin), or erythromycin solution; and administering a systemic antibiotic (cephalosporin or dicloxacillin) if the patient has extensive infection and carbunculosis. If MRSA is the causative organism, topical mupirocin and an appropriate antibiotic may be used, depending on the sensitivity panel.

Patients with furunculosis may also require incision and drainage of ripe lesions after application of warm, wet compresses and a systemic antibiotic after drainage. Carbuncles require systemic antibiotic therapy as well as incision and drainage.

NURSING CONSIDERATIONS

▶ Be alert for possible reactions to systemic antibiotic therapy, which may include gastric disturbances and sensitivity reactions.
◗ Change the dressing frequently, and maintain aseptic technique. To prevent the spread of infection, properly dispose of contaminated dressings and use standard precautions; use contact precautions if draining skin abscesses are present.
▶ Assess the patient for discomfort, and apply warm, moist compresses to aid suppuration.
▶ Encourage the patient to verbalize feelings about his or her appearance. Recognize the importance of body image.
▶ Assist with general hygiene and comfort measures as needed.
▶ Administer an analgesic and an antibiotic, as ordered, and monitor the patient's response.

Patient teaching

▶ Teach the patient about prescribed medications, including dosage, administration, and possible adverse effects.

▶ Instruct the patient and family to complete the entire course of the prescribed antibiotic, even if the lesions appear to have healed. Advise them to notify the physician if adverse reactions to systemic antibiotic therapy occur.
▶ Teach the patient and family how to apply warm compresses, change dressings with aseptic technique, and properly dispose of contaminated dressings.

 PREVENTION To prevent the spread of infection, teach the patient and family meticulous handwashing technique and encourage the patient to take daily showers with antibacterial soap. Also, urge the patient not to share clothes, towels, washcloths, or bed linens and to launder these items in hot water before reusing. Tell the patient to change his or her clothes and bedsheets daily. To prevent the spread of infection to surrounding areas and minimize scarring, stress the importance of not squeezing lesions.

Gas gangrene

Gas gangrene is caused by local infection with the anaerobic, spore-forming, gram-positive rod *Clostridium perfringens* (or another clostridial species). It occurs in devitalized tissue and results from compromised arterial circulation after trauma, surgery, compound fracture, or laceration. Gas gangrene is rare, with only 1,000 to 3,000 cases occurring in the United States each year. The infection carries a high mortality rate unless therapy begins immediately after diagnosis; however, with prompt treatment, 80% of patients with gas gangrene of the extremities survive. The prognosis is poorer for patients with gas gangrene in other sites, such as the abdominal wall or the bowel. The usual incubation period is 1 to 4 days, but it can vary from 3 hours to 6 weeks or longer.

CAUSES

C. perfringens is a normal inhabitant of the GI and female genital tracts; it's also prevalent in soil. Transmission of infection occurs by entry of organisms during trauma or surgery. Because *C. perfringens* is anaerobic and spore forming, gas gangrene is usually found in deep wounds, especially those in which tissue necrosis further reduces the oxygen supply. Clostridial bacteria produce four different toxins (alpha, beta, epsilon, and iota) that can cause potentially fatal symptoms. When *C. perfringens* invades soft tissue, it produces thrombosis of regional blood vessels, tissue necrosis, localized edema, and damage to the myocardium, liver, and kidneys. Such necrosis releases both carbon dioxide and hydrogen subcutaneously, producing interstitial gas bubbles. Gas gangrene usually occurs in the extremities and in abdominal wounds; it's less common in the uterus.

COMPLICATIONS

Possible complications of gas gangrene include renal failure, hypotension, hemolytic anemia, shock, and tissue death, requiring amputation of the affected body part. If left untreated, gas gangrene leads to death.

ASSESSMENT FINDINGS

True gas gangrene produces myositis and anaerobic cellulitis, another form of the condition that involves only soft tissue. Most signs of infection develop within 72 hours of trauma or surgery. The hallmark of gas gangrene is crepitation (a crackling sensation when the skin is touched), which is a result of carbon dioxide and hydrogen accumulation as a metabolic by-product in necrotic tissue. Other typical indications are severe localized and progressive pain, swelling, and discoloration (initially pale, later orange tinted, dusky brown, or reddish), with bullae formation and necrosis within 36 hours of the onset of symptoms. The skin over the wound may rupture, revealing dark red or black necrotic muscle, a foul-smelling watery or frothy discharge, intravascular hemolysis, thrombosis of blood vessels, and evidence of infection spread.

In addition to these local symptoms, gas gangrene produces early signs of toxemia and hypovolemia (tachycardia, tachypnea, and hypotension), with moderate fever that usually does not exceed 101° F (38.3° C). Although pale, prostrate, and motionless, patients with gas gangrene may exhibit toxic delirium and are extremely apprehensive. Possible sudden death is preceded by delirium and coma and, in some cases, vomiting, profuse diarrhea, and circulatory collapse.

DIAGNOSTIC TESTS

▶ A history of recent surgery or a deep puncture wound and the rapid onset of pain and crepitation around the wound suggest gas gangrene. Diagnosis must rule out synergistic gangrene and necrotizing fasciitis; unlike gas gangrene, these disorders both anesthetize the skin around the wound.
▶ Anaerobic cultures of wound drainage show *C. perfringens*.
▶ Gram stain of wound drainage reveals large, gram-positive, rod-shaped bacteria.

▶ Radiography displays gas in body tissue; computed tomography or magnetic resonance imaging detects gas in the deeper tissue.
▶ Blood work may show leukocytosis and, later, hemolysis.

TREATMENT

Treatment of gas gangrene includes careful observation for signs of myositis and cellulitis followed by immediate treatment if these signs appear; immediate wide surgical excision of all affected tissue and necrotic muscle in myositis (delayed or inadequate surgical excision is a fatal mistake); I.V. administration of high-dose penicillin; and, after adequate debridement, hyperbaric oxygenation if available. Every 6 to 8 hours, the patient is placed in a hyperbaric chamber for 1 to 3 hours, exposing him or her to pressures designed to increase oxygen tension and prevent multiplication of the anaerobic clostridia. Surgery may be performed within the hyperbaric chamber if the chamber is large enough.

NURSING CONSIDERATIONS

▶ Careful observation may result in early diagnosis. Look for signs and symptoms of ischemia (cool skin; pallor or cyanosis; sudden, severe pain; sudden edema; and loss of pulses in involved limb).
▶ After the diagnosis:
- Provide adequate fluid replacement, and assess pulmonary and cardiac function often. Maintain airway and ventilation.
- To prevent skin breakdown and further infection, give good skin care. After surgery, provide meticulous wound care.

- Before penicillin administration, obtain a patient history of allergies; afterward, watch closely for signs of hypersensitivity.
- Psychological support is critical because these patients can remain alert until death, knowing that death is imminent and unavoidable.
- Deodorize the room to control foul odor emanating from the wound. Prepare the patient emotionally for a large wound after surgical excision, and refer him or her for physical rehabilitation as necessary.
- Maintain standard precautions. Dispose of drainage material properly, and wear sterile gloves when changing dressings. Spore-forming bacteria aren't destroyed by ordinary disinfecting methods. Contaminated items should be cleaned and disinfected or sterilized, as appropriate.

 PREVENTION Routinely take precautions to render all wound sites unsuitable for growth of clostridia by attempting to keep granulation tissue viable; adequate debridement is imperative to reduce anaerobic growth conditions. The surgeon may delay closure of wounds. Be alert for devitalized tissue, and notify the surgeon promptly. Position the patient to facilitate drainage, and eliminate all dead spaces in closed wounds.

Patient teaching

▶ Tell any patient who reports sudden, severe, and persistent pain at a wound site to consult a physician at once.
▶ Teach the patient with a cast or covered wound to report any foul odor or drainage.

CONTACT PRECAUTIONS

Gastroenteritis

Gastroenteritis (also called intestinal flu, traveler's diarrhea, dysentery, viral or bacterial enteritis, and food poisoning) is an inflammation of the stomach and small intestine that is usually self-limiting. The bowel reacts to any of the varied causes of gastroenteritis with hypermotility, producing severe diarrhea and secondary depletion of intracellular fluid. Nausea, vomiting, and acute or chronic abdominal cramping are also common.

Gastroenteritis occurs in people of all ages. In the United States, this disorder ranks second to the common cold as a cause of lost work time and fifth as a cause of death among young children. It can be life-threatening in elderly and debilitated people. Traveler's diarrhea affects 20% to 25% of people traveling from industrialized countries to developing countries.

CAUSES

Gastroenteritis has many possible causes, including bacteria, such as *Staphylococcus aureus, Salmonella, Shigella, Clostridium botulinum, Clostridium perfringens, Escherichia coli, Campylobacter, Aeromonas,* and *Yersinia*; protozoans such as *Giardia lamblia* and *Cryptosporidium*; amoebae, especially *Entamoeba histolytica*; parasites, such as *Ascaris, Enterobius,* and *Trichinella spiralis*; viruses (may be responsible for traveler's diarrhea), such as rotaviruses, noroviruses, adenoviruses, echoviruses, and coxsackieviruses; ingestion of toxins, such as poisonous plants and toadstools; drug reactions, for example, to antibiotics; enzyme deficiencies; and food allergens.

Chronic gastroenteritis may be the result of another GI disorder, such as ulcerative colitis. Diarrhea outbreaks in day-care facilities are typically due to viral gastroenteritis.

COMPLICATIONS

In most patients, the disorder resolves with no sequelae. However, persistent or untreated gastroenteritis can cause severe dehydration and loss of crucial electrolytes, which can lead to shock, vascular collapse, renal failure and, rarely, death. Typically, infants, elderly people, and debilitated patients are at greatest risk because of their immature or impaired immune systems.

ASSESSMENT FINDINGS

Patient history commonly reveals the acute onset of diarrhea accompanied by abdominal pain and discomfort. The patient may complain of cramping, nausea, and vomiting. He or she may also report malaise, fatigue, anorexia, fever, abdominal distention, and rumbling in the lower abdomen. If diarrhea is severe, the patient may experience rectal burning, tenesmus, and bloody, mucoid stools.

Investigate the patient's history to try to determine the cause of the signs and symptoms. Ask about ingestion of contaminated food or water. The cause may be apparent if the patient reports that others who ingested the same food or water have similar signs and symptoms. Also ask about the health of other family members and about recent travels.

Inspection may reveal slight abdominal distention. On palpation, the patient's skin turgor may be poor, a sign of dehydration. Auscultation may disclose hyperactive bowel sounds and, if the patient is dehydrated, orthostatic hypotension or generalized hypotension. Temperature may be either normal or elevated.

DIAGNOSTIC TESTS

‣ A stool sample can be used to check for occult blood and can be cultured to determine a suspected bacterial or fungal cause of symptoms. Routine stool cultures only identify *Campylobacter, Shigella, Salmonella, Aeromonas,* and *Yersinia* species. Specialized media will be needed to test for other pathogens.

▸ Enzyme-linked immunosorbent assay can detect *Giardia* and *Cryptosporidium* microorganisms. *Clostridium difficile* toxin assays can be performed when antibiotic-associated diarrhea is suspected.

TREATMENT

Medical management is usually supportive, consisting of bed rest, nutritional support, increased fluid intake and, occasionally, antidiarrheal therapy. If gastroenteritis is severe or affects a young child or an elderly or debilitated person, hospitalization may be required. Treatment may include I.V. fluid and electrolyte replacement and administration of antidiarrheals, antiemetics, and antimicrobials.

Antidiarrheals, such as bismuth subsalicylate, are typically used as the first line of defense against diarrhea. If necessary, other antidiarrheals, such as camphorated tincture of opium (paregoric), diphenoxylate with atropine (Lomotil), and loperamide (Imodium), may be ordered.

Oral, I.V., or rectal suppository antiemetics, such as prochlorperazine (Compro) and trimethobenzamide (Tigan), may be prescribed for severe vomiting. Antiemetics should be avoided in patients with viral or bacterial gastroenteritis.

Specific antibiotic administration is restricted to patients who have bacterial gastroenteritis, as identified by diagnostic testing.

NURSING CONSIDERATIONS

▸ Monitor fluid status carefully. Take vital signs at least every 4 hours, weigh the patient daily, monitor for fluid and electrolyte balance, and record intake and output.
▸ Watch for signs of dehydration, such as dry skin and mucous membranes, fever, and sunken eyes.
▸ Administer oral and I.V. fluids and electrolytes as ordered. Administer medications as ordered.
◆ To prevent the spread of infection, wash your hands thoroughly after providing care and use standard precautions when handling emesis or stools. Contact precautions should be followed for diapered or incontinent patients.
▸ If food poisoning is probable, contact public health authorities so they can interview patients and food handlers and take samples of the suspected contaminated food.

Patient teaching

▸ Teach the patient about gastroenteritis, including its symptoms and varied causes.
▸ Instruct the patient about dietary recommendations of clear liquids progressing to bland, soft foods, such as cooked cereal, rice, and applesauce. Tell the patient to avoid foods that are spicy, greasy, or high in roughage, such as whole-grain products and raw fruits or vegetables.
▸ Carefully review prescribed medications, including dosage, administration, and possible adverse effects.

 PREVENTION Patients who expect to travel should be advised to pay close attention to what they eat and drink, especially in developing nations. Review proper hygiene measures to prevent recurrence. Instruct the patient to cook foods thoroughly, especially pork, and to drink only bottled or boiled water; refrigerate perishable foods, such as milk, mayonnaise, potato salad, and cream-filled pastry; always wash hands with warm water and soap before handling food and after using the bathroom; clean utensils thoroughly; and eliminate flies and roaches in the home. If traveler's diarrhea occurs despite precautions, bismuth subsalicylate, kaolin or pectin preparations, diphenoxylate with atropine, or loperamide can be used to relieve the symptoms. Packets of oral rehydration solution powder can be purchased commercially and added to boiled water to avoid dehydration.

CONTACT PRECAUTIONS

Giardiasis

Giardiasis (also called *Giardia* enteritis) is an infection of the small bowel caused by the symmetrical flagellate protozoan *Giardia (duodenalis) lamblia*. A mild infection may not produce intestinal symptoms, and asymptomatic carriage is common. In untreated giardiasis, symptoms wax and wane; with treatment, recovery is complete. Giardiasis doesn't confer immunity, so re-infections may occur. People infected with human immunodeficiency virus may have more serious and prolonged giardiasis.

CAUSES

G. lamblia has two stages: the cystic stage and the trophozoite stage. Ingestion of *G. lamblia* cysts in fecally contaminated water or the fecal-oral transfer of cysts by an infected person results in giardiasis. Giardiasis may be transmitted through sexual contact (direct or indirect fecal-oral contact). When cysts enter the small bowel, they become trophozoites and attach themselves with their sucking disks to the bowel's epithelial surface. The trophozoites then encyst again, travel down the colon, and are excreted. Unformed feces that pass quickly through the intestine may contain trophozoites as well as cysts.

Giardiasis occurs worldwide but is most common in developing countries and other areas where sanitation and hygiene are poor. In the United States, giardiasis is most common in travelers who have recently returned from endemic areas and in campers who drink unpurified water from contaminated streams. Probably because of frequent hand-to-mouth activity, children are more likely to become infected with *G. lamblia* than are adults. Hypogammaglobulinemia also appears to predispose people to this disorder.

Those at risk for acquiring giardiasis include employees and children in day-care settings, especially if diaper-age children are present; close contacts, family members, and caregivers of an infected person; people who imbibe contaminated water or ice (including water that has not been boiled, filtered, or disinfected with chemicals); campers or hikers who drink unpurified water or do not practice good handwashing technique; swimmers who swallow contaminated water from lakes, streams, ponds, rivers, and recreational settings; international travelers; and people participating in sexual practices that expose them to feces, such as anal intercourse.

COMPLICATIONS

The mucosal destruction caused by the protozoa decreases food transit time through the small intestine and results in malabsorption. Other complications include dehydration and lactose intolerance. Giardiasis can be life-threatening in patients with hypogammaglobulinemia. It can also complicate conditions such as cystic fibrosis.

ASSESSMENT FINDINGS

Attachment of *G. lamblia* to the intestinal lumen causes superficial mucosal invasion as well as destruction, inflammation, and irritation. All of these destructive effects decrease food transit time through the small intestine and result in malabsorption. Such malabsorption produces chronic GI complaints—such as abdominal cramps—and pale, loose, greasy, malodorous, and frequent stools (from 2 to 10 daily) with concurrent nausea. Stools may contain mucus but not pus or blood. Nausea may also occur. Chronic giardiasis may produce fatigue, dehydration, and weight loss in addition to these typical signs and symptoms. Suspect giardiasis when travelers to endemic areas or campers who may have drunk unpurified water develop symptoms. Symptoms generally begin 1 to 2 weeks after infection occurs and last approximately 2 to 6 weeks.

DIAGNOSTIC TESTS

▶ Examination of a fresh stool specimen shows cysts; examination of duodenal aspirate or biopsy shows trophozoites. Multiple stool specimens may be needed over several days to obtain a diagnosis. Three negative specimens are needed to rule out the infection.

◗ Antigen tests using enzyme-linked immunosorbent assay or direct fluorescent antibody are diagnostic. These tests are best used for screening in settings where infection is common, such as day-care centers, or during an epidemic.

◗ A small bowel biopsy shows *Giardia*.

◗ A barium radiograph of the small bowel may show mucosal edema and barium segmentation.

TREATMENT

Giardiasis responds readily to a 10-day course of metronidazole (Flagyl). Severe diarrhea may require parenteral fluid replacement to prevent dehydration if oral fluid intake is inadequate.

NURSING CONSIDERATIONS

◗ If hospitalization is required, use standard precautions. Contact precautions should be used for diapered or incontinent patients or to control an institutional outbreak.

◗ A child or an incontinent adult with giardiasis should be placed in a private room or be grouped with persons with similar diagnoses.

◗ Pay strict attention to hand hygiene, particularly after handling feces. Quickly dispose of fecal material. (Normal sewage systems can remove and process infected feces adequately.)

◗ Monitor electrolyte levels for abnormal values. Administer electrolyte replacements as needed.

◗ Administer medications as ordered, and monitor for adverse reactions.

◗ Collect stool specimens for culture as ordered.

◗ Encourage oral fluid intake and monitor the patient for signs of dehydration, such as thirst, decreased urine output, tenting of skin, and hypotension.

◗ Report all cases of giardiasis to the state health department or the Centers for Disease Control and Prevention. Report epidemic situations to public health authorities.

PATIENT TEACHING

◗ Inform patients who are receiving metronidazole (Flagyl) about the possible adverse effects of this drug, which commonly include headache, anorexia, and nausea and, less commonly, vomiting, diarrhea, and abdominal cramps. Warn against drinking alcoholic beverages because metronidazole may provoke a disulfiram-like reaction. If the patient is a woman, ask if she's pregnant because metronidazole is contraindicated during pregnancy.

◗ When talking to family members and other suspected contacts, emphasize the importance of stool examinations for *G. lamblia* cysts.

◗ Teach good personal hygiene, particularly proper handwashing technique. Stress the need to wash hands after changing diapers or assisting children with toileting.

◗ Advise patients not to swim in pools or use hot tubs until 1 week after diarrhea has stopped to prevent contamination of the water, which can cause infection in others.

◗ Tell parents to keep their child out of day-care facilities until diarrhea is resolved.

◗ Recommend the use of a barrier during oral-anal sex and stress the need for handwashing after removing a condom following anal sex or if touching the rectal area.

 PREVENTION To help prevent giardiasis, warn travelers to endemic areas not to drink untreated water or eat uncooked or unpeeled fruits or vegetables (they may have been rinsed in contaminated water) and to drink and use ice made only from bottled or boiled water. Prophylactic drug therapy isn't recommended. Advise campers to purify all stream water before drinking it.

Gingivitis

Gingivitis is inflammation of the gingiva, which is part of the soft-tissue lining (gums) of the mouth that surrounds the teeth. Gingivitis is classified according to its appearance (ulcerative, purulent, hemorrhagic, or necrotizing), cause (hormonal, nutritional, drug- or plaque-induced), and whether it is acute or chronic. The most common type of gingivitis is chronic gingivitis, which results when plaque and tartar accumulate between the teeth. Acute necrotizing ulcerative gingivitis (ANUG) is also known as trench mouth. (See *Acute necrotizing ulcerative gingivitis (ANUG)*.)

Gingivitis may progress to parodontitis, which is gum disease that spreads below the gum line and affects the tissue and bones that support the teeth.

CAUSES

Chronic gingivitis is generally caused by inadequate oral hygiene, which allows bacteria to remain between the teeth and plaque to build up on the teeth. ANUG is caused by organisms in the tissue and is not contagious. It may be a complication of chronic gingivitis, or it may be due to decreased immune defenses. Gingivitis may also be caused by drugs, such as anticoagulants, oral contraceptives, or calcium channel blockers; poor nutrition; allergic reactions; chronic disease; or lack of dental care. Tobacco use, diabetes mellitus, and human immunodeficiency virus infection may increase the incidence of gingivitis. Gingivitis may also be an early sign of hypovitaminosis, diabetes mellitus, and blood dyscrasias.

Risk factors involved in developing gingivitis include poor dental hygiene; smoking or use of tobacco products; a family history of gum disease; high levels of stress; a history of diabetes, acquired immunodeficiency syndrome, or leukemia; poor diet; pregnancy and puberty (due to hormonal changes); misaligned teeth or teeth with rough edges; ill-fitting or unclean dentures, bridges, or crowns; and ingestion of heavy metals (such as lead or bismuth). Gingivitis is also associated with the severe periodontal decay disease that results from use of the drug methamphetamine, known as "meth mouth."

Acute necrotizing ulcerative gingivitis (ANUG)

Acute necrotizing ulcerative gingivitis (ANUG), also known as trench mouth, Vincent's stomatitis, or Vincent's infection, after French physician Jean Hyacinthe Vincent, is an acute infectious type of gingivitis. It was common among trench-bound soldiers in World War II.

ANUG is caused by an abundance of oral bacteria, such as *Prevotella intermedia*, alpha-hemolytic streptococci, or *Actinomyces* species, among others. Contributing factors include poor diet, smoking, oral hygiene, lifestyle, stress, chemotherapy, diabetes, and an impaired immune system. If left untreated, necrotizing stomatitis may cause destruction of the periodontium, cheek tissue, lips, or bones of the jaws. The infection can also spread systemically to any other part of the body.

With ANUG, bleeding of the gums occurs spontaneously or with minimal local trauma. The patient may experience a metallic taste and have offensive breath. Local pain, fever, and malaise may also be reported. A gray pseudomembrane may be present on the gums, along with ulceration. ANUG is not contagious.

Salt water and hydrogen peroxide rinses, along with chlorhexidine or metronidazole, may help reduce oral bacteria. An antibiotic, such as penicillin, is also prescribed. Dental cleaning improves the condition, but ANUG will recur if causative factors are not removed or adjusted.

COMPLICATIONS

Gingivitis can lead to periodontal disease and tooth loss. Dental abscesses may occur. Left untreated, ANUG can lead to systemic infection and even death.

ASSESSMENT FINDINGS

Oral inspection reveals inflammation of the gums with painless swelling, redness, and a change in the normal contour of the gum line. Bleeding may occur with brushing, flossing, or eating. Gum tenderness and itchy gums may be noted in some patients, and mouth sores may be present. Gum detachment from the teeth can be measured by a dental professional. Teeth may be loose and may not fit together properly when biting. Pockets between teeth may contain pus, and bad breath may occur. ANUG may cause local pain, an alteration in taste, and foul breath.

DIAGNOSTIC TESTS

▶ Evaluation by a dentist of the patient's history and symptoms will lead to diagnosis.
▶ If the cause is unknown, the dentist may recommend a medical evaluation in addition to the dental assessment.

TREATMENT

Treatment of gingivitis includes removal of irritating factors in the mouth, such as tartar or faulty dentures. Good oral hygiene, including flossing, is important, along with rinsing with chlorhexidine or other rinses. Saline rinses may also be helpful. Nonsteroidal anti-inflammatory drugs may help reduce pain and inflammation. A topical anesthetic, such as viscous lidocaine, may be applied prior to brushing to reduce pain. Regular dental checkups and cleanings help minimize plaque and tartar. It takes approximately 3 months for bacteria buildup in the gum pockets to start the inflammatory process again, although plaque begins to grow within hours after cleaning and tartar may start to re-form within 24 hours.

Antibiotics, such as penicillin and erythromycin, are used to treat ANUG and may be prescribed prior to dental surgery.

 ALERT According to the Pennsylvania Medical Society, good oral health may reduce the risk of cardiac events by helping to prevent bacteria from entering the bloodstream.

NURSING CONSIDERATIONS

▶ Monitor gums for bleeding when assisting with or performing mouth care on patients.
▶ Apply an anesthetic to the gums prior to performing mouth care if the patient complains of pain.
▶ Encourage patients to perform mouth care twice daily, if they are able to do so independently. For patients who need dependent oral care, perform twice daily. If the patient is on a ventilator, perform oral care every 4 hours.
▶ Provide information for smoking cessation, if appropriate.

Patient teaching

▶ Recommend use of an electric toothbrush along with fluoride toothpaste.
▶ Advise the patient to have a professional dental cleaning every 6 months, or as recommended by a dentist. Dental cleanings every 3 months may be recommended for some patients.
▶ Encourage patients to floss the teeth after brushing. If this is not possible, recommend use of a plaque-removing rinse.
▶ Teach patients about any medication that is prescribed, including dosage, administration, and possible adverse effects. Tell them to take medication for the entire time it is prescribed.

 PREVENTION To prevent gingivitis, teach patients to control underlying illness, brush and floss twice daily, and follow up with regular dental checkups. Encourage smoking cessation or discontinuing use of tobacco products.

CONTACT PRECAUTIONS

Gonorrhea

Gonorrhea is a common sexually transmitted infection that usually starts as an infection of the genitourinary tract, especially the urethra and cervix. It can also cause infection in the eyes (conjunctivitis), pharynx, and anorectal area; pharyngeal and anorectal infections are not uncommon in females and homosexual males. Left untreated, gonorrhea spreads through the blood to the joints, tendons, meninges, and endocardium; in females, it also can lead to chronic pelvic inflammatory disease (PID) and sterility. Gonorrhea is especially prevalent among young people and those who have multiple sexual partners. With adequate treatment, the prognosis is excellent, although re-infection is common.

CAUSES

Gonorrhea is caused by the bacterial organism *Neisseria gonorrhoeae* (gonococcus), which is transmitted almost exclusively through sexual contact with an infected person. A child born to an infected mother can contract gonococcal ophthalmia neonatorum during passage through the birth canal. A patient with gonorrhea can contract gonococcal conjunctivitis by touching the eyes with a contaminated hand. Genitourinary gonorrhea in a child is considered an indicator of possible sexual abuse.

COMPLICATIONS

Gonorrhea can lead to PID, acute epididymitis, proctitis, salpingitis, septic arthritis, dermatitis, and perihepatitis. Severe gonococcal conjunctivitis can lead to corneal ulceration and, possibly, blindness. Rare complications include meningitis, osteomyelitis, pneumonia, and acute respiratory distress syndrome.

ASSESSMENT FINDINGS

The patient may report unprotected sexual contact (vaginal, oral, or anal) with an infected person, an unknown partner, or multiple sex partners. He or she may also have a history of sexually transmitted infection.

After a 3- to 6-day incubation period, male patients may complain of dysuria, although patients of both genders can remain asymptomatic. Patients with rectal infection may be asymptomatic or may complain of anal pruritus, burning, and tenesmus and pain with defecation. Patients with pharyngeal infection may be asymptomatic or may complain of a sore throat. Some females may suffer uterine invasion, often around menstruation.

Assessment of a patient with gonorrhea reveals a low-grade fever. If the disease has become systemic, or if the patient has developed PID or acute epididymitis, the fever is higher. Other assessment findings vary with the infection site.

Inspection of the male patient's urethral meatus reveals a purulent discharge; such discharge may be expressed from a female patient's urethra, and her meatus may appear red and edematous. Inspection of the cervix with a speculum discloses a friable cervix and a greenish yellow discharge, the most common sign in females. Vaginal inspection reveals engorgement, redness, swelling, and a profuse purulent discharge (The vagina is the most common infection site in girls over age 1.)

If the patient has a rectal infection, inspection may reveal a purulent discharge or rectal bleeding. With an ocular infection, inspection may show a purulent discharge from the conjunctiva; with a pharyngeal infection, redness and a purulent discharge may be noted.

Palpation of the patient with PID reveals tenderness over the lower quadrant, abdominal rigidity and distention, and adnexal tenderness (usually bilateral). In a patient with perihepatitis, palpation discloses right upper quadrant tenderness.

If the infection has become systemic, papillary skin lesions—possibly pustular, hemorrhagic, or necrotic—may appear on the hands and feet.

Assessment of a patient with a systemic infection may also reveal pain and a cracking noise when moving an involved joint. Asymmetrical involvement of only a few joints—typically the knees, ankles, and elbows—may differentiate gonococcal arthritis from other forms of arthritis.

Signs of gonococcal ophthalmia neonatorum include lid edema, bilateral conjunctival infection, and abundant purulent discharge 2 to 3 days after birth. Adult conjunctivitis, most common in males, causes unilateral conjunctival redness and swelling. Untreated gonococcal conjunctivitis can progress to corneal ulceration and blindness.

DIAGNOSTIC TESTS

▶ A culture from the infection site (the urethra, cervix, rectum, or pharynx), grown on a Thayer-Martin medium, usually establishes the diagnosis. A culture of conjunctival scrapings confirms gonococcal conjunctivitis. In male patients, a Gram stain that shows gram-negative diplococci may confirm gonorrhea.

▶ Diagnosis of gonococcal arthritis requires identification of gram-negative diplococci on a smear from joint fluid or skin lesions.

▶ Complement fixation and immunofluorescent assays of serum reveal antibody titers four times the normal rate.

TREATMENT

Ceftriaxone (Rocephin) by I.M. injection is recommended by the Centers for Disease Control and Prevention (CDC) for all types of gonorrhea; presumptive treatment of concurrent *Chlamydia trachomatis* infection is oral doxycycline (Doryx). Uncomplicated urogenital or rectal gonorrhea may be treated with a single oral dose of cefixime (Suprax). Gonorrhea may also be treated with a single dose of azithromycin (Zithromax), per CDC guidelines. Resistance to penicillin and tetracycline is common, and some resistance to quinolones and cephalosporins has been documented, which underscores the need for follow-up testing after treatment.

Treatment for gonococcal conjunctivitis requires a single dose of ceftriaxone I.M. and one lavage of the infected eye with normal saline solution. Routine instillation of 1% silver nitrate drops or erythromycin ointment into the eyes of neonates has greatly reduced the incidence of gonococcal ophthalmia neonatorum.

NURSING CONSIDERATIONS

▶ Use standard precautions when obtaining specimens for laboratory examination and when caring for the patient. Carefully place all soiled articles in containers, and dispose of them according to facility policy.

◗ Use contact precautions for patients with an eye infection.

▶ Report all cases of gonorrhea to the local public health authorities. Report all cases of gonorrhea in children to child abuse authorities.

▶ Routinely instill prophylactic medications, according to facility protocol, in the eyes of all neonates on admission to the nursery.

▶ Report all cases of gonorrhea to the state health department or the CDC.

Patient teaching

▶ Urge the patient to inform all sexual partners about the infection so that they can seek treatment.

▶ Instruct the patient to take the antibiotics as prescribed, even if feeling better and symptoms have resolved.

 PREVENTION To prevent re-infection, tell the patient to avoid sexual contact with anyone suspected of being infected, to use condoms during intercourse, and to wash genitalia with soap and water before and after intercourse.

DROPLET PRECAUTIONS

Haemophilus influenzae infection

H. influenzae can cause diseases in many organ systems but usually attacks the respiratory system. *H. influenzae* is one of the three most common organisms causing community-acquired pneumonia. It is also a common cause of epiglottiditis, laryngotracheobronchitis, bronchiolitis, otitis media, and meningitis. Less commonly, it causes bacterial endocarditis, conjunctivitis, facial cellulitis, septic arthritis, and osteomyelitis.

H. influenzae type b (Hib) infection predominantly affects children, at a rate of 3% to 5% in the United States. This incidence was higher before vaccinations were widely used. The Hib vaccine is administered to children at ages 2, 4, 6, and 15 months. In Native American and Alaska Native populations, the incidence of Hib infection exceeds 5%, possibly due to exposure, socioeconomic conditions, and/or genetic differences in immune response. Hib infection is fatal in 3% to 6% of cases; up to 20% of patients suffer permanent hearing loss or other long-term sequelae.

CAUSES

A small, gram-negative, pleomorphic aerobic bacillus, *H. influenzae* appears predominantly in coccobacillary exudates. It is usually found in the pharynx and, less commonly, in the conjunctiva and genitourinary tract. Transmission occurs by direct contact with nasopharyngeal secretions or respiratory droplets.

COMPLICATIONS

The microorganism can cause subdural effusions and permanent neurologic sequelae from meningitis; complete upper airway obstruction from epiglottiditis, cellulitis, and pericarditis; pleural effusion; and respiratory failure from pneumonia.

ASSESSMENT FINDINGS

The patient may report a recent viral infection. Onset of *H. influenzae* infection is usually sudden with progressive symptoms. Generalized malaise is a common complaint, along with a high fever. *H. influenzae* provokes a characteristic tissue response—acute suppurative inflammation. When *H. influenzae* infects the larynx, trachea, or bronchial tree, it leads to irritable cough, dyspnea, mucosal edema, and thick, purulent exudate. When it invades the lungs, it causes bronchopneumonia. In the pharynx, *H. influenzae* usually produces no remarkable changes, except when it causes epiglottiditis, which generally affects both the laryngeal and pharyngeal surfaces. The pharyngeal mucosa may be reddened, rarely with a soft yellow exudate, although it usually appears normal or shows only slight diffuse redness, even while severe pain makes swallowing difficult or impossible. Meningitis, the most serious infection caused by *H. influenzae*, is indicated by fever and altered mental status. In young children, nuchal rigidity may be absent.

 ALERT Take steps to prevent airway obstruction in acute epiglottiditis. If a child develops symptoms of acute epiglottiditis, don't attempt to examine the throat or obtain a throat culture—either could lead to a fatal airway obstruction. Only an experienced professional, such as an anesthetist or anesthesiologist, should perform such a procedure and only with emergency airway equipment nearby.

DIAGNOSTIC TESTS

▶ Blood culture isolating *H. influenzae* confirms infection.
▶ Laboratory tests may reveal polymorphonuclear leukocytosis or leukopenia in young children with severe infection.
▶ *H. influenzae* bacteremia is found in many patients with meningitis.

TREATMENT

H. influenzae infections usually respond to a course of ampicillin, cefotaxime, gatifloxacin, moxifloxacin (Avelox), or ceftriaxone (Rocephin) as an initial treatment, although resistant strains are becoming more common. As an alternative, a combination of chloramphenicol and ampicillin is prescribed. If the strain proves susceptible to ampicillin, chloramphenicol is discontinued. Other measures are supportive, such as airway maintenance and ventilation support.

NURSING CONSIDERATIONS

⬥ Maintain droplet precautions, and practice strict handwashing. The patient is no longer considered infectious after 24 to 48 hours of effective antibiotic therapy.

❱ Maintain adequate respiratory function through proper positioning, humidification (croup tent) in children, and suctioning, as needed. Monitor the rate and type of respirations. Watch for signs of cyanosis and dyspnea, which require intubation or a tracheotomy. Monitor the patient's level of consciousness (LOC) as a decreased LOC may indicate hypoxemia. For home treatment, suggest using a room humidifier or breathing moist air from a shower or bath as needed.

❱ Check the patient's history for drug allergies before administering antibiotics. Monitor the complete blood count for signs of bone marrow depression when therapy includes ampicillin or chloramphenicol.

❱ Monitor the patient's intake (including I.V. infusions) and output. Watch for signs of dehydration, such as decreased skin turgor, parched lips, concentrated urine, decreased urine output, and increased pulse rate.

❱ Provide a quiet, calm, environment. Organize your physical care measures before you enter the patient's room, and perform them quickly so as not to disrupt the patient's rest.

❱ Avoid fluid overload in patients with meningitis because of the danger of cerebral edema. Perform neurologic assessments, and monitor for changes in LOC.

❱ Report all cases of *H. influenzae* infection to the local health department. Antibiotic prophylaxis for household and day-care contacts may be indicated for Hib, although not for other serotypes.

Patient teaching

❱ Explain the infection to the patient or the patient's parents. Review how the infection may have been acquired as well as diagnostic tests and treatment.

❱ Inform the parents of a child infected with *H. influenzae* about the high risk of acquiring this infection at day-care centers.

❱ Ensure that the patient or the patient's parents understand the importance of continuing the prescribed antibiotic until the entire prescription is finished, even if feeling better.

❱ Teach patients with pneumonia how to cough and perform deep-breathing exercises to clear secretions.

❱ Teach the patient to control spread of the infection by performing proper handwashing and appropriate disposal of secretions.

 PREVENTION Advise the patient or the patient's parents about preventive measures, such as vaccinating infants, maintaining droplet precautions, performing proper hand hygiene, properly disposing of respiratory secretions by placing soiled tissues in a plastic bag, and decontaminating all equipment.

Haverhill fever

Haverhill fever—also known as rat-bite fever, sodoku, streptobacillary fever, streptobacillosis, spirillary fever, and epidemic arthritic erythema—is an infection that usually results from handling or being bitten by an infected rat, although outbreaks have also been associated with ingestion of milk or water contaminated with rat urine or feces. Haverhill fever is not a notifiable disease in the United States, so its exact incidence is not known. It is found worldwide but is uncommon in North and South America and most of Europe.

CAUSES

Haverhill fever is caused by *Actinobacillus muris* (formerly known as *Streptobacillus moniliformis*) and *Spirillum minus*. People at risk for contracting this infection include animal handlers and veterinarians, people who have pet rodents, and people living in rat-infested dwellings. Haverhill fever is not transmitted from person to person. More often, it is transmitted through contact with the urine or secretions from the mouth, eyes, or nose of an infected animal. Besides rats, other rodents that may transmit the infection include mice, squirrels, gerbils, and weasels.

COMPLICATIONS

Complications of Haverhill fever include endocarditis, pericarditis, and meningitis. Abscesses of the brain or soft tissue, parotitis, and tenosynovitis may also occur. Mortality can be as high as 13% without appropriate treatment.

ASSESSMENT FINDINGS

Signs and symptoms of Haverhill fever begin 2 to 10 days after exposure. Symptoms are flu-like, including chills and fever (101° to 104° F or 38.3° to 40° C), muscle aches, and sore throat. Joints may become red, swollen, and painful. (See *Causes, signs, and symptoms of Haverhill fever.*) A rash often occurs on the hands and feet within 2 to 4 days. If infection

---

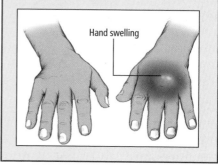

Causes, signs, and symptoms of Haverhill fever

It has been estimated that about 10% of rat bites result in some form of Haverhill fever. The condition has also been associated with the bites of mice, squirrels, and gerbils as well as with exposure to animals that prey on these rodents. Cases of Haverhill fever have also been reported in children with no history of direct rodent contact but who live in rat-infested dwellings.

With Haverhill fever, joints may become red, swollen, and painful. A roseolarurticarial rash sometimes develops on the hands and feet.

Hand swelling

---

is with *S. minus*, an open-crusted sore may form around the area of a rat bite. This form of Haverhill fever is called sodoku.

DIAGNOSTIC TESTS

▶ A history of exposure to infected rodents or rodent droppings narrows the list of diagnostic differentials.
▶ Blood cultures identify the causative organism.
▶ Cultures of joint fluid, lymph nodes, or skin help identify the causative organism.

TREATMENT

Haverhill fever is treated with antibiotics, although the infection may resolve with no treatment. Penicillin is the antibiotic of choice; if allergy is present, then tetracycline or erythromycin (E-Mycin) may be prescribed. Acetaminophen (Tylenol) or ibuprofen (Motrin) may be given for fever and pain. Fluid intake should be increased and rest encouraged until symptoms resolve. The bite area should be cleaned with soap and water.

Nursing considerations

▶ Maintain standard precautions, and teach visitors proper handwashing technique.
▶ Monitor vital signs as well as intake and output. Encourage fluid intake, especially for patients with fever.
▶ After checking for allergies, administer antibiotics as ordered. Administer analgesics and antipyretics as needed, and evaluate their effects.
▶ Provide comfort measures, such as tepid baths and muscle massage.

Patient teaching

▶ Teach the patient about the infection, including how it is acquired and the treatment prescribed.
▶ Explain all medications, including administration, dosage, and possible adverse effects. Tell the patient to be sure to complete all prescribed medication, even if feeling better.

▶ Describe any complications that the patient should report to the physician immediately, such as a change in level of consciousness, chest pain, difficulty breathing, and any unusual swelling that may indicate an abscess.
▶ If exposure was caused by a family pet, such as a gerbil, obtain information from the local animal control department about removing the animal from the home.
▶ Teach the patient and family about proper wound care if the illness is caused by a rat bite.

 PREVENTION Teach the patient and family to avoid contact with rodents, especially rats, and to avoid rodent-infested dwellings. If contact with rodents cannot be avoided, as with pet store employees, veterinary personnel, or other animal handlers, encourage the use of gloves and proper handwashing after handling rodents. Stress the importance of avoiding hand-to-mouth contact after handling rodents or cleaning rodent cages.

Helicobacter pylori infection

The bacterial infection *H. pylori* is most commonly recognized for causing circumscribed lesions in the mucosal membrane, or peptic ulcers. *H. pylori* releases a toxin that promotes mucosal inflammation and ulceration. It is thought to be present in 50% of the population and is detected in approximately 90% of patients with peptic ulcer disease. However, it is also thought to be associated with some other illnesses, such as mucosa-associated lymphoid tissue (MALT) lymphomas, iron deficiency anemia, GI reflux disease, skin disease, and rheumatologic disorders, although confirmation of the association between *H. pylori* infection and these conditions is still being investigated.

CAUSES

The bacteria *H. pylori* (formerly known as *Campylobacter pylori*) is passed via person-to-person contact; although the exact mechanism of transmission is not known, the microorganism has been isolated in saliva, in dental plaque, and in stool (in children). Risk factors for *H. pylori* infection may include crowded living conditions and living with someone who is infected with *H. pylori*.

COMPLICATIONS

H. pylori infection is the predominant cause of ulcers. Ulceration may lead to GI hemorrhage, which can progress to hypovolemic shock, perforation, and obstruction. Obstruction of the pylorus may cause the stomach to become distended with food and fluid, leading to abdominal or intestinal infarction. A fairly common occurrence in patients with duodenal ulcer is penetration, in which the ulcer crater extends beyond the duodenal walls into attached structures, such as the pancreas, biliary tract, liver, and gas-

trohepatic omentum. *H. pylori* infection is also considered a risk factor for stomach cancer.

ASSESSMENT FINDINGS

Typically, patients with *H. pylori* infection do not display symptoms. Instead, symptoms result from the complication of peptic ulcer or gastritis, and this is when the infection is detected. Patients with a gastric ulcer may report recent weight loss or decreased appetite. They may not feel like eating or may have developed an aversion to food because eating causes discomfort. There may be pain in the left epigastrium, often described by the patient as heartburn or indigestion. Discomfort may be accompanied by a feeling of fullness or distention. Commonly, the onset of pain signals the start of an attack.

Patients with a duodenal ulcer may have epigastric pain that they describe as sharp, gnawing, or burning. Alternatively, they may describe the pain as boring or aching and poorly defined, or they may liken it to a sensation of hunger, abdominal pressure, or fullness. Typically, pain occurs 90 minutes to 3 hours after eating. Because eating often reduces the pain of a duodenal ulcer, the patient may report a recent weight gain. Vomiting and other digestive disturbances are rare in patients with *H. pylori* duodenal ulcer.

DIAGNOSTIC TESTS

▶ Immunoglobulin A anti–*H. pylori* testing on a venous blood sample detects antibodies to *H. pylori*.
▶ Carbon-13 (^{13}C) urea breath test results reflect activity of *H. pylori*. (*H. pylori* contains the enzyme urease, which breaks down orally administered urea containing the radioisotope ^{13}C before it's absorbed systemically. Low levels of ^{13}C in exhaled breath point to *H. pylori* infection.)
▶ *H. pylori* fecal antigen testing identifies antigens associated with *H. pylori*.
▶ Tissue biopsy of the gastric mucosa may identify *H. pylori*.

TREATMENT

Current recommendations are to treat *H. pylori* infection only in patients who also have ulcers or low-grade gastric MALT lymphoma and in those who have had an early gastric cancer removed. The goal of drug therapy is to eradicate *H. pylori*, reduce gastric secretions, protect the mucosa from further damage, and relieve pain. Triple therapy is recommended for patients with peptic ulcer disease resulting from *H. pylori* and may include bismuth and two other antimicrobial agents, usually tetracycline or amoxicillin and metronidazole (Flagyl). Other combinations can include a proton pump inhibitor, such as omeprazole (Nexium) or lansoprazole (Prevacid), with an anti-infective, such as amoxicillin or clarithromycin (Biaxin).

For patients with gastric involvement, standard therapy also includes rest and decreased activity, which help to decrease gastric secretions. Diet therapy may consist of eating six small meals daily (or small hourly meals) rather than three regular meals. If GI bleeding occurs, emergency treatment begins with passage of a nasogastric tube to allow iced saline lavage, possibly containing norepinephrine. Gastroscopy allows visualization of the bleeding site and coagulation by laser or cautery to control bleeding. This therapy allows surgery to be postponed until the patient's condition stabilizes. Surgery is indicated for perforation, unresponsiveness to conservative treatment, suspected cancer, and other complications.

NURSING CONSIDERATIONS

▶ Support the patient emotionally, and offer reassurance if gastric complications occur.

 SAFETY Maintain standard precautions.

▶ Administer prescribed medications. Monitor the patient for the desired effects, and watch for adverse reactions. Most medications should alleviate the patient's discomfort, so ask whether the pain is relieved.

▶ Patients with *H. pylori* infection do not have dietary restrictions. If gastric complications are present, advise the patient to eat slowly, chew thoroughly, and have small snacks between meals, or provide six small meals or small hourly meals as ordered.

▶ Schedule the patient's care so that he or she can get plenty of rest.

Patient teaching

▶ Teach the patient about the infection, including the diagnostic and treatment plan. Help patients with peptic ulcer disease to recognize its signs and symptoms. Review symptoms associated with complications, and urge the patient to notify the physician if any of these complications occur. Emphasize the importance of complying with treatment, even after symptoms have subsided.

▶ Review the proper use of prescribed medications, including the desired actions and possible adverse reactions of each drug.

▶ Stress to the patient that over-the-counter medications, such as cimetidine (Tagamet), famotidine (Pepcid), and other histamine-receptor antagonists, shouldn't be taken without consulting the physician. These drugs may duplicate prescribed medications or suppress important symptoms.

Hemolytic-uremic syndrome

Hemolytic-uremic syndrome (HUS) is a disorder that involves blood clotting within the capillaries, resulting in progressive renal failure. HUS is also related to thrombotic thrombocytopenic purpura and has been associated with *Escherichia coli* O157:H7 infection resulting from food poisoning. It is classified as two types—one associated with diarrhea (D+) and the other not associated with diarrhea (D–).

Originally described in 1955, HUS was once commonly fatal. A patient with HUS now has a better prognosis due to the availability of dialysis and kidney transplantation. HUS is the most common cause of acute renal failure in children, but it has also been recognized in adults.

Causes

HUS is believed to result from an inflammatory reaction in the blood that causes platelets to sludge and form clots, leading to decreased platelets elsewhere in the body. The triggering event for HUS may be a bacterial infection, such as *E. coli* or *Streptoccoccus pneumoniae*; a rickettsial infection, such as Rocky Mountain spotted fever; a viral infection, such as human immunodeficiency virus or influenza virus; or a fungal infection, such as *Aspergillus fumigatus*. Other possible triggers include pregnancy, cancer (and chemotherapy), vaccinations, transplantation, and medications. The trigger for HUS may also be idiopathic. There is also an inherited form of HUS that affects the normal clotting mechanism.

D+HUS more frequently affects children younger than age 5 and is more common than D–HUS. However, mortality in patients with D–HUS is higher than that in patients with D+HUS.

Complications

Complications of HUS include renal failure, stroke, coma, seizures, and bleeding complications. Irreversible brain damage can occur, as can death. Complications associated with HUS caused by *E. coli* include dehydration and electrolyte imbalances. HUS has also been associated with prostatic, gastric, and pancreatic cancers. Cardiac dysfunction and fluid overload may occur. Death may occur if the patient is not treated and the disease has progressed.

Assessment findings

HUS associated with *E. coli* infection initially presents with abdominal cramping and vomiting along with watery diarrhea, which becomes bloody after 1 to 2 days in 70% of cases, and decreased urine output. After resolution of these symptoms, signs of anemia may be present, including weakness, lethargy, and sleepiness. There may also be signs of a low platelet count, including purpura and bleeding. Other signs include hypertension, edema, pallor, and anuria. Seizures may also occur, along with irritability or altered mental status.

Diagnostic tests

▶ Urinalysis may reveal hematuria and proteinuria.

▶ Blood urea nitrogen and creatinine levels will be elevated in patients with renal failure. Lactate dehydrogenase and indirect bilirubin levels are elevated and reflect intravascular hemolysis. A complete blood count shows decreased hemoglobin (typically < 8 g/dl) and thrombocytopenia (platelet count < 60,000 per ml). Prothrombin time, activated partial thromboplastin time, D-dimer, and fibrinogen values are usually normal.

▶ A peripheral blood smear shows schistocytes and may contain giant platelets.

▶ Stool culture may identify *E. coli* O157:H7 or *Shigella* bacteria.

▶ Pathologic findings for kidney tissue reveal occlusive lesions of the arterioles and small arteries along with tissue microinfarctions.

TREATMENT

Treatment of HUS is supportive and may include blood and platelet transfusions, I.V. fluids, and electrolyte replacement. Plasmapheresis or plasma exchange may be performed daily until remission and is the treatment of choice. Hemodialysis may be performed to treat renal failure. Antidiarrheal medications should be avoided. Use of antibiotics has been shown to increase the risk of severe HUS and should only be used in cases of sepsis. Hypertension should be controlled with antihypertensive medication. For children with end-stage renal disease, renal transplantation may be performed.

NURSING CONSIDERATIONS

▶ Maintain standard precautions. Urge all visitors to perform proper handwashing technique.
▶ Monitor lab studies, including complete blood counts (especially platelet count), electrolytes, and blood urea nitrogen and creatinine levels.
▶ Monitor intake and output as well as vital signs. Especially watch blood pressure for hypertension. If renal function diminishes, the patient may need dialysis.
▶ Watch for signs of bleeding, especially from puncture sites and in the urine.
▶ Provide I.V. fluids and electrolyte replacement therapy as indicated.
▶ Administer blood products as indicated.
▶ Provide emotional support for the patient and family. If the patient is a child, provide diversional activities when possible.

▶ Provide fluids and a renal diet if the patient is in renal failure. Maintain fluid restrictions as ordered, and monitor diet for protein and high-potassium foods.
▶ If the patient is experiencing severe diarrhea, parenteral nutrition may be needed.
▶ Provide meticulous skin care, especially for patients with profuse diarrhea.
▶ If the patient is receiving dialysis treatments, provide care to the access site per facility policy.
▶ Report all cases of HUS to the state health department or the Centers for Disease Control and Prevention.

Patient teaching

▶ Teach the patient about the disorder, including diagnostic tests and treatment.
▶ Teach the patient about medications, including dosage, administration, and possible adverse effects.
▶ Advise the patient to look for signs of bleeding, such as bruising or overt bleeding from puncture sites, and to report these signs to the physician immediately.
▶ Show the patient how to monitor urine output. If the patient is receiving dialysis, monitor vital signs during treatment and lab values before and after treatment.

 PREVENTION To help prevent *E. coli* infection, teach patients how to handle food properly, and stress the importance of thoroughly cooking hamburger products. Remind patients to defrost meat in the refrigerator and not on the counter or in the microwave. Teach patients about the proper treatment of drinking water and to avoid ingestion of unpasteurized milk and juice. Teach proper handwashing technique.

Hemorrhagic fever with renal failure syndrome

Hemorrhagic fever with renal failure syndrome (HFRS) is a group of clinically similar illnesses found throughout the world. It is caused by a hantavirus, which is transmitted through aerosolized urine, droppings, saliva, or dust from the nests of infected rodents. Transmission from person to person is rare. HFRS is characterized by fever and renal failure associated with hemorrhagic manifestations. The severity of the virus is related to the specific type of viral infection. HFRS occurs more often in males and in people older than age 15.

CAUSES

HFRS is caused by hantaviruses from the Bunyaviridae family, specifically Hantaan virus, which is widely distributed in Asia; Dobrava virus, found in the Balkans; Puumala virus, found in Scandinavia, Western Europe, and Russia; and Seoul virus, which occurs worldwide and has been found in many cities in the eastern part of the United States.

COMPLICATIONS

Complications of HFRS include retroperitoneal bleeding, intraventricular bleeding, renal rupture, pulmonary edema, neurologic and renal tubular defects, hepatomegaly and liver dysfunction, chronic renal insufficiency, and hypertension from renal disease. Hypovolemic shock may result from severe fluid loss. Hypopituitarism may occur but is usually temporary. The Dobrava virus causes a severe form of HFRS and may result in death.

ASSESSMENT FINDINGS

Signs and symptoms of HFRS appear 2 to 8 weeks after infection. There are five stages

to the illness: febrile, hypotensive, oliguric, diuretic, and convalescent:

1. The initial febrile stage includes high fevers (up to 104° F [40° C]). Other signs include the following, which occur suddenly and last 4 to 6 days: chills, blurred vision, subconjunctival hemorrhage, back and abdominal pain, and headache. Flushing of the face, neck, and chest may be present.
2. The hypotensive stage includes tachycardia, hypotension, and possibly convulsions and lasts a few hours to 2 days. Paralytic ileus may occur, causing an acute abdomen.
3. The oliguric stage lasts 3 to 6 days and includes oliguria, hypertension, edema, and bleeding tendencies. During this phase, thrombocytopenia may resolve.
4. In the diuretic stage, which can last 2 to 3 weeks, urine output increases to 3 to 6 L per day. Signs of dehydration and hypovolemic shock may occur at this time due to fluid loss.
5. The convalescent stage may last 3 to 6 months and generally starts in the second week of the illness.

DIAGNOSTIC TESTS

▶ Anti-hantaviral immunoglobulin G (IgG and immunoglobulin M (IgM) titers are elevated in patients with HFRS.
▶ Immunohistochemical staining and microscopic examination identify hantavirus antigen.
▶ Urinalysis shows proteinuria and hematuria during the initial phase; these conditions may resolve within 2 weeks.
▶ Coagulation studies are abnormal and include prolonged prothrombin time and activated partial thromboplastin time; fibrin degradation product is elevated. Leukocytosis and thrombocytopenia may also be present. Chemistry levels may be abnormal during the oliguric and diuretic stages.

TREATMENT

Treatment for HFRS is mainly supportive and based on the stage of illness. Fluid and electrolyte maintenance is essential to recovery. Dialysis may be necessary to control fluid overload and acidosis if diuretics are ineffective. Continuous arteriovenous hemofiltration may be the most effective overall treatment, based on the patient's condition. Vasopressors and albumin may be needed to maintain blood pressure during the hypotensive stage; if hypertension occurs during the oliguric phase, antihypertensives may be needed. If bleeding occurs, administration of blood products is appropriate. An antiviral drug, I.V. ribavirin, may be given. Bed rest is recommended during the acute phase. Fluid restriction, a low-sodium diet, and furosemide administration are appropriate during the oliguric phase. Increased fluid intake, oral and parenteral, should be monitored closely during the diuretic stage.

NURSING CONSIDERATIONS

▶ Maintain standard precautions. Encourage proper handwashing for all visitors.

▶ Monitor vital signs and temperature. Administer medications as indicated for fever, hypotension, or hypertension.

▶ Monitor laboratory values. Administer electrolyte replacement therapy as indicated. Administer blood products if indicated.

▶ Monitor intake and output closely, especially during the diuretic phase. Administer fluid replacement as ordered. Look for signs of edema, bleeding, and hypovolemic shock.

▶ Provide comfort measures, such as tepid baths, position changes, and analgesics, and note the effects of each.

▶ Monitor the patient during dialysis treatments. Provide emotional support during all treatments.

▶ Monitor for signs of complications, such as bleeding, respiratory failure, and shock.

Patient teaching

▶ Teach about the illness, including how it was acquired and any diagnostic tests. Explain all treatment measures and prescribed medications.

▶ Explain dialysis treatments and why they are needed. Tell the patient when dialysis treatments will occur and what to expect during a session.

▶ Stress the need for follow-up care during the convalescent stage. Instruct the patient about signs and symptoms of electrolyte imbalance, dehydration, and other complications and when to report them to the physician.

▶ Advise the patient to comply with follow-up care as recommended by the physician; weekly visits may be required initially, progressing to monthly visits once creatinine clearance is normal. Long-term monitoring of renal function and blood pressure may be necessary.

 PREVENTION Teach the patient and family about proper food storage to prevent contact with rodents. Stress the need for rodent control in living and work areas. Teach safety techniques when cleaning areas with rodent droppings or rodent nests, including the use of rubber, vinyl, or latex gloves; wetting contaminated areas with bleach solution (do not sweep), using paper towels to pick up debris, then mopping the area with a bleach solution; and spraying dead rodents with bleach or disinfectant and double bagging them along with any cleaning materials used. Stress proper handwashing after these measures.

CONTACT PRECAUTIONS

Hepatitis

Viral hepatitis is a fairly common systemic disease. It is marked by hepatic cell destruction, necrosis, and autolysis leading to anorexia, jaundice, and hepatomegaly. In most patients, hepatic cells eventually regenerate with little or no residual damage, allowing complete recovery. However, old age and serious underlying disorders make complications more likely. The prognosis is poor if edema and hepatic encephalopathy develop.

Today, six types of viral hepatitis are recognized:

▶ Type A (infectious or short-incubation hepatitis) is on the rise in homosexuals and in people with immunosuppression related to human immunodeficiency virus (HIV) infection. It's usually self-limiting and without a chronic form.

▶ Type B (serum or long-incubation hepatitis) is also increasing among HIV-positive individuals. Hepatitis B is considered a sexually transmitted infection because of the high incidence and rate of transmission by this route. Routine screening of donor blood for hepatitis B surface antigen (HBsAg) has decreased the incidence of posttransfusion-related cases, but transmission via needles shared by drug abusers remains a major problem.

▶ Type C hepatitis accounts for about 20% of all viral hepatitis cases and is transmitted primarily through blood and body fluids or during tattooing.

▶ Type D (delta hepatitis) is confined to people who are frequently exposed to blood and blood products, such as I.V. drug users and hemophiliacs. It's transmitted parenterally and, less commonly, sexually. It occurs only in those who have hepatitis B virus.

▶ Types C and E hepatitis occur primarily in people who have recently returned from an endemic area (such as India, Africa, Asia, or Central America).

▶ Type G is a newly discovered form of hepatitis. Transmission is by the bloodborne route, and it occurs more commonly in those who receive blood transfusions.

CAUSES

The six major forms of viral hepatitis—A, B, C, D, E, and G—result from infection with causative viruses.

Type A hepatitis is highly contagious and is usually transmitted by the fecal-oral route, commonly within institutions or families. However, it may also be transmitted parenterally. Hepatitis A usually results from ingestion of contaminated food, milk, or water. Outbreaks of this type are often traced to ingestion of seafood from polluted water.

Type B hepatitis is transmitted by the direct exchange of contaminated blood as well as by contact with contaminated human secretions and stools. Transmission of hepatitis B also occurs during intimate sexual contact and through perinatal transmission.

Type C hepatitis is a blood-borne illness transmitted primarily via sharing of needles by I.V. drug users, through unsanitary tattooing, and through blood transfusions. People with chronic hepatitis C are considered infectious.

Type D hepatitis is found only in patients with an acute or a chronic episode of hepatitis B. Type D infection requires the presence of HBsAg; the type D virus depends on the double-shelled type B virus to replicate. For this reason, type D infection can't outlast a type B infection.

Type E hepatitis is transmitted enterically and is usually waterborne, much like type A. Because this virus is inconsistently shed in stools, detection is difficult. Outbreaks of type E hepatitis have occurred in developing countries. Hepatitis G is thought to be blood-borne, with transmission similar to that of hepatitis C.

COMPLICATIONS

Life-threatening fulminant hepatitis—the most feared complication—develops in about 1% of patients. Fulminant hepatitis causes unremitting liver failure with encephalopathy, progresses to coma, and commonly leads to death within 2 weeks.

Other complications may be specific to the type of hepatitis:

▶ Chronic active hepatitis may occur as a late complication of hepatitis B.

▶ During the prodromal stage of acute hepatitis B, a syndrome resembling serum sickness, characterized by arthralgia or arthritis, rash, and angioedema, may occur. This syndrome can lead to misdiagnosis of hepatitis B as rheumatoid arthritis or lupus erythematosus.

▶ Primary liver cancer may develop after infection with hepatitis B or C.

▶ Type D hepatitis can cause a mild or asymptomatic form of hepatitis B to flare into severe, progressive, chronic active hepatitis and cirrhosis.

▶ Weeks to months after apparent recovery from acute hepatitis A, relapsing hepatitis may develop.

Hepatitis may also lead to pancreatitis, cirrhosis, myocarditis, pneumonia, aplastic anemia, transverse myelitis, or peripheral neuropathy.

ASSESSMENT FINDINGS

The patient's history may reveal the source of transmission (for example, recent ear piercing or tattooing, travel to a foreign country where hepatitis is endemic, or living conditions that are, or were, overcrowded). The patient's employment history—such as work in a hospital or laboratory where the risk of viral exposure from contaminated instruments or waste could be high—may indicate occupational exposure. Also, the patient's background may show possible exposure to toxic chemicals, such as carbon tetrachloride, which can cause nonviral hepatitis.

Assessment findings are similar for the different types of hepatitis. Typically, signs and symptoms progress in several stages. In the prodromal (preictal) stage, the patient generally complains of easy fatigue and anorexia, possibly with mild weight loss. Generalized malaise, depression, headache, weakness, arthralgia, myalgia, photophobia, and nausea with vomiting may also be reported. The patient may describe changes in the senses of taste and smell.

Assessment of vital signs may reveal fever, with a temperature of 100° to 102° F (37.8° to 38.9° C). As the prodromal stage draws to a close, usually 1 to 5 days before the onset of the clinical jaundice stage, inspection of urine and stool specimens may reveal dark urine and clay-colored stools.

If the patient has progressed to the clinical jaundice stage, he or she may report pruritus, abdominal pain or tenderness, and indigestion. Early in this stage, the patient may complain of anorexia; later, the appetite may return. Inspection of the sclerae, mucous membranes, and skin may show jaundice, which can last for 1 to 2 weeks. Jaundice indicates that the damaged liver can't remove bilirubin from the blood; it doesn't indicate disease severity. Occasionally, hepatitis occurs without jaundice.

During the clinical jaundice stage, skin inspection may reveal rashes, erythematous patches, or hives, especially if the patient has hepatitis B or C. Palpation may disclose abdominal tenderness in the right upper quadrant, an enlarged and tender liver and, in some cases, splenomegaly and cervical adenopathy.

Patient assessment during the recovery or posticteric stage will reveal that most symptoms are decreasing or have subsided. On palpation, a decrease in liver enlargement may be noted. The recovery phase generally lasts from 2 to 12 weeks, sometimes longer in patients with hepatitis B, C, or E.

DIAGNOSTIC TESTS

▶ In suspected viral hepatitis, a hepatitis profile is routinely performed. This study identifies antibodies specific to the causative virus, establishing the type of hepatitis:

- Type A: Detection of an antibody to hepatitis A virus confirms the diagnosis.
- Type B: The presence of HBsAg and hepatitis B antibodies confirms the diagnosis.

- Type C: Diagnosis depends on serologic testing for the specific antibody 1 or more months after the onset of acute illness. Until then, the diagnosis is principally established by obtaining negative test results for hepatitis A, B, and D.
- Type D: Detection of intrahepatic delta antigens or immunoglobulin (Ig) M antidelta antigens in acute disease (or IgM and IgG in chronic disease) establishes the diagnosis.
- Type E: Detection of hepatitis E antigens supports the diagnosis; however, the diagnosis may also consist of ruling out hepatitis C.
- Type G: Detection of hepatitis G ribonucleic acid supports the diagnosis. Serologic assays are being developed.

▶ Liver biopsy is performed if chronic hepatitis is suspected. (This study is performed for acute hepatitis only if the diagnosis is questionable.)

TREATMENT

Persons believed to have been exposed to hepatitis A virus and the household contacts of patients with confirmed cases should be treated with standard immunoglobulin. Travelers planning to visit areas known to harbor such viruses should receive hepatitis A vaccine.

Hepatitis B immunoglobulin and hepatitis B vaccine are given to individuals exposed to blood or body secretions of infected individuals. The immunoglobulin is effective but very expensive. In addition to its administration as part of the routine childhood immunization schedule, hepatitis B vaccine is now recommended for everyone. There is no vaccine against hepatitis C, but it is usually treated with interferon alpha-2b (Intron A) and the more recently Food and Drug Administration–approved peginterferon alpha-2a (Pegasys). In the early stages of the disease, the patient is advised to rest and combat anorexia by eating small, high-calorie, high-protein meals. (Protein intake should be reduced if signs of precoma—lethargy, confusion, mental changes—develop.)

With acute viral hepatitis, hospitalization usually is required only for patients with severe symptoms or complications. Parenteral nutrition may be required if the patient has persistent vomiting and is unable to maintain oral intake. Antiemetics (trimethobenzamide [Tigan] or benzquinamide) may be given to relieve nausea and prevent vomiting. For severe pruritus, the cholestyramine resin (Questran), which sequesters bile salts, may be given.

NURSING CONSIDERATIONS

▶ Observe standard precautions to prevent transmission of the disease.
◐ Maintain contact precautions with diapered or incontinent patients.
▶ Provide rest periods throughout the day.
▶ If symptoms are severe and the patient can't tolerate oral intake, provide I.V. therapy and parenteral nutrition as ordered.
▶ Provide adequate fluid intake. The patient should consume at least 4 L of liquid per day to maintain adequate hydration.
▶ Administer antiemetics as ordered. Observe the patient for the desired effects, and note any adverse reactions.
▶ Record the patient's weight daily, and keep accurate intake and output records. Observe the stools for color, consistency, and amount.
▶ Monitor for signs of complications.
▶ Report all cases of hepatitis to the state health department or the Centers for Disease Control and Prevention.

Patient teaching

▶ Teach the patient about viral hepatitis, including its signs and symptoms, diagnostic tests, and recommended treatments.
▶ Explain that the liver takes 3 weeks to regenerate and up to 4 months to return to normal functioning. Advise the patient to avoid contact sports until the liver returns to its normal size. Instruct the patient to check with the physician before performing any strenuous activity.

❯ Instruct the patient to eat high-calorie, high-protein foods in small meals. Also stress the need for adequate fluid intake and abstinence from alcohol.

❯ Explain to the patient and family that anyone exposed to the disease through contact with the patient should receive prophylaxis as soon as possible after exposure.

❯ Stress the need for continued medical care.

PREVENTION Instructing patients about the following measures can help prevent the spread of viral hepatitis:

- Stress the importance of thorough and frequent handwashing.

- Tell infected patients not to share food, eating utensils, or toothbrushes.

- Warn patients with hepatitis A or E not to contaminate food or water with fecal matter because these forms of the disease are transmitted by the fecal-oral route.

- Explain to patients with hepatitis B, C, D, or G that transmission occurs through exchange of blood or body fluids that contain blood. While infected, patients shouldn't donate blood or have unprotected sexual relations.

CONTACT PRECAUTIONS

Herpes simplex

Herpes simplex virus (HSV) is a recurrent viral infection. HSV type I (HSV-1), which is transmitted by oral and respiratory secretions, affects the skin and mucous membranes, commonly producing cold sores. HSV type 2 (HSV-2) primarily affects the genital area and is transmitted by sexual contact. However, cross-infection may result from oral-genital sex or via autoinoculation from one site to the other.

CAUSES

HSV is caused by *Herpesvirus hominis* (HVH), a widespread infectious agent that causes two serologically distinct HSV types. HSV-1 is transmitted primarily by contact with oral secretions. It mainly affects oral, labial, ocular, or skin tissue. HSV-2, transmitted primarily by contact with genital secretions, mainly affects genital structures. Infection with HSV-1 occurs more frequently and earlier in life than infection with HSV-2. More than 90% of adults have antibodies to HSV-1 by age 40. However, in lower socioeconomic groups, most people acquire HSV-1 by age 20. Antibodies to HSV-2 aren't routinely detected before puberty.

About 85% of all HVH infections are subclinical; the others produce localized lesions and systemic reactions. After the first infection, the patient is a carrier and susceptible to recurrent infections, which may be provoked by fever, menses, stress, heat, and cold. However, the patient usually has no constitutional signs and symptoms in recurrent infections.

COMPLICATIONS

Primary (or initial) HSV infection during pregnancy can lead to abortion, premature labor, microcephaly, and uterine growth retardation. Congenital herpes transmitted during vaginal birth may produce a subclinical neonatal infection or severe infection with seizures, chorioretinitis, skin vesicles, and hepatosplenomegaly.

In infants, HSV-1 can cause life-threatening nonepidemic encephalitis. Primary HSV infection is a leading cause of gingivostomatitis in children ages 1 to 3.

Blindness may result from ocular infection. Females with HSV-2 may be at increased risk for cervical cancer. Urethral stricture may result from recurrent genital herpes.

Perianal ulcers, colitis, esophagitis, pneumonitis, and various neurologic disorders resulting from HSV infection are serious complications in patients with AIDS and other immunocompromised conditions. Viremia can occur, with multiple-organ involvement.

ASSESSMENT FINDINGS

In neonates, HVH symptoms usually appear 1 to 2 weeks after birth. Symptoms range from localized skin lesions to a disseminated infection of organs, such as the liver, lungs, or brain.

Primary infection in childhood may be localized or generalized and occurs after an incubation period of 2 to 12 days. After brief prodromal tingling and itching, localized infection causes typical primary lesions, which erupt as vesicles on an erythematous base; vesicles eventually rupture, leaving a painful ulcer followed by a yellowish crust. Vesicles may form on any part of the oral mucosa, especially the tongue, gingiva, and cheeks. Healing begins 7 to 10 days after onset and is complete in 3 weeks.

Generalized infection begins with fever, pharyngitis, erythema, and edema. Vesicles occur with submaxillary lymphadenopathy, increased salivation, halitosis, anorexia, and a fever of up to 105° F (40.6° C). Herpetic stomatitis may lead to severe dehydration in children. A generalized infection usually runs its course in 4 to 10 days. In this form, virus reactivation causes cold sores—a single or group of vesicles in and around the mouth.

Genital herpes usually affects adolescents and young adults. Typically painful, the initial attack produces fluid-filled vesicles that ulcerate and heal in 1 to 3 weeks. Fever, regional lymphadenopathy, and dysuria may also occur.

Usually, herpetic keratoconjunctivitis is unilateral and causes only local signs and symptoms: conjunctivitis, regional adenopathy, blepharitis, and vesicles on the lid. Other ocular effects may include excessive lacrimation, edema, chemosis, photophobia, and purulent exudate.

Both types of HVH can cause acute sporadic encephalitis with altered levels of consciousness, personality changes, and seizures. Other effects may include smell and taste hallucinations and neurologic abnormalities such as aphasia.

Herpetic whitlow, an HVH finger infection, affects many nurses. First the finger tingles and then it becomes red, swollen, and painful. Vesicles with a red halo erupt and may ulcerate or coalesce. Other effects may include satellite vesicles, fever, chills, malaise, and a red streak up the arm.

Diagnosis

❱ Typical lesions may suggest HVH infection.
❱ Isolation of the virus from local lesions confirms the diagnosis.
❱ A rise in antibodies and moderate leukocytosis may support the diagnosis.

Treatment

No cure exists for herpes; however, recurrences tend to be milder and of shorter duration than the primary infection. Symptomatic and supportive therapy is essential. Generalized primary infection usually requires an analgesic-antipyretic to reduce fever and relieve pain. Anesthetic mouthwashes, such as viscous lidocaine, may reduce the pain of gingivostomatitis, enabling the patient to eat and preventing dehydration. Drying agents, such as calamine lotion, ease the pain of labial or skin lesions. Avoid petroleum-based ointments, which promote viral spread and slow healing. Acyclovir may bring relief to patients with genital herpes, rectal herpes, and herpetic whitlow.

Nursing considerations

❱ Follow standard precautions, such as wearing gloves, for contact with mucous membranes to prevent acquisition of herpetic whitlow.
◗ Maintain contact precautions until lesions are crusted and dried.
❱ Patients with central nervous system infection (encephalitis) alone need no isolation.

Patient teaching

❱ Teach patients with genital herpes to use warm compresses or take sitz baths several times per day; to use a drying agent, such as povidone-iodine solution; to increase fluid intake; and to avoid all sexual contact during the active stage.

 SAFETY Instruct patients with herpetic whitlow not to share towels or eating utensils. Educate staff members and other susceptible people about the risk of contagion. Abstain from direct patient care if you have herpetic whitlow. Tell patients with cold sores not to kiss people.

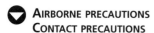

Herpes zoster

Herpes zoster (also called shingles) is an acute unilateral and segmental inflammation of the dorsal root ganglia caused by infection with the herpes varicella-zoster virus, which also causes chickenpox. Herpes zoster infection usually occurs in adults. It produces localized vesicular skin lesions, confined to a dermatome, and severe neuralgic pain in peripheral areas innervated by the nerves arising in the inflamed root ganglia.

The prognosis in patients with herpes zoster is good unless the infection spreads to the brain. Eventually, most patients recover completely, except for possible scarring and, in those with corneal damage, visual impairment. Occasionally, neuralgia may persist for months or years.

CAUSES

Herpes zoster results from reactivation of varicella virus that has lain dormant in the cerebral ganglia (extramedullary ganglia of the cranial nerves) or in the ganglia of posterior nerve roots since a previous episode of chickenpox. Exactly how or why this reactivation occurs isn't clear. Some believe that the virus multiplies as it is reactivated and that antibodies remaining from the initial infection neutralize it. However, if effective antibodies aren't present, the virus continues to multiply in the ganglia, destroy the host neuron, and spread down the sensory nerves to the skin.

COMPLICATIONS

In rare cases, herpes zoster infection leads to generalized central nervous system infection, muscle atrophy, motor paralysis (usually transient), acute transverse myelitis, and ascending myelitis. More commonly, generalized infection causes acute urine retention and unilateral diaphragm paralysis. In postherpetic neuralgia, which is most common in elderly persons, intractable neurologic pain may persist for years. Scars may be permanent.

ASSESSMENT FINDINGS

Herpes zoster infection begins with fever and malaise. Within 2 to 4 days, severe deep pain, pruritus, and paresthesia or hyperesthesia develop, usually on the trunk and occasionally on the arms and legs in a dermatomal distribution. Pain may be continuous or intermittent and usually lasts from 1 to 4 weeks. In some cases, small, red, nodular skin lesions erupt on the painful areas up to 2 weeks after the first symptoms. These lesions typically spread unilaterally around the thorax or vertically over the arms or legs. When these nodules appear, they quickly become vesicles filled with clear fluid or pus. About 10 days later, the vesicles dry and form scabs. Intense pain may occur before the rash appears and after the scabs form.

Occasionally, herpes zoster involves the cranial nerves, especially the trigeminal and geniculate ganglia or the oculomotor nerve. Geniculate zoster may cause vesicle formation in the external auditory canal, ipsilateral facial palsy, hearing loss, dizziness, and loss of taste. Trigeminal ganglion involvement causes eye pain and may cause corneal and scleral damage as well as impaired vision. Rarely, oculomotor involvement causes conjunctivitis, extraocular weakness, ptosis, and paralytic mydriasis.

Patients with immunodeficiency disorders may develop disseminated zoster. Lesions are bilateral and not limited to dermatomal distribution. (See *Herpes zoster lesions.*)

DIAGNOSTIC TESTS

▶ Characteristic skin lesions identify the illness.

▶ Examination of vesicular fluid and infected tissue shows eosinophilic intranuclear inclusions and varicella virus.

▶ Lumbar puncture shows increased pressure; examination of cerebrospinal fluid shows increased protein levels and, possibly, pleocytosis.

Herpes zoster lesions

Herpes zoster infection produces local-ized vesicular skin lesions and severe neuralgic pain in peripheral areas inner-vated by the nerves arising in the in-flamed root ganglia.

Lesions occur most often on the trunk, but they can sometimes be found on the arms and legs. Lesions rarely cross the midline, although they can involve ad-joining dermatomes.

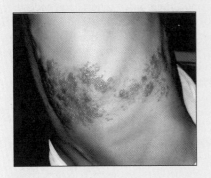

▶ Differentiation of herpes zoster from localized herpes simplex virus requires stain-ing antibodies from vesicular fluid and iden-tification under fluorescent light.

TREATMENT

Antiviral therapy is the mainstay of treat-ment. Acyclovir seems to stop the rash's pro-gression and prevent visceral complications. Capsaicin, transcutaneous electrical nerve stimulation, and low-dose amitriptyline are the current treatments of choice for posther-petic neuralgia. Topical antiviral ointment is helpful if started early in the disease process.

Herpes zoster infection can resolve spon-taneously and may only require sympto-matic treatment, the goal of which is to re-lieve itching and neuralgic pain. Such treatments include calamine lotion or anoth-er antipruritic; aspirin, possibly with codeine or another analgesic; and, occasionally, collo-dion or compound benzoin tincture applied to unbroken lesions.

Trigeminal herpes zoster with corneal in-volvement calls for instillation of idoxuridine (Dendrid) ointment or another antiviral agent. For post-herpetic pain, corticosteroids, tranquilizers, sedatives, or tricyclic antide-pressants with phenothiazine may be pre-scribed. In some immunocompromised patients—both children and adults—I.V. acyclovir appears to prevent disseminated, life-threatening disease. High doses of inter-feron (an antiviral glycoprotein) have been used in patients with cancer when the herpetic lesions are limited to the dermatome.

NURSING CONSIDERATIONS

◔ Airborne and contact precautions are rec-ommended for any patient with disseminat-ed disease and for localized disease in any immunocompromised patient.
▶ If vesicles rupture, apply a cold compress as ordered.
▶ To decrease the pain of oral lesions, tell the patient to use a soft toothbrush, eat soft foods, and use a saline or bicarbonate mouthwash.
▶ To minimize neuralgic pain, administer analgesics as ordered and evaluate their effect.

Patient teaching

▶ Teach the patient about the disorder, in-cluding diagnostic tests and treatment.
▶ Advise the patient and family about air-borne and contact precautions and how to prevent the spread of the disease.
▶ Instruct the patient to avoid scratching the lesions.

 PREVENTION Vaccination with Zostavax is recommended to prevent the occur-rence of shingles in adults over age 60.

Histoplasmosis

Histoplasmosis is a fungal infection caused by *Histoplasma capsulatum*. This disease may also be called Ohio Valley, Central Mississippi Valley, Appalachian Mountain, or Darling's disease. In the United States, it occurs in three forms: primary acute histoplasmosis, progressive disseminated histoplasmosis (acute disseminated or chronic disseminated disease), and chronic pulmonary (cavitary) histoplasmosis, which produces cavitations in the lung similar to those seen in pulmonary tuberculosis.

A fourth form, African histoplasmosis, occurs only in Africa and is caused by the fungus *Histoplasma capsulatum* var. *duboisii*.

The prognosis varies with each form. The primary acute disease is benign; the progressive disseminated disease is fatal in approximately 90% of patients; and, without proper chemotherapy, chronic pulmonary histoplasmosis is fatal in 50% of patients within 5 years.

CAUSES

H. capsulatum is found in the feces of birds and bats or in soil contaminated by their feces, such as that found near roosts, chicken coops, barns, or caves or underneath bridges. Transmission occurs through inhalation of *H. capsulatum* or *H. duboisii* spores or through the invasion of spores after minor skin trauma. Possibly, oral ingestion of spores may cause the disease.

The incubation period is from 5 to 18 days, although chronic pulmonary histoplasmosis may progress slowly for many years. Histoplasmosis is more common in adult men, likely due to occupational exposure. Fatal disseminated disease, however, is more common in infants and elderly men.

Histoplasmosis occurs worldwide, especially in the temperate areas of Asia, Africa, Europe, and North and South America. In the United States, it's most prevalent in the central and eastern states, especially in the Mississippi and Ohio River Valleys.

COMPLICATIONS

Possible complications include vascular or bronchial obstruction, acute pericarditis, pleural effusion, mediastinal fibrosis or granuloma, intestinal ulceration, Addison's disease, endocarditis, and meningitis.

ASSESSMENT FINDINGS

The patient may have a history of an immunocompromised condition or exposure to contaminated soil in an endemic area. The severity of symptoms depends on the size of the inhaled inoculums and the immune condition of the host.

Symptoms vary with each form of this disease. Primary acute histoplasmosis may be asymptomatic or may cause symptoms of a mild respiratory illness similar to those seen with a severe cold or influenza. Typical clinical effects may include fever, malaise, headache, myalgia, anorexia, cough, chest pain, anemia, leukopenia, thrombocytopenia, and oropharyngeal ulcers.

Progressive disseminated histoplasmosis causes hepatosplenomegaly, general lymphadenopathy, anorexia, weight loss, fever and, possibly, ulceration of the tongue, palate, epiglottis, and larynx with resulting pain, hoarseness, and dysphagia. It may also cause endocarditis, meningitis, pericarditis, and adrenal insufficiency.

Chronic pulmonary histoplasmosis mimics pulmonary tuberculosis and causes a productive cough, dyspnea, and occasional hemoptysis. Eventually, it produces weight loss, extreme weakness, breathlessness, and cyanosis.

African histoplasmosis produces cutaneous nodules, papules, and ulcers; lesions of the skull and long bones; lymphadenopathy; and visceral involvement without pulmonary lesions.

DIAGNOSTIC TESTS

▶ Blood cultures conducted using the lysis-centrifugation technique reveal the causative organism.

▶ With disseminated histoplasmosis, culture of bone marrow, mucosal lesions, liver, and bronchoalveolar lavage may show the organism causing infection.

▶ Sputum cultures are preferred in chronic pulmonary histoplasmosis and may take 2 to 4 weeks to show growth of the organism.

▶ Radioactive assay for *Histoplasma* antigen in blood or urine shows the presence of *Histoplasma* antigen.

▶ Rising complement fixation and agglutination titers (more than 1:32) strongly suggest histoplasmosis.

TREATMENT

Treatment consists of antifungal therapy, surgery, and supportive care. Antifungal therapy is most important. Except for asymptomatic primary acute histoplasmosis (which resolves spontaneously) and the African form, histoplasmosis requires high-dose or long-term (10-week) therapy with amphotericin B (Abelcet), fluconazole (Diflucan), ketoconazole (Extina), or itraconazole (Sporanox). For a patient who also has acquired immunodeficiency syndrome, lifelong therapy with fluconazole is indicated.

Supportive care usually includes oxygen for respiratory distress, glucocorticoids for adrenal insufficiency, and parenteral fluids for dysphagia due to oral or laryngeal ulcerations. Histoplasmosis doesn't require isolation, as it is not transmitted from person to person.

NURSING CONSIDERATIONS

▶ Give medications as ordered, and watch for possible adverse effects. Because amphotericin B (Abelcet) may cause chills, fever, nausea, and vomiting, give appropriate antipyretics and antiemetics, as ordered.

▶ Perform a respiratory assessment every shift and as needed. Note diminished breath sounds or pleural friction rub, and evaluate for effusion. Refer to chest radiographs to determine whether the patient has pulmonary or pleural effusions.

▶ Provide oxygen therapy as needed, and monitor pulse oximetry. Plan rest periods.

▶ Perform a cardiovascular assessment every shift. Report muffled heart sounds, jugular vein distention, pulsus paradoxus, or other signs of cardiac tamponade to the physician immediately.

▶ Provide psychological support because of long-term hospitalization. As needed, refer the patient to a social worker or occupational therapist. Help the parents of children with this disease arrange for a visiting teacher.

Patient teaching

▶ Teach the patient about drug therapy, including possible adverse effects.

▶ Inform the patient about the need for follow-up care on a regular basis for at least 1 year.

 PREVENTION Teach patients in endemic areas to watch for early signs of this infection and to seek treatment promptly. Instruct a patient who's at risk for occupational exposure to contaminated soil to avoid areas that may harbor fungus.

Human immunodeficiency virus infection

A retrovirus—human immunodeficiency virus (HIV) type 1—is the primary causative agent of acquired immunodeficiency syndrome (AIDS). The natural history of AIDS begins with infection by the HIV retrovirus, which is detectable only by laboratory tests, and ends with the severely immunocompromised, terminal stage of this disease. Depending on individual variations and the presence of cofactors that influence progression, the time elapsed from acute HIV infection to the appearance of symptoms (mild to severe) to the diagnosis of AIDS and, eventually, to death varies greatly. Transmission of HIV occurs by contact with infected blood or body fluids and is associated with identifiable high-risk behaviors.

CAUSES

HIV is transmitted by direct inoculation during intimate sexual contact, especially with the mucosal trauma of receptive anal intercourse; transfusion of contaminated blood or blood products (a risk diminished by routine testing of all blood products); sharing of contaminated needles; and transplacental or postpartum transmission from infected mother to fetus (by cervical or blood contact at delivery and in breast milk).

HIV is not transmitted by casual household or social contact. The average time between exposure to the virus and the diagnosis of AIDS is 8 to 10 years, but shorter and longer incubation times have been recorded. Most people develop antibodies within 6 to 8 weeks of contracting the virus.

COMPLICATIONS

Complications from AIDS include immunodeficiency, which may cause opportunistic infections and unusual cancers; autoimmunity, which may lead to lymphoid interstitial pneumonia, arthritis, hypergammaglobulinemia, and production of autoimmune antibodies; and neurologic dysfunction, which results in AIDS dementia complex, HIV encephalopathy, and peripheral neuropathies.

ASSESSMENT FINDINGS

HIV infection manifests itself in many ways. The infected person usually experiences a mononucleosis-like syndrome, which may be attributed to flu or other virus and then may remain asymptomatic for years. In this latent stage, the only sign of HIV infection is laboratory evidence of seroconversion.

When signs and symptoms appear, they may present as persistent generalized adenopathy, nonspecific signs and symptoms (weight loss, fatigue, night sweats, and fevers), neurologic symptoms resulting from HIV encephalopathy, or opportunistic infection or cancer.

The clinical course of AIDS varies slightly in children. Signs and symptoms resemble those seen in adults, except for findings related to sexually transmitted infections.

DIAGNOSTIC TESTS

▶ A CD4+ T-cell count of 200 cells/ml or an associated clinical condition or disease can be diagnostic.
▶ Enzyme-linked immunosorbent assay, in addition to a confirmatory test, usually the Western blot or an immunofluorescence assay, identifies HIV antibodies.
▶ Direct tests include antigen tests (p24 antigen), HIV cultures, nucleic acid probes of peripheral blood lymphocytes with determination of HIV-1 RNA levels, and polymerase chain reaction.

TREATMENT

No cure has yet been found for AIDS; however, primary therapy for HIV infection includes three types of antiretroviral agents: protease inhibitors (PIs), such as atazanavir (Reyataz), ritonavir (Norvir), fosamprenavir (Lexiva), darunavir (Prezista), and saquinavir (Invirase); nucleoside reverse transcriptase inhibitors (NRTIs), such as emtricitabine + efavirenz + tenofovir (Atripla), abacavir + zidovudine + lamivudine (Trizivir), lamivudine (Epivir), and lamivudine + zidovudine (Combivir); and nonnucleoside reverse transcriptase inhibitors (NNRTIs), such as nevirapine (Viramune) and efavirenz (Sustiva).

Treatment protocols combine two or more agents in an effort to gain the maximum benefit with the fewest adverse reactions. Such regimens typically include one PI plus two NRTIs, or one NNRTI plus two NRTIs. Many variations and drug interactions are under investigation. Combination therapy helps to inhibit the production of resistant, mutant strains. Supportive treatments help to maintain nutritional status and relieve pain and other distressing physical and psychological symptoms.

NURSING CONSIDERATIONS

▶ Maintain standard precautions. Insist that visitors adhere to proper handwashing technique.
▶ Provide emotional support to the patient and family. Recognize that a diagnosis of AIDS is profoundly distressing because of the disease's social impact and the discouraging prognosis.
▶ Monitor the patient for fever, noting any pattern, and for signs of skin breakdown, cough, sore throat, and diarrhea. Assess the patient for swollen, tender lymph nodes, and check laboratory values regularly.
▶ Encourage the patient to maintain as much physical activity as he or she can tolerate. Make sure the patient's schedule includes time for both exercise and rest.
▶ Ensure adequate fluid intake, and monitor intake and output.
▶ If the patient develops Kaposi's sarcoma, monitor the progression of lesions.

▶ Monitor opportunistic infections or signs of disease progression, and treat infections as ordered.
▶ Provide meticulous skin care, especially if the patient is debilitated.
▶ Report all cases of HIV to the state health department or the Centers for Disease Control and Prevention.

 PREVENTION Health care workers and visitors should diligently practice standard precautions.

Patient teaching

▶ Teach the patient about the infection and how it is transmitted. Urge the patient to inform potential sexual partners and health care workers that he or she has HIV infection.
▶ Inform the patient not to donate blood, blood products, organs, tissue, or sperm.
▶ If the patient uses I.V. drugs, caution him or her not to share needles.
▶ Teach the patient about the medications, including dosage, administration, and potential adverse effects. Stress the importance of adhering to the prescribed regimen.
▶ Teach the patient how to identify signs of impending infection, and stress the importance of seeking immediate medical attention at the first sign of infection.

 PREVENTION Discuss safer sexual practices. Inform the patient that high-risk sexual practices for AIDS transmission are those that exchange body fluids, such as vaginal or anal intercourse without a condom. Abstaining is the best way to prevent transmission of the disease. Advise women of childbearing age with HIV/AIDS to avoid pregnancy. Explain that an infant may become infected before birth, during delivery, or during breastfeeding.

Human papillomavirus

Human papillomavirus (HPV) is a group of more than 100 strains of viruses that cause epithelial tumors of the skin and mucous membranes. There are three types of HPV infection: nongenital, anogenital, and epidermodysplasia verruciformis (EV). HPV is further classified as clinical (grossly apparent), subclinical (visualized with application of acetic acid), or latent (asymptomatic and detected with testing). Examples of conditions associated with nongenital HPV include common warts, plantar warts, and squamous cell carcinoma of the lungs; anogenital HPV includes genital warts and cervical cancer; EV includes skin cancer. HPV infection does not cause cancerous tissue; rather, coexisting conditions, such as tobacco use, ultraviolet radiation exposure, folate deficiency, and immune suppression, along with HPV, have been associated with malignant cell formation.

CAUSES

HPV is transmitted via skin-to-skin contact and enters the body through a break in the tissue or outer layer of the skin. Genital warts are transmitted through sexual contact and are the most common sexually transmitted infection (STI). HPV 16 is associated with carcinoma of the vulva, vagina, cervix, anus, and penis. Risk factors include having multiple sexual contacts at a young age and an impaired immune system. It is estimated that approximately 50% of sexually active adults acquire HPV at some point in their lives.

COMPLICATIONS

Complications of HPV infection include scarring with wart removal and conversion to cancerous cells in the presence of coexisting factors. Seventy percent of cervical cancers are associated with HPV. Large genital warts may cause urinary obstruction during pregnancy; warts in the vagina can decrease elasticity of the vaginal wall and cause obstruction during childbirth.

ASSESSMENT FINDINGS

Signs and symptoms of HPV vary according to which virus is present. Many patients are asymptomatic. Common warts appear as skin-colored papules and nodules and are usually found on the feet and hands. Plantar warts are solitary painful lesions that have a small, black center (thrombosed capillaries). Genital warts develop on moist areas: in males, on the subpreputial sac, within the urethral meatus and, less commonly, on the penile shaft; in females, on the vulva and on vaginal and cervical walls. In both genders, papillomas spread to the perineum and the perianal area. These painless warts start as tiny red or pink swellings that grow (sometimes up to 10 cm) and become pedunculated. Typically, multiple swellings give them a cauliflower-like appearance. If infected, the warts become malodorous. EV typically arises as premalignant lesions on the forehead and other sun-exposed areas and may appear as polymorphic, wartlike, red to brownish plaques. (See *Genital warts*.)

DIAGNOSTIC TESTS

▶ Physical examination identifies skin lesions and often may be the only diagnostic determination of HPV.
▶ HPV DNA testing is diagnostic.
▶ Tissue biopsy confirms HPV infection.
▶ A Papanicolaou (Pap) test identifies abnormal cells, which may or may not be caused by HPV. Further testing should be done to confirm HPV.

TREATMENT

No treatment exists to eradicate HPV—a normal immune system can fight off infection. Treatment is aimed at removal of the lesions or treatment of specific diseases caused by HPV. For common warts, plaster patches impregnated with acid (such as 40% salicylic acid plasters) or acid drops (such as 5% to 16.7% salicylic acid in flexible collodion or trichloroacetic acid) are appropriate. A

Genital warts

Genital warts are transmitted through sexual contact and are the most common sexually transmitted infection. Risk factors include having multiple sexual contacts at a young age and having an impaired immune system. There are more than 40 types of HPV that can infect the genital areas of both men and women. You cannot see HPV. The majority of people who become infected with HPV don't even know they have it. It is estimated that approximately 50% of sexually active adults acquire HPV at some point in their lives.

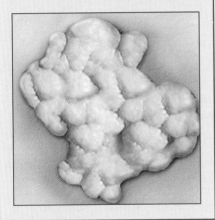

25% podophyllin solution may be used for venereal warts. Topical medication may take several applications and may cause scarring. Cryotherapy, electrosurgery, laser surgery, or simple surgical excision may also be performed to remove warts. Medications used for genital warts include immune response modifiers, such as interferon alpha-2b; antimitotic agents, such as podofilox (Condylox); or antimetabolites, such as fluorouracil (Carac).

 PREVENTION The papillomavirus vaccine is recommended to prevent HPV in females ages 9 to 26. It is indicated to prevent cervical cancer, genital warts, and precancerous genital lesions. It is given as a series of three injections and is most effective if given before the female becomes sexually active.

NURSING CONSIDERATIONS

▶ Maintain standard precautions.
▶ Encourage the patient's sexual partners to be examined for HPV and other STIs.
▶ Assist with pelvic examination and acquisition of specimens for Pap smear.
▶ Provide emotional support as needed. Young girls may be anxious about undergoing a gynecologic examination. Answer all questions concerning the procedure and why it needs to be done. Have the patient's mother stay with her, if desired, to provide additional emotional support.

Patient teaching

▶ If the patient has an STI, provide information regarding medication, including possible adverse effects.
▶ Advise female patients to have a Pap test every year.
▶ Discuss the type of HPV that is present, including treatment options and route of transmission.
▶ If age appropriate, encourage having the vaccine administered, per physician recommendation.
▶ Stress the importance of wearing sunscreen when outdoors during the day.
▶ Teach patients how to care for lesions and what complications to report to the physician.

 PREVENTION Having sexual intercourse at a young age increases the risk for contracting HPV. Advise your patients that delaying first intercourse may help reduce the risk of infection, as will having fewer sexual partners. Stress the use of condoms during sexual intercourse, and tell the patient that abstinence is the only sure way to avoid genital warts and other STIs.

CONTACT PRECAUTIONS

Impetigo, bullous

Impetigo (impetigo contagiosa) is a vesiculo-pustular eruptive disorder that spreads most easily among infants, young children, and elderly people. It appears most commonly on the face (usually around the nose and mouth) and other exposed areas.

Infants and young children may develop aural impetigo, or otitis externa. These lesions usually clear without treatment in 2 to 3 weeks unless an underlying disorder, such as eczema, is present. Candidal organisms, additional bacteria, fungi, or viruses may complicate lesions in the diaper area. In addition, impetigo may complicate chickenpox, eczema, and other skin disorders that are marked by open lesions.

CAUSES

Caused by coagulase-positive *Staphylococcus aureus*, bullous impetigo starts as a blister. Beta-hemolytic streptococci produce the nonbullous form of impetigo, which later also may harbor staphylococci, producing a mixed-organism infection. Predisposing factors, such as poor hygiene, anemia, malnutrition, and a warm climate, favor outbreaks of this infection, which is more prevalent in late summer and early fall. Methicillin-resistant *S. aureus* (MRSA) is becoming a common cause of impetigo.

COMPLICATIONS

Complications of impetigo include glomerulonephritis (rare), which is caused by a nephritogenic strain of beta-hemolytic streptococci, and ecthyma. If the infection becomes systemic, meningitis, bacteremia, and osteomyelitis may result. Since the epidermal layer of the skin sloughs, large areas of skin loss and permanent scarring may also occur.

ASSESSMENT FINDINGS

The patient history discloses exposure to insect bites or other predisposing factors.

Recognizing impetigo

In impetigo, when the vesicles break, crust forms from the exudate. This infection is especially contagious among young children.

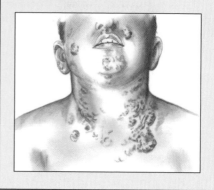

Additionally, the patient may relate a history of painless pruritus and burning.

In patients with streptococcal (nonbullous) impetigo, inspection typically reveals a small, red macule that has turned into a vesicle, becoming pustular within a few hours. When the vesicle breaks, a characteristic thick, honey-colored crust forms from the exudate. Autoinoculation may cause satellite lesions to appear.

In patients with staphylococcal (bullous) impetigo, a thin-walled vesicle opens. Inspection finds a thin, clear crust forming from the exudate and a lesion that appears as a central clearing circumscribed by an outer rim—much like a ringworm lesion. Observation typically reveals these lesions on the face or other exposed areas. Bullous and nonbullous impetigo may appear simultaneously and can be clinically indistinguishable. (See *Recognizing impetigo*.)

Ecthyma is a skin infection that resembles impetigo but extends into the dermis and takes longer to resolve. Ecthyma lesions are more common on distal extremities.

DIAGNOSTIC TESTS

❱ Gram stain reveals neutrophils with gram-positive cocci in chains or clusters.

❱ Culture and sensitivity testing of fluid or denuded skin reveals the causative organism and may indicate the most appropriate antibiotic therapy.

 ALERT Therapy shouldn't be delayed for laboratory results, which can take up to 3 days.

❱ Laboratory tests may reveal an elevated white blood cell count if impetigo is present.

TREATMENT

Topical agents, particularly mupirocin (Bactroban), have been used successfully in combination with crust removal prior to each application. A broad-spectrum systemic antibiotic may be needed for extensive or nonresolving lesions. Treatment also includes removal of the exudate by washing the lesions two or three times a day with soap and water; warm soaks or compresses of normal saline or diluted soap solution can be used to remove stubborn crusts. An antihistamine can help alleviate itching. If there are large areas of ruptured bullae, fluid resuscitation may be indicated with I.V. fluid at a volume and rate similar to the volume replacement used for burns.

NURSING CONSIDERATIONS

➲ In hospitalized patients, contact precautions should be maintained until 24 hours after effective treatment has been initiated.

❱ Use meticulous handwashing technique and standard precautions to prevent the infection from spreading.

❱ Cut the patient's fingernails short to prevent scratching, which can cause new skin breaks and autoinoculation.

❱ Remove the crusts by gently washing with antibacterial soap and water. Soften stubborn crusts with warm compresses; scrub gently to aid crust removal before applying a topical antibiotic.

❱ Give medications as ordered, and monitor the patient's response. Remember to check for penicillin allergy.

❱ Encourage the patient to verbalize feelings about his or her appearance, and acknowledge the importance of body image.

Patient teaching

PREVENTION To prevent contagion, emphasize to the patient and family the importance of meticulous handwashing technique. Advise parents to cut their child's fingernails short. Encourage frequent bathing with an antibacterial soap. Tell the patient not to share towels, washcloths, or bed linens, which should be kept separate and laundered in hot water before reuse.

❱ Teach the family how to identify and care for characteristic lesions. Encourage regular whole-body inspections, especially of children, to identify new lesions. If the patient is a school-age child, notify the school nurse about the condition.

❱ Stress the need to continue taking prescribed medications for 7 to 10 days, even after lesions have healed. Instruct the patient and family to notify the physician if adverse reactions occur.

❱ Provide written instructions for the care of impetiginous lesions, including crust removal, application of topical medications, and dressing change technique.

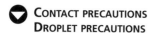

CONTACT PRECAUTIONS
DROPLET PRECAUTIONS

Influenza, H1N1

Influenza H1N1 is a highly contagious respiratory disease in pigs that is caused by one of several swine influenza (flu) type A viruses. Transmission to humans occurs when a person comes in contact with infected pigs or environments contaminated with a swine influenza virus. Once a person becomes infected, the virus can be spread to other humans by coughing or sneezing.

Influenza H1N1 causes acute febrile illness and other systemic symptoms ranging from mild fatigue to respiratory failure and death. In the Northern and Southern hemispheres, the virus is more prevalent in the winter months. In April 2009, U.S. public health officials declared swine influenza A (H1N1) virus a nationwide public health emergency. By early January 2010, the World Health Organization announced that 208 countries and territories had reported laboratory-confirmed cases of influenza H1N1, including 12,799 deaths worldwide. However, this number of reported cases undervalues the true number because many countries are no longer required to test and report individual cases.

CAUSES

Influenza virus may be one of three basic types (A, B, or C), depending on the number of gene segments surrounding the RNA viral core. H1N1, commonly referred to as swine flu virus, is one of the most common prevailing subtypes of influenza A, a zoonotic infection with over 100 types infecting most species of birds, pigs, horses, dogs, and seals. In humans, it is spread by respiratory secretions from an infected person. The virus then invades and replicates in the airway and respiratory tract cells, causing systemic symptoms from inflammatory mediators. The incubation period of influenza ranges from 18 to 72 hours.

COMPLICATIONS

Complications from influenza H1N1 include acute respiratory distress, conjunctivitis, myocarditis, pericarditis, pneumonia, sepsis, organ failure, and death.

ASSESSMENT FINDINGS

Patients infected with influenza H1N1 may present with mild symptoms or severe illness. Initial symptoms may include high fever (as high as 104° F [40° C]), mild to severe myalgia, rhinorrhea, and sore throat. Tachycardia may occur from hypoxia, fever, or both. The skin may be warm or hot, depending on temperature status. Nausea and vomiting may occur, and diarrhea is common in children. This may produce signs of dehydration. Frontal orbital headache is often severe and accompanied by photophobia, burning sensations, or pain upon motion. Weakness and severe fatigue may prevent patients from performing their activities of daily living and lead to the need for bed rest. A nonproductive cough, pleuritic chest pain, and dyspnea may occur. Acute encephalopathy may occur in patients with influenza A virus, producing altered mental status, coma, seizures, and ataxia.

DIAGNOSTIC TESTS

▶ Viral culture of nasopharyngeal or throat samples reveals the type of influenza, and staining the infected cultured cell lines with fluorescent antibody confirms the diagnosis.
▶ Other tests that can reveal the type of influenza include direct immunofluorescent assays (which are labor intensive and less sensitive than culture methods), serologic studies (which are quick but expensive to perform and may produce false-negative results for influenza A and B; test sensitivities range from 60% to 70%), and office tests, including the 10-minute QuickVue bedside test with a sensitivity of 70% to 80%.

ALERT Because of the high cost, limited availability, and lack of sensitivity of available testing methods, most health care providers will base a diagnosis of influenza on clinical criteria alone. Upon suspicion of influenza H1N1, however, a respiratory swab should be placed in a refrigerator (not a freezer) for collection and testing by the state or local health department.

▶ Chest radiography may reveal bilateral symmetrical interstitial infiltrates indicative of pneumonia.

▶ Arterial blood gas testing may reveal hypoxemia in severe cases.

▶ Laboratory tests may reveal leukopenia, lymphopenia, and/or thrombocytopenia.

TREATMENT

Influenza H1N1 is resistant to the antiviral agents amantadine (Symmetrel) and rimantadine (Flumadine) but is sensitive to oseltamivir (Tamiflu) and zanamivir (Relenza). Antiviral agents should be initiated within 48 hours of symptom onset. The usual vaccine for influenza administered at the beginning of the flu season is not effective against this viral strain. Treatment is otherwise supportive, with bed rest, fluids, and administration of antipyretics or analgesics. Malaise may persist for weeks after the illness has cleared.

NURSING CONSIDERATIONS

◉ Maintain contact and droplet precautions.

▶ Watch for signs and symptoms of complications.

▶ Teach the patient about proper disposal of tissues and good handwashing technique.

 SAFETY Shedding of the virus occurs at or just before (up to 24 hours) the onset of illness and continues for 5 to 10 days. Young children may shed virus longer, placing others at increased risk. Infection control precautions include handwashing and encouraging the patient to cover the mouth with a tissue when sneezing or coughing.

▶ Advise the patient to increase fluid intake. Warm baths or heating pads may relieve myalgia. Give the patient nonopioid analgesics-antipyretics as ordered.

▶ Watch for signs and symptoms of developing pneumonia, such as crackles, another temperature increase, or coughing accompanied by purulent or bloody sputum. Assist the patient to resume his or her normal activities gradually.

Patient teaching

▶ Educate patients about influenza immunizations.

 PREVENTION For high-risk patients (such as infants, children and adolescents, pregnant women, new mothers, the elderly, and those who are immunocompromised) and health care personnel, suggest annual inoculations at the start of the flu season (late autumn). The vaccination becomes effective 10 to 14 days after administration.

▶ Teach good handwashing technique to prevent the spread of infection, and discuss proper disposal of tissues and cleansing of surfaces.

▶ Teach the patient and family about the infection, including how it is transmitted, possible cause, and treatment plan.

▶ Teach the patient about prescribed medications, including the drug dosage and schedule of administration. Review signs of adverse effects, and outline which symptoms should be reported to the health care provider.

▶ Encourage adequate fluid intake and proper nutrition, and highlight the importance of rest during the convalescent phase.

▶ Instruct patients who are sick with flu-like symptoms to avoid contact with others for at least 24 hours.

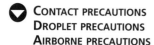

CONTACT PRECAUTIONS
DROPLET PRECAUTIONS
AIRBORNE PRECAUTIONS

Influenza, H5N1

Influenza H5N1, also known as avian influenza (flu), mainly infects birds but is also of concern to humans, who have no immunity against it. The virus that causes this infection in birds can mutate and easily infect humans and potentially start a deadly worldwide epidemic. The first avian flu virus to infect humans directly occurred in Hong Kong in 1997 and has since spread across Asia. Prognosis depends on the severity of infection as well as the type of avian flu virus that caused it.

CAUSES

Highly infective avian flu viruses, such as H5N1, have been shown to survive in the environment for long periods of time, with infection being spread simply by touching contaminated surfaces. Birds who recover from flu can continue to shed the virus in their feces and saliva for as long as 10 days.

Those at risk include farmers, agricultural workers, travelers visiting affected countries, people who eat raw or undercooked poultry, immunocompromised individuals, and health care workers and others who come in contact with patients who have avian flu.

COMPLICATIONS

Complications from avian influenza include conjunctivitis, pneumonia, acute respiratory distress, viral pneumonia, sepsis, organ failure, and death.

ASSESSMENT FINDINGS

Symptoms of avian flu infection in humans depend on the particular strain of virus present. With the H5N1 virus, infection causes more classic flu-like symptoms, which might include headache, malaise, dry or productive cough, sore throat, fever above 100.4° F (38° C), runny nose, difficulty breathing, diarrhea, and muscle aches. The patient may also exhibit signs of upper respiratory tract infection, including coryza, pharyngitis and, less commonly, conjunctivitis.

DIAGNOSTIC TESTS

▶ Nasal wash specimens detect the virus and allow viral subtyping.

 SAFETY Many laboratories are not equipped with the isolation needed to safely contain avian influenza. It is classified as category 3+ containment, higher than that used for human immunodeficiency virus. If a sample is sent, the laboratory may need to be shut down for decontamination. Samples should be sent to the Centers for Disease Control and Prevention (CDC), which will perform antiviral sensitivity testing as well as subtyping of the virus. If the CDC is able to handle testing, personnel should be called ahead of time before specimens are obtained. The specimen should then be transported by hand using a leak-proof specimen bag. The specimen should be clearly labeled as "suspected avian influenza," and the person who transports the specimen should wear appropriate personal protective equipment.

▶ Chest radiography can also aid in diagnosis.

▶ Blood work may reveal leukopenia (usually a lymphopenia); thrombocytopenia is common. Elevated liver enzyme levels are common.

▶ Disseminated intravascular coagulation may be evident.

▶ Other tests, including blood cultures, lumbar puncture for cerebrospinal fluid analysis (including polymerase chain reaction), and sputum cultures, assist in diagnosis.

TREATMENT

Supplemental oxygenation may be necessary to manage respiratory symptoms or hypoxia. In cases of respiratory failure, ventilatory support and intubation may be required. Supportive therapy should also include I.V. administration of crystalloids to support hemodynamic stability. If started within

48 hours after symptoms begin, the antiviral medications oseltamivir (Tamiflu) and, perhaps, zanamivir (Relenza) may decrease the severity of the disease. Oseltamivir may also be prescribed for household contacts of people diagnosed with avian flu. Supportive treatment, including mechanical ventilation, I.V. fluids, and symptomatic treatment, should be provided as needed.

It's currently recommended that contact, droplet, and airborne precautions be used with people diagnosed with H5N1 infection.

A vaccine designed to be effective against H5N1 is available. It is indicated for active immunization of adults who are at increased risk of exposure to the influenza H5N1 virus subtype.

NURSING CONSIDERATIONS

▶ Assess vital signs as well as pulmonary, cardiac, and neurologic status; administer oxygen as ordered and monitor response; encourage deep breathing and coughing. If the patient is on a ventilator, suction as needed and turn the patient every 2 hours.
▶ Monitor fluid intake and output, maintain I.V. therapy as ordered, report laboratory results, and monitor trends.
▶ Tell patients to call their health care provider if they develop flu-like symptoms within 10 days of handling infected birds or traveling to an area with a known avian flu outbreak.
▶ Travelers should avoid visits to live-bird markets in areas where there is an avian flu outbreak.
▶ Those who work with birds that might be infected should wear protective clothing and special breathing masks.

▶ Watch for signs and symptoms of complications.
▶ Teach the patient how to dispose of tissues properly, and explain good handwashing technique.
▶ Advise the patient to increase fluid intake. Warm baths or heating pads may relieve myalgia. Give the patient nonopioid analgesics-antipyretics as ordered.
▶ Maintain contact, droplet, and airborne precautions to reduce the risk of spreading the infection.

Patient teaching

▶ Educate patients about influenza immunizations. For high-risk patients and health care personnel, suggest annual vaccinations at the start of the flu season (late autumn). The vaccination becomes effective 10 to 14 days after administration.

 PREVENTION Tell patients that avoiding undercooked or uncooked meat reduces the risk of exposure to avian flu and other foodborne illnesses. Also, teach the patient about proper disposal of tissues and good handwashing technique.

▶ Teach the patient about the infection, including how it is transmitted, possible causes, and treatment plan.
▶ Teach the patient about prescribed medications, including the drug dosage and schedule of administration. Review signs of adverse effects as well as which symptoms to report to the health care provider.
▶ Encourage adequate fluid intake and proper nutrition, and stress the importance of rest during the convalescent phase.

DROPLET PRECAUTIONS

Influenza, seasonal

Influenza (also called the grippe or the flu) is an acute, highly contagious infection of the respiratory tract caused by influenza viruses from the family Orthomyxoviridae. Influenza viruses, which are usually seen during the colder months, are classified into three groups: Type A, the most prevalent, strikes every year, with new serotypes causing epidemics every 3 years; type B strikes annually and causes epidemics every 4 to 6 years; and type C is endemic and causes only sporadic cases. Epidemics tend to peak within 2 to 3 weeks after initial cases are diagnosed and subside within a month.

Although influenza affects all age groups, its incidence is highest in school-age children. However, its effects are most severe in persons who are young, elderly, or suffering from chronic disease. In these groups, influenza may lead to death.

CAUSES

Transmission of influenza occurs through inhalation of respiratory droplets from an infected person or by indirect contact with an object, such as a drinking glass or other item, that has been contaminated with respiratory secretions. The influenza virus then invades the epithelium of the respiratory tract, causing inflammation and desquamation.

One of the remarkable features of the influenza virus is its capacity for antigenic variation into numerous distinct strains, allowing it to infect new populations that have little or no immunologic resistance. Antigenic variation is characterized as antigenic drift (minor changes that occur yearly or every few years) and antigenic shift (major changes that lead to pandemics).

COMPLICATIONS

Complications that may occur with seasonal influenza include pneumonia, myositis, exacerbation of chronic obstructive pulmonary disease, Reye syndrome, myocarditis (rare), pericarditis (rare), transverse myelitis (rare), and encephalitis (rare).

ASSESSMENT FINDINGS

After an incubation period of 24 to 48 hours, flu symptoms begin to appear: sudden onset of chills, fever of 101° to 104° F (38.3° to 40° C), headache, malaise, myalgia (particularly in the back and limbs), a nonproductive cough and, occasionally, laryngitis, hoarseness, conjunctivitis, rhinitis, and rhinorrhea. These symptoms usually subside within 3 to 5 days, but cough and weakness may persist. Fever is usually higher in children than in adults. Also, cervical adenopathy and croup are likely to be associated with influenza in children. In some patients (especially elderly patients), lack of energy and easy fatigability may persist for several weeks. Fever that persists longer than 5 days signals the onset of complications.

DIAGNOSTIC TESTS

▶ Isolation of the virus through nose and throat cultures and increased serum antibody titers help confirm the diagnosis. Rapid diagnostic methods for detecting influenza are now available.

▶ Blood work shows a decreased white blood cell count with an increase in lymphocytes.

TREATMENT

Treatment of uncomplicated influenza includes bed rest, adequate fluid intake, antipyretics and analgesics to relieve fever and muscle pain, and antitussives to relieve nonproductive coughing. Prophylactic antibiotics aren't recommended because they have no effect on the influenza virus.

The antiviral agents amantadine (Symmetrel) and rimantadine (Flumadine) are no longer recommended due to resistance of the virus to these agents. The neuraminidase inhibitors oseltamivir (Tamiflu) and zanamivir (Relenza) are currently recommended for the treatment of influenza A and B. In influenza complicated by pneumonia, supportive care (fluid and electrolyte supplements, oxygen, and assisted ventilation) and treatment of bacterial super-infection with appropriate antibiotics are necessary. No specific therapy exists for cardiac, central nervous system, or other complications.

NURSING CONSIDERATIONS

▶ Unless complications occur, influenza doesn't require hospitalization; patient care focuses on relief of symptoms.
▶ Monitor fluid intake and output; advise the patient to increase fluid intake.
▶ Warm baths or heating pads may relieve myalgia. Administer nonopioid analgesics-antipyretics as ordered.

 SAFETY Visitors should be screened to protect the patient from bacterial infection and the visitors from influenza. Use droplet precautions. Teach the patient proper disposal of tissues and good handwashing technique to prevent the virus from spreading.

▶ Watch for signs and symptoms of developing pneumonia, such as crackles, another temperature rise, or coughing accompanied by purulent or bloody sputum. Assist the patient to gradually resume normal activities.

Patient teaching

 PREVENTION Educate patients about influenza immunizations. For high-risk patients and health care personnel, suggest annual vaccinations at the start of the flu season (late autumn). Remember, however, that influenza vaccines are made from chicken embryos and must not be given to people who are hypersensitive to eggs. The vaccine administered is based on the previous year's virus and is usually about 75% effective.

▶ Inform people receiving the vaccine about possible adverse effects, such as discomfort at the vaccination site, fever, malaise and, rarely, Guillain-Barré syndrome. An inactivated influenza vaccine is recommended for women who are pregnant and who will be in the second or third trimester during influenza season.

▶ Live-attenuated influenza vaccine is also available as a nasal spray. Criteria and contraindications for use vary from those for the inactivated, injectable vaccine. Recipients of live-attenuated influenza vaccine may shed influenza virus for up to 21 days after immunization.
▶ Teach good handwashing technique, and discuss proper disposal of tissues and cleansing of surfaces.
▶ Teach the patient and family about the infection, including how it is transmitted, possible causes, and treatment plan.
▶ Teach the patient about prescribed medications, including the drug dosage and schedule of administration. Review signs of adverse effects, and identify which symptoms should be reported to the health care provider.
▶ Encourage adequate fluid intake and proper nutrition, and stress the importance of rest during the convalescent phase.

Legionellosis

Infections caused by species of the genus *Legionella* are collectively termed legionellosis, or Legionnaires' disease. Legionellosis is an acute bronchopneumonia produced by the gram-negative bacillus *L. pneumophila*. Outbreaks usually occur in late summer and early fall and may be either epidemic or confined to a few cases. The infection may range from a mild illness (with or without pneumonitis) to serious multilobed pneumonia with mortality as high as 15%. Legionellosis is most likely to affect middle-aged or elderly people as well as immunocompromised patients and those with a chronic underlying disease, such as diabetes or chronic renal failure.

Pontiac fever is a less severe, self-limiting form of legionellosis that subsides within 2 to 5 days but leaves the patient fatigued for several weeks. This disorder is caused by the same microorganism that causes legionellosis but produces few or no respiratory symptoms, no pneumonia, and no fatalities.

Causes

Legionellosis infections are caused by *L. pneumophila*, an aerobic, gram-negative bacillus that's probably transmitted by air. The primary reservoir for the microorganism seems to be water distribution systems, such as humidifiers, whirlpool spas, decorative water fountains, respiratory therapy devices, and shower heads. The infection isn't spread from person to person. The *Legionella* microorganisms enter the lungs after aspiration or inhalation and then migrate to the pili. Although alveolar macrophages phagocytize the *Legionella*, the microorganisms aren't killed and proliferate intracellularly. The cells rupture, releasing the *Legionella* microorganisms, and the cycle starts again.

Lesions develop a nodular appearance and the alveoli become filled with fibrin, neutrophils, and alveolar macrophages. Conditions impairing mucociliary clearance (such as smoking, lung disease, or alcoholism) predispose the patient to infection.

Complications

Patients in whom pneumonia develops may experience hypoxia and acute respiratory failure. Other complications include hypotension, delirium, seizures, heart failure, arrhythmias, renal failure, and shock, which is usually fatal.

Assessment findings

The patient's history may include proximity to a suspected source of infection. Onset of illness may be gradual or sudden. After a 2- to 10-day incubation period (or a 1- to 2-day incubation period in Pontiac fever), the patient may report nonspecific prodromal symptoms, including diarrhea, anorexia, malaise, diffuse myalgia and generalized weakness, headache, and recurrent chills. He or she may also complain of a cough (initially nonproductive but eventually productive), dyspnea and chest pain, nausea, vomiting, and abdominal pain. Sputum is grayish or rust-colored, nonpurulent and, occasionally, streaked with blood. Some patients demonstrate tachypnea, bradycardia (about 50% of patients), and neurologic signs, especially an altered level of consciousness. Chest percussion may disclose dullness over areas of secretions and consolidation or pleural effusions. Auscultation may reveal fine crackles that develop into coarse crackles as the disease progresses.

With Pontiac fever, the patient may complain of myalgia, malaise, chills, headache, a nonproductive cough, and nausea. Fever is present. Complete recovery in patients with Pontiac fever occurs within a few days without antibiotic therapy, although some patients may experience lassitude for a few weeks after other symptoms subside.

Diagnostic tests

▶ Isolation of *Legionella* microorganisms from respiratory secretions or bronchial washings or through thoracentesis is a definitive method of diagnosis.

▶ Immunofluorescent antibody (IFA) and enzyme-linked immunosorbent assay serum antibody testing, performed twice 4 to 8 weeks apart, confirms infection with *Legionella* when it consistently reveals a single increased antibody titer when the IFA titer is 1:256 or higher. A single elevated titer does not necessarily confirm a diagnosis of legionellosis: titers of 1:256 or higher can be found in 1% to 16% of healthy people.

▶ The urinary antigen assay can be used to detect *L. pneumophila.*

▶ Chest radiography typically shows patchy, localized infiltration that progresses to multilobed consolidation (usually involving the lower lobes) and pleural effusion. In fulminant disease, chest radiography reveals opacification of the entire lung.

▶ Blood work may reveal leukocytosis, an increased erythrocyte sedimentation rate, a moderate increase in liver enzyme (alkaline phosphatase, alanine aminotransferase, and aspartate aminotransferase) levels, decreased partial pressure of oxygen and, initially, decreased partial pressure of carbon dioxide. Hyponatremia (serum sodium level less than 131 mg/L) is evident on blood chemistry analysis.

TREATMENT

Antibiotic treatment begins as soon as infection is suspected and diagnostic material is collected. Doxycycline (Doryx), azithromycin (Zithromax), macrolides, and quinolones are more effective against legionellosis than is erythromycin. Supportive therapy includes administration of antipyretics, fluid replacement, circulatory support with pressor drugs if necessary, and oxygen administration by mask or cannula or by mechanical ventilation with positive end-expiratory pressure.

NURSING CONSIDERATIONS

▶ Monitor the patient's respiratory status. Evaluate chest wall expansion, depth and pattern of respirations, cough, and chest pain. Watch the patient for restlessness, which may indicate hypoxemia. A patient with legionellosis may need suctioning, repositioning, postural drainage, chest physiotherapy, or aggressive oxygen therapy. Provide mechanical ventilation or other respiratory therapy, if ordered. Administer antianxiety medication to decrease oxygen requirements and improve tolerance of mechanical intervention.

▶ Continually evaluate vital signs, arterial blood gas levels, hydration, and color of lips and mucous membranes. Be alert for signs of shock, such as decreased blood pressure; tachycardia; weak, thready pulse; diaphoresis; and clammy skin.

▶ Administer antipyretics and antibiotic therapy as ordered. Keep the patient comfortable and protected from drafts; give tepid sponge baths or use cooling blankets to lower fever.

▶ Replace fluids and electrolytes as needed. If renal failure develops, prepare the patient for dialysis.

▶ Report all cases of legionellosis to the state health department or the Centers for Disease Control and Prevention.

Patient teaching

▶ Instruct the patient to take medication as ordered, even if feeling better.

▶ Remind the patient about the importance of keeping follow-up appointments with the physician.

 SAFETY Maintain standard precautions. Remember to teach the patient and family how to dispose of soiled tissues to prevent disease transmission.

Leishmaniasis

Leishmaniasis is a protozoal disease that manifests in cutaneous, mucocutaneous, visceral, and viscerotropic forms. Cutaneous disease may be classified as localized, diffuse, leishmaniasis recidivans or post-kala-azar dermal leishmaniasis. The extent of disease depends on the immunity of the host, the virulence of the species, and the parasite burden. Travelers, government workers, and military personnel are at risk due to environmental exposure to the habitat of the sandfly.

CAUSES

Inoculation occurs after an infected sandfly bites an exposed part of the body (usually the legs, arms, neck, or face). Rare cases have occurred through needle sharing, transfusions, pregnancy, and sexual intercourse. Female sandflies transmit the parasite 7 to 10 days after feeding on an infected person or animal. Once inside the body, the parasites infect the reticuloendothelial system, incubating for weeks to months before symptoms begin to occur.

COMPLICATIONS

Complications of leishmaniasis include disfiguring lesions, respiratory compromise, dysphagia, airway obstruction, aspiration, amyloidosis, glomerulonephritis, and cirrhosis. Death usually results from malnutrition, airway obstruction from lesions, aspiration, and secondary infection.

ASSESSMENT FINDINGS

Cutaneous leishmaniasis develops weeks to months after a bite and is detected by the presence of a firm, nontender, nonpruritic, erythematous papule measuring several centimeters with central ulceration, serous crusting, granuloma formation, and a raised erythematous border (volcano sign). Multiple wet or dry lesions may occur with localized lymphangitic spread. Diffuse spreading develops in those with a poor immune response. Healed lesions leave a characteristic retracted, hypopigmented scar.

Leishmaniasis recidivans follows the development of new ulcers and papules over the edge of the old scar, proceeding inward to form a lesion, usually on the cheek. In post-kala-azar dermal leishmaniasis, multiple hypopigmented, erythematous macules develop over the face or trunk, coalescing to form large, raised growths.

Patients with mucocutaneous leishmaniasis may have rhinorrhea, epistaxis, and nasal congestion due to tissue obstruction and perforation. The oral cavity may exhibit granulation, erosion, and ulceration. Involvement of the nasal cartilage produces a parrot's beak or camel's nose. Hoarseness indicates laryngeal involvement. Gingivitis, periodontitis, and localized lymphadenopathy may occur; optical and genital mucosal involvement has been reported in severe cases.

Visceral disease (kala-azar or black fever) results from systemic infection of the liver, spleen, and bone marrow. The patient is often cachetic, with abdominal distention, massive hepatosplenomegaly, epistaxis, petechiae, fever, weight loss, night sweats, weakness, anorexia, lymphadenopathy, hair changes, and skin hyperpigmentation (patchy darkening of the face and trunk). In patients with human immunodeficiency virus and visceral leishmaniasis co-infection, GI ulcerations, masses, pleural effusions, and odynophagia can occur.

Viscerotropic disease can occur 1 month to 2 years after exposure, with symptoms of malaise, fatigue, intermittent fever, cough, diarrhea, abdominal pain, rigors, fatigue, malaise, nonproductive cough, headache, arthralgia, myalgia, nausea, adenopathy, and transient hepatosplenomegaly.

DIAGNOSTIC TESTS

▶ Leishmaniasis is confirmed by tissue biopsy and culture of the parasite from infected tissue (cutaneous), dental scrapings or mucosal granuloma biopsy (mucocutaneous), bone marrow or splenic aspiration (visceral), or liver biopsy and lymph node dissection.

ALERT Contraindications for bone marrow or splenic aspiration include a low platelet count, abnormal prothrombin time, and a spleen that is palpable 4 cm or less below the costophrenic angle.

▶ Polymerase chain reaction or serologic detection of antibodies [direct agglutination test, immunofluorescence assay, or enzyme-linked immunosorbent assay] can assist in diagnosing visceral leishmaniasis.

▶ Blood work may reveal normocytic-normochromic anemia, leukopenia with decreased neutrophils, and thrombocytopenia in parasitic bone marrow infiltration (visceral leishmaniasis). An elevated serum immunoglobulin level and elevations in alkaline phosphatase, aspartate aminotransferase, and alanine aminotransferase levels are found in patients with visceral involvement.

TREATMENT

Sodium stibogluconate is available from the Centers for Disease Control and Prevention as an investigational drug and is currently used in the military. Amphotericin B (Abelcet) is effective against resistant mucocutaneous disease and visceral leishmaniasis; I.M. pentamidine is effective against visceral leishmaniasis but is associated with persistent diabetes mellitus and disease recurrence. Other agents include ketoconazole (Extina), itraconazole (Sporanox), fluconazole (Diflucan), allopurinol (Aloprim), and dapsone (Aczone). Cutaneous disease may be treated topically with paromomycin; smaller lesions may be treated by cryotherapy or radiofrequency ablation. Severe mucocutaneous leishmaniasis may require surgery.

 ALERT Surgical removal is not recommended for cutaneous lesions because recurrence often occurs at the excision site. In addition, the disease may be exacerbated by surgery.

NURSING CONSIDERATIONS

▶ Administer medications and treatments as ordered, and monitor for adverse effects.
▶ Provide wound care, and monitor for infection and progression of the disease.
▶ Provide emotional support.

Patient teaching

▶ Tell the patient that re-treatment may be required with resistant disease. Successful treatment results in immunity from the species causing the infection.

 PREVENTION Leishmaniasis may be reduced by reservoir eradication, vector control, and mass treatment of infected individuals. Insect repellent, protective clothing, and permethrin-impregnated mosquito nets should be used in endemic areas.

▶ Educate patients about recurrent disease, and encourage follow-up visits to assess for complications and monitor for recurrence.
▶ Review with patients the risk factors and routes of transmission for leishmaniasis.
▶ Review medication dosage and adverse effects as well as treatment regimen and skin care, as appropriate.
▶ Review signs and symptoms of infection, poor healing, or progression of the disease.

CONTACT PRECAUTIONS

Leprosy

Leprosy, also known as Hansen's disease, is a chronic, systemic infection characterized by progressive cutaneous lesions. With timely and appropriate treatment, leprosy has a good prognosis; left untreated, however, it can cause severe disability. Leprosy occurs in three distinct forms. Lepromatous leprosy causes damage to the upper respiratory tract, eyes, testes, nerves, and skin and can lead to blindness and deformities. Tuberculoid leprosy affects the peripheral nerves and surrounding skin, especially the face, arms, legs, and buttocks. Borderline (dimorphous) leprosy has characteristics of both lepromatous and tuberculoid leprosy, with diffuse, poorly defined lesions.

CAUSES

Leprosy is caused by *Mycobacterium leprae*, an acid-fast bacillus that attacks cutaneous tissue and peripheral nerves, producing a cellular immune response that results in skin lesions, anesthesia, infection, and deformities. Leprosy isn't highly contagious, but transmission can occur from continuous, close contact, possibly via nasal droplets or by skin breaks (with a contaminated hypodermic or tattoo needle, for example). The incubation period ranges from 2 to 40 years, with an average of 5 to 7 years. Early clinical indications of skin lesions and muscular and neurologic deficits are usually sufficiently diagnostic in patients from endemic areas.

COMPLICATIONS

Complications of leprosy include fever, malaise, lymphadenopathy, ulceration into muscle and fascia, secondary bacterial infection, and amyloidosis.

ASSESSMENT FINDINGS

M. leprae attacks the peripheral nervous system, especially the ulnar, radial, facial, deep fibular, and posterior popliteal nerves. Bacilli

damage the skin's fine nerves, causing anesthesia, anhidrosis, and dryness. If a large nerve trunk is infected, motor nerve damage, weakness, and pain occur, followed by peripheral anesthesia, muscle paralysis, or atrophy. In later stages, clawhand, footdrop, and ocular complications (corneal insensitivity and ulceration, conjunctivitis, photophobia, and blindness) can occur. Injury, ulceration, infection, and disuse of the deformed parts cause scarring and contracture. Neurologic complications occur in both lepromatous and tuberculoid leprosy but are less extensive and develop more slowly in the lepromatous form. Lepromatous leprosy can invade tissue in every organ of the body, but the organs remain functional.

In lepromatous disease, early lesions are multiple, symmetrical, and erythematous, appearing as macules or papules with smooth surfaces. Later, they enlarge and form plaques or nodules (lepromas) on the earlobes, nose, eyebrows, and forehead, giving a characteristic leonine appearance. In advanced stages, *M. leprae* may infiltrate the entire skin surface. Lepromatous leprosy also causes loss of eyebrows, eyelashes, sebaceous and sweat gland function and, in advanced stages, conjunctival and scleral nodules. Upper respiratory lesions cause epistaxis, ulceration of the uvula and tonsils, septal perforation, and nasal collapse. Lepromatous leprosy can lead to hepatosplenomegaly and orchitis. Fingertips and toes deteriorate when bone resorption follows trauma and infection in these insensitive areas.

When tuberculoid leprosy affects the skin, it produces raised, large, erythematous plaques or macules with clearly defined borders. As lesions grow, they become rough, hairless, and hypopigmented and leave anesthetic scars. In borderline leprosy, skin lesions are numerous but smaller, less anesthetic, and less sharply defined than tuberculoid lesions. Untreated borderline leprosy may deteriorate into lepromatous disease.

Occasionally, acute episodes intensify leprosy's slowly progressing course. Erythema nodosum leprosum, seen in lepromatous leprosy, produces fever, malaise, lymphadenopathy, and painful red skin nodules, usually during antimicrobial treatment, although it may occur in untreated people. In Mexico and other Central American countries, some patients with lepromatous disease develop Lucio's phenomenon, a malady producing generalized punched-out ulcers that may extend into muscle and fascia.

DIAGNOSTIC TESTS

▶ Biopsies of skin lesions, peripheral nerve biopsy, or smears of the skin or ulcerated mucous membranes help confirm the diagnosis.

▶ Blood work may reveal an increased erythrocyte sedimentation rate; decreased albumin, calcium, and cholesterol levels; and, possibly, anemia.

TREATMENT

Treatment consists of antimicrobial therapy using dapsone (Aczone), which may cause hypersensitivity reactions.

🔴 **ALERT** Hepatitis and exfoliative dermatitis, although uncommon, are especially dangerous reactions. If they occur, sulfone therapy should be stopped immediately. Alternative therapy includes either rifampin in combination with minocycline (Arestin) or ciprofloxacin (Cetraxal).

When a patient's disease becomes inactive, treatment is discontinued according to a specific schedule. Lepromatous disease requires lifetime therapy. Clawhand, wristdrop, or footdrop may require surgical correction.

NURSING CONSIDERATIONS

▶ Give antipyretics, analgesics, and sedatives as needed. Watch for and report complications.

▶ Report all cases of leprosy to the state health department or Centers for Disease Control and Prevention.

▶ Provide emotional support throughout treatment.

▶ Provide skin care and assist with treatment and rehabilitation of affected extremities.

▶ Stress the importance of adequate nutrition and rest. Watch for fatigue, jaundice, and other signs of anemia and hepatitis.

◐ Maintain contact precautions.

Patient teaching

▶ Patients with eye dryness need to use a tear substitute daily and protect their eyes to prevent corneal irritation and ulceration.

▶ Tell the patient with an anesthetized leg to avoid injury by not putting too much weight on the leg, testing water before entering to prevent scalding, and wearing appropriate footwear.

▶ Instruct the patient about medication dosage and adverse effects as well as treatments and the need for follow-up.

▶ Review with the patient possible symptoms of complications, and indicate which should be reported to the health care provider.

 SAFETY Tell the patient to practice respiratory etiquette by covering coughs or sneezes with a tissue and promptly disposing of the tissue.

CONTACT PRECAUTIONS

Leptospirosis

Leptospirosis is caused by *Leptospira* spirochetes and is considered the most common zoonosis in the world. The disease usually involves an acute phase with severe illness, followed by an anicteric phase that lasts 1 to 3 days without fever, and progresses to an immune (delayed) phase. Leptospires can remain in organs and other body tissue, such as the renal tubules, brain, and anterior chamber of the eye, for weeks to months. The extent of the disease is influenced by the patient's health, nutritional status, age, and time to treatment.

CAUSES

Leptospirosis is transmitted by direct contact with the body fluid of an acutely infected animal or by exposure to soil or water that has been contaminated with urine from an animal (bovine, murine, or canine) that is a chronic carrier. The disease can be acquired occupationally, during travel or vacations that involve water sports or hiking, or as a consequence of flooding. The leptospires enter the host through skin abrasions, intact mucous membranes or conjunctiva, the nasal mucosa and cribriform plate, the lungs (after inhalation of aerosolized body fluid), or the placenta during pregnancy. Organisms travel to the bloodstream through the lymphatics and can multiply in the small blood vessel endothelium, resulting in leptospiremia and multiorgan involvement. The incubation period is generally 5 to 14 days but can be as short as 72 hours or as long as a month or more.

COMPLICATIONS

Complications include interstitial nephritis, tubular necrosis, septicemia, hypovolemia, shock, vasculitis, secondary infection, disseminated intravascular coagulation (DIC), hemolytic-uremic syndrome, thrombotic thrombocytopenic purpura, and multiorgan failure. Pulmonary involvement results in hemorrhage and is the major cause of leptospirosis-associated death.

ASSESSMENT FINDINGS

Initially, an acute illness begins with high fever, rigors, sudden headache, nausea and vomiting, anorexia, diarrhea, cough, pharyngitis, nonpruritic skin rash, and muscle pain. Myalgia often affects the calf and lumbar areas. This phase lasts 5 to 7 days and either regresses to a relatively asymptomatic period or progresses to a more severe illness. When fever is severe and prolonged, hypotension and shock can occur. Petechial eruptions of the palate, jaundice, purpura, reddened conjunctiva (without exudate), and uveitis follow acute leptospirosis. Signs of meningitis (neck stiffness and rigidity, photophobia) and cardiac-related pulmonary edema (rales and wheezes) can occur. Myocarditis may occur in severe disease, with signs of biventricular heart failure and arrhythmias. Abdominal examination may reveal liver enlargement and tenderness due to hepatitis; cholecystitis and pancreatitis may also be present in severe cases. Heme-positive stool and bleeding on rectal examination occurs with DIC. Delirium may be an early finding in severe disease; depression, anxiety, irritability, psychosis, and even dementia can persist in the convalescent phase.

DIAGNOSTIC TESTS

▶ Isolation of the leptospires from tissue or body fluids (urine, blood, or cerebrospinal fluid) confirms the diagnosis.
▶ Blood work may indicate significant anemia due to pulmonary and GI hemorrhage; the platelet count may be diminished in DIC. Blood urea nitrogen and serum creatinine may be profoundly elevated in patients with anuric or oliguric renal failure. Serum bilirubin levels become elevated in obstructive disease due to capillaritis in the liver. Alkaline phosphatase levels may be elevated 10-fold. Coagulation times may be elevated in patients with hepatic dysfunction or DIC. Serum creatine kinase levels (MM fraction) are elevated with muscular involvement.

TREATMENT

Leptospirosis is treated with antimicrobial therapy: Doxycycline [Doryx] or I.V. penicillin G is the treatment of choice, but third-generation cephalosporins are also effective.

Treatment is supportive in patients with multiorgan involvement. Treatment for cardiovascular collapse and shock includes fluids and vasopressor agents. If the patient develops renal failure, dialysis may be necessary. For respiratory compromise, maintain a patent airway and provide endotracheal intubation and mechanical ventilation as needed to maintain oxygenation. Treatment of arrhythmias will depend on the type of arrhythmia present. Plasma exchange, corticosteroids, and I.V. immunoglobulin have been used in patients who have not responded to conventional therapy.

 PREVENTION Chemoprophylaxis with doxycycline is effective and may be used for military troops traveling to endemic areas or for vacationers engaging in aquatic recreation. It is not recommended for long-term or repeated use.

NURSING CONSIDERATIONS

▶ Maintain a patent airway; monitor oxygenation status; and assist with mechanical ventilation.

▶ Assess vital signs, and monitor for arrhythmias.

▶ Auscultate breath and heart sounds, and report alterations from normal.

▶ Administer I.V. fluids and vasopressor agents as ordered; monitor intake and output as well as peripheral perfusion and cardiovascular and renal status.

▶ Assist with dialysis treatments as ordered; monitor laboratory results.

▶ Monitor for complications, such as signs of overt or covert hemorrhage and other organ involvement.

▶ Before administering antibiotics, check the patient history for allergies; monitor for adverse reactions to antibiotics.

⊗ Maintain contact precautions.

Patient teaching

▶ Review the disorder with the patient, including the treatment plan, medication regimen, and signs and symptoms to report.

 SAFETY To prevent the spread of leptospirosis, tell the patient to avoid or reduce contact with potentially affected animals or contaminated soil or water. Those at risk for exposure should wear protective garments (footwear, gloves, and eye protection). Rodent control, decontamination of affected surfaces, and control of livestock infection are imperative to reduce the incidence in high-risk areas.

 PREVENTION No vaccine is currently available for high-risk groups. Immunization of livestock is available to prevent the spread of leptospires to other animals or humans.

Listeriosis

Listeriosis is an infection caused by the weakly hemolytic, gram-positive bacillus *Listeria monocytogenes*, which has been found in soil, wood, and decaying plant matter in the natural environment. The principal route of infection, however, is through the ingestion of contaminated food products. *Listeria* has been found in meat products, such as hot dogs and deli meat; in dairy products, including mostly soft cheeses and unpasteurized milk; and in unwashed raw vegetables and seafood. Listeriosis occurs most commonly in fetuses, in neonates (during the first 3 weeks of life), during pregnancy, and in older or immunosuppressed adults. Infected fetuses are usually stillborn or are born prematurely, almost always with lethal listeriosis. However, the infection produces milder illness in pregnant women and varying degrees of illness in older and immunosuppressed patients. The prognosis depends on the severity of illness.

CAUSES

The primary method of person-to-person transmission of listeriosis is neonatal infection either in utero (through the placenta) or during passage through an infected birth canal. Transmission may also occur by inhaling contaminated dust; drinking contaminated, unpasteurized milk; eating unprocessed soft cheeses or deli meats; and coming in contact with infected animals, contaminated sewage or mud, or soil contaminated with feces containing *L. monocytogenes*.

COMPLICATIONS

Complications of listeriosis include sepsis, diffuse clotting dyscrasias, respiratory insufficiency, circulatory insufficiency, meningitis, cerebritis, nonpurulent conjunctivitis, and granulomatous skin infection.

ASSESSMENT FINDINGS

Contact with *L. monocytogenes* commonly causes a transient asymptomatic carrier state, but it may produce bacteremia and a febrile, generalized illness. In a pregnant woman, especially during the third trimester, listeriosis causes a mild illness with malaise, chills, fever, and back pain. Her fetus may suffer severe uterine infection, however, potentially resulting in spontaneous abortion, premature delivery, or stillbirth. Transplacental infection may also cause early neonatal death or granulomatosis infantiseptica, which produces organ abscesses in infants.

Infection with *L. monocytogenes* commonly causes meningitis (especially in immunocompromised patients), resulting in tense fontanels, irritability, lethargy, seizures, and coma in neonates and low-grade fever and personality changes in adults. Fulminant manifestations with coma are rare. Infants may be poor feeders, appear lethargic, and have temperature instability and seizures. If granulomatosis infantisepticum is present, an erythematous rash appears with small, pale nodules or granulomas.

DIAGNOSTIC TESTS

▶ *L. monocytogenes* is identified by its diagnostic tumbling motility on a wet mount of the culture.
▶ Positive blood culture, cerebrospinal fluid culture, drainage from cervical or vaginal lesions, or lochia from a mother with an infected infant assist with diagnosis, but isolation of the organism from these specimens is generally difficult. Other tests that may aid in diagnosis include respiratory tract culture, histopathology and culture of the rash, and culture of other infected tissue (joint fluid, pericardial fluid, pleural fluid, amniotic fluid, placenta, gastric aspirate).
▶ Computed tomography or magnetic resonance imaging can detect abscesses in the brain or liver.

TREATMENT

The treatment of choice is an I.V. infusion of ampicillin or penicillin for 3 to 6 weeks, possibly with gentamicin to increase its effectiveness. Alternative treatments include ciprofloxacin (Cetraxal), trimethoprim-sulfamethoxazole (Bactrim), and chloramphenicol. Ampicillin or penicillin G is best for treating meningitis due to *L. monocytogenes* because the microorganisms can easily cross the blood-brain barrier. Pregnant women require prompt, vigorous treatment to combat fetal infection. For an infected newborn with *Listeria*, antibiotics as well as careful monitoring of the patient's temperature, respiratory system, fluid and electrolyte balance, nutrition, and cardiovascular support are necessary. Critically ill newborns are best treated in a specialized neonatal intensive care unit.

NURSING CONSIDERATIONS

▶ Deliver specimens to the laboratory promptly. Because few organisms may be present, take at least 10 ml of spinal fluid for culture.
▶ Report all cases of listeriosis to the state health department or the Centers for Disease Control and Prevention.

 SAFETY Maintain standard precautions until a series of cultures are negative. Be especially careful when handling lochia from an infected mother and secretions from her infant's eyes, nose, mouth, and rectum, including meconium.

▶ Evaluate neurologic status at least every 2 hours. In an infant, check the fontanels for bulging.
▶ Maintain adequate I.V. fluid intake; measure intake and output accurately.
▶ If the patient has central nervous system depression and becomes apneic, provide respiratory assistance, monitor respirations, and obtain frequent arterial blood gas measurements.

▶ Provide adequate nutrition by total parenteral nutrition, nasogastric tube feedings, or a soft diet, as ordered.
▶ Allow the patient's parents to see and, if possible, hold their infant in the neonatal intensive care unit. Be flexible about visiting privileges. Keep the parents informed of the infant's status and prognosis at all times.
▶ Reassure the parents of an infected neonate who may feel guilty about the infant's illness.
▶ Review the patient's history for any allergies prior to administration of antibiotics; monitor for adverse effects.

Patient teaching

▶ To reduce the incidence of infection, advise pregnant women to avoid infective materials on farms where listeriosis is endemic among livestock.

 PREVENTION To avoid infection, instruct the patient and family to avoid soft cheeses and to cook such foods as hot dogs thoroughly. Immunocompromised patients should avoid soft cheeses and deli meats.

▶ Teach the patient about possible complications, including signs and symptoms to report to the health care provider.
▶ Teach the patient about any prescribed medications, including drug, dosage, schedule of administration, and duration of therapy.
▶ Encourage the patient to maintain adequate nutrition and fluid intake and to rest during convalescence.

Lyme disease

A multisystemic disorder, Lyme disease is caused by the spirochete *Borrelia burgdorferi*, which is carried by *Ixodes scapularis, Ixodes pacificus,* and other ticks in the Ixodidae family. The infection commonly begins with a painless papule that becomes red and warm. This classic skin lesion is called erythema chronicum migrans (ECM). Weeks or months later, cardiac or neurologic abnormalities sometimes develop, possibly followed by arthritis of the large joints. Because isolation of *B. burgdorferi* is difficult in humans and serologic testing isn't standardized, diagnosis is usually based on the characteristic ECM lesion and related clinical findings, especially in endemic areas.

CAUSES

Lyme disease occurs when a tick injects spirochete-laden saliva into the bloodstream while feeding. After incubating for 3 to 32 days, the spirochetes migrate out to the skin, causing ECM. They then disseminate to other skin sites or organs via the bloodstream or lymph system. The spirochetes may survive for years in the joints, or they may trigger an inflammatory response in the host and then die.

COMPLICATIONS

Complications from Lyme disease include myocarditis, pericarditis, arrhythmias, heart block, meningitis, encephalitis, cranial or peripheral neuropathies, and arthritis.

ASSESSMENT FINDINGS

Typically, Lyme disease has three stages. ECM occurs in about 75% of the cases and heralds stage one with a red macule or papule, commonly at the site of a tick bite. This lesion typically feels hot and itchy and may grow to more than 20 inches (50.8 cm) in diameter; it resembles a bull's eye or target. Within a few days, more lesions may erupt and a migratory, ringlike rash, conjunctivitis, or diffuse urticaria occurs. In 3 to 4 weeks, lesions are replaced by small red blotches that persist for several more weeks. Malaise and fatigue are constant, but other findings are intermittent: headache, neck stiffness, fever, chills, achiness, and regional lymphadenopathy. Less common effects are meningeal irritation, mild encephalopathy, migrating musculoskeletal pain, hepatitis, and splenomegaly. A persistent sore throat and dry cough may appear several days before ECM.

Weeks to months later, the second stage (disseminated infection) begins, during which patients may develop additional symptoms depending on the system affected. Neurologic abnormalities—fluctuating meningoencephalitis with peripheral and cranial neuropathy—usually resolve after days or months. Facial palsy is especially noticeable. Cardiac abnormalities, such as a brief, fluctuating atrioventricular heart block, left ventricular dysfunction, or cardiomegaly may also develop. Cardiac involvement lasts only a few weeks but can be fatal.

Stage three (persistent infection) usually begins weeks or years later and is characterized by arthritis in about 80% of patients. Migrating musculoskeletal pain leads to frank arthritis with marked swelling, especially in the large joints. Recurrent attacks may precede chronic arthritis with severe cartilage and bone erosion.

DIAGNOSTIC TESTS

▶ Antibodies to *B. burgdorferi* are identified by immunofluorescence or enzyme-linked immunosorbent assay (ELISA). ELISAs are confirmed with Western blot tests.
▶ Blood work results, including mild anemia, an elevated erythrocyte sedimentation rate and leukocyte count, and increased serum immunoglobulin M and aspartate aminotransferase levels, may support the diagnosis.

TREATMENT

Animal studies have shown that transmission of infection is unlikely unless the infected tick is remains attached to the body for at least 24 hours. However, transmission is very likely when ticks are attached for longer than 72 hours. A 3-week course of an antibiotic, such as doxycycline (Doryx), is the treatment of choice for nonpregnant adults. Alternatives include amoxicillin, cefuroxime (Ceftin), erythromycin, azithromycin (Zithromax), and amoxicillin-clavulanic acid (Augmentin). When given in the early stages of infection, these drugs can minimize later complications. During the late stages of infection, high-dose I.V. ceftriaxone (Rocephin) may be successful. In patients with renal impairment, dosage adjustment may be required. Supportive therapy is given otherwise for symptoms and other organ and system involvement.

Nursing considerations

▶ Take a detailed patient history, asking about travel to endemic areas and exposure to ticks.

▶ Report all cases of Lyme disease to the state health department or the Centers for Disease Control and Prevention.

▶ Check for drug allergies, and administer antibiotics carefully; monitor for adverse effects.

▶ If the patient is receiving doxycycline, photosensitivity may occur with prolonged exposure to sunlight or tanning equipment.

▶ Monitor for therapeutic drug levels in patients receiving prolonged therapy with antibiotics.

▶ For a patient with arthritis, help with range-of-motion and strengthening exercises, but avoid overexertion. Ibuprofen helps relieve joint stiffness. Refer the patient for physical and occupational therapy as needed.

▶ Assess the patient's neurologic function and level of consciousness frequently. Watch for signs of increased intracranial pressure and cranial nerve involvement, such as ptosis, strabismus, and diplopia. Also check for cardiac abnormalities, such as arrhythmias and heart block.

▶ Monitor vital signs, and report changes in trends.

▶ Provide emotional support for the patient.

Patient teaching

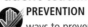 **PREVENTION** Advise the patient about ways to prevent contracting Lyme disease.

▶ Inform the patient that avoiding areas where deer ticks and western black-legged ticks live can reduce the chance of infection. Ticks live in wooded, brushy, and grassy areas, including lawns and gardens. Advise the patient to protect skin by wearing long pants and long shirts, and by using tick and insect repellent with N,N-diethyl-*meta*-toluamide (DEET) or permethrin on exposed skin when outdoors.

▶ Review with the patient the early stages of Lyme disease as well as symptoms that can develop later; encourage follow-up visits.

▶ Teach the patient about the disorder, including how it is transmitted, the cause, and the treatment required.

▶ Teach the patient about prescribed medications, including drug, dosage, schedule of administration, and duration of therapy.

▶ Teach the patient about possible complications that may occur, and specify signs that should be reported to the health care provider.

▶ Because Lyme disease is often chronic and treatment failure is a possibility, encourage follow-up with the health care provider.

Lymphangitis

The lymphatic system consists of a network of vessels, glands, and organs and functions as part of the immune system. The lymphatic system is also responsible for transporting fluids, fats, proteins, and other substances throughout the body. Lymph nodes or glands act as filters for the lymph fluid and are able to detect foreign bodies, such as bacteria or viruses. When bacteria or viruses are detected, an immune response is then triggered to fight infection.

Lymphangitis is an inflammation of the lymphatic channels that occurs as a result of an infection at a site distal to the channel. The pathogenic microorganisms invade the lymphatic vessels and spread to regional lymph nodes. Bacteria grow rapidly in the lymphatic system, resulting in inflammation of the lymphatic vessels. However, with prompt treatment, the prognosis for patients with uncomplicated lymphangitis is good.

CAUSES

Lymphangitis occurs when microorganisms enter the lymphatic channels directly through an abrasion or wound. It can also occur as a complication of infection. The more common causes in those with normal host defenses are the group A beta-hemolytic streptococcal species. Other offending microorganisms include *Staphylococcus aureus* and *Pseudomonas* species. The microorganisms enter the lymphatic channels, causing local inflammation and infection, producing red streaks on the skin, and then extending proximally toward regional lymph nodes.

COMPLICATIONS

Complications of lymphangitis include bacteremia, sepsis, cellulitis that may extend along the channels, necrosis, and ulceration. Without prompt treatment, lymphangitis caused by group A beta-hemolytic streptococci rapidly progresses to bacteremia, sepsis, and death.

ASSESSMENT FINDINGS

Patients with lymphangitis may have a history of minor trauma to an area distal to the site of infection. The primary site may be an abscess, an infected wound, or an area of cellulitis. Upon examination, tender, warm, erythematous and irregular linear streaks extend from the primary infection site toward draining regional nodes, which are often swollen and tender. Blistering of the affected skin may also occur. In addition, the patient may be febrile and tachycardic. (See *Evaluating the lymph nodes*.)

DIAGNOSTIC TESTS

▶ Culture and gram staining of an aspirate from the infection site assists in identifying the causative agent and determining appropriate antimicrobials.
▶ Laboratory tests often reveal marked leukocytosis.
▶ Blood cultures may reveal that infection has spread to the bloodstream, but results are rarely positive.

TREATMENT

Lymphangitis is treated with an appropriate antimicrobial agent, which is effective in more than 90% of cases. Common agents for outpatient therapy include penicillinase-resistant synthetic penicillin or a first-generation cephalosporin. Inpatient therapy may include a second- or third-generation cephalosporin, such as cefuroxime (Ceftin), ceftriaxone (Rocephin), or penicillinase-resistant synthetic penicillin.

 ALERT In areas of the country where rates of methicillin-resistant *S. aureus* (MRSA) are high, alternative antimicrobial agents such as clindamycin or trimethoprim-sulfamethoxazole (Bactrim) should be considered.

Analgesics and anti-inflammatory medications can help reduce pain and inflammation, as can the use of hot, moist compresses on the affected area. Abscessed areas may require surgical incision and drainage.

Evaluating the lymph nodes

The lymphatic system acts as a filter for foreign matter, such as bacteria and viruses. Palpable lymph nodes often result from an inflammatory response to infection, such as occurs in lymphangitis. To palpate the lymph nodes, begin in the preauricular or parotid gland area in the patient's temporal region. Proceed downward from the head and neck to the axillary and inguinal areas.

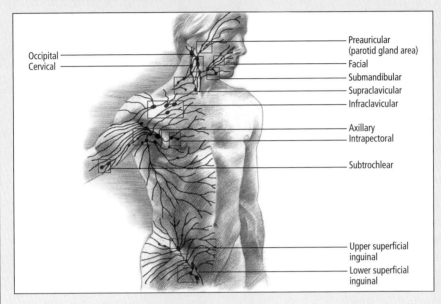

Occipital
Cervical

Preauricular (parotid gland area)
Facial
Submandibular
Supraclavicular
Infraclavicular
Axillary
Intrapectoral
Subtrochlear
Upper superficial inguinal
Lower superficial inguinal

NURSING CONSIDERATIONS

▶ Give prescribed medications; ensure patent I.V. access as appropriate.
▶ Monitor vital signs, and report changes in trends.
▶ Monitor intake and output, and assess hydration status; encourage fluids as ordered.
▶ Monitor laboratory studies and note trends.
▶ Assess the patient for response to treatment as well as adverse effects of medications.
▶ Provide comfort measures for pain and temperature; assess response to antipyretics and analgesics.
▶ Provide emotional support for the patient and family.
▶ Administer wound care, as appropriate, and report signs of infection or complications. Consult with wound care specialists as indicated.

Patient teaching
▶ Teach the patient about the infection, including how it is transmitted, possible cause, and treatment.
▶ Teach the patient about the prescribed medications, including drug dosage, schedule of administration, and duration of therapy.
▶ Review signs of adverse reactions to medications.
▶ Teach the patient about possible complications, including signs and symptoms to report to the health care practitioner.
▶ Encourage the patient to maintain adequate nutrition and hydration; encourage frequent rest periods during convalescence.

Malaria

Malaria, an acute infectious disease, is caused by protozoa of the genus *Plasmodium*—*P. falciparum*, *P. vivax*, *P. malariae*, *P. ovale*, and a more recent species, *P. knowlesi*—all of which are transmitted to humans by mosquito vectors. Falciparum malaria is the most severe form of the disease. When treated, malaria is rarely fatal; left untreated, it's fatal in 10% of patients, usually as a result of complications such as disseminated intravascular coagulation (DIC).

Untreated primary attacks last from a week to a month or longer. Relapses are common and can recur sporadically over several years. Susceptibility to the disease is universal.

CAUSES

Malaria is transmitted by the bite of female *Anopheles* mosquitoes, which abound in humid, swampy areas. When an infected mosquito bites, it injects *Plasmodium* sporozoites into the wound. The infective sporozoites migrate through the blood to parenchymal cells in the liver; there they form cystlike structures containing thousands of merozoites.

Upon release, each merozoite invades a red blood cell (RBC) and feeds on hemoglobin. Eventually, the RBC ruptures, releasing heme (malaria pigment), cell debris, and more merozoites, which, unless destroyed by phagocytes, enter other RBCs. (See *What happens in malaria.*)

At this point, the infected person becomes a reservoir of malaria and infects any mosquito that feeds on him or her, thus beginning a new cycle of transmission. Each *Plasmodium* species has a specific incubation period: *P. falciparum* infection typically develops within 1 month of exposure but has been known to develop after a year, whereas *P. vivax* and *P. ovale* may emerge weeks to months after inoculation.

Because blood transfusions and street-drug paraphernalia can also spread malaria, there is a higher incidence of the disease in drug addicts. The outcome of infection depends on host immunity: Parasites are cleared spontaneously in those with immunity, while in those without immunity the parasites continue to expand the infection.

COMPLICATIONS

Complications of malaria include renal failure, liver failure, heart failure, pulmonary edema, DIC, seizures, hypoglycemia, splenic rupture, cerebral dysfunction, and death.

ASSESSMENT FINDINGS

The patient history usually reveals travel to an area known to harbor malaria parasites. Some patients may present with only splenomegaly and no overt symptoms. An acute infection may present with flu-like symptoms, including chills, fever, fatigue, headache, and myalgia. Some may present with GI symptoms (diarrhea, nausea, vomiting), while others present with only anemia. Acute attacks (paroxysms) occur when RBCs rupture. There are three stages of paroxysms:

▶ Cold stage, lasting 1 to 2 hours, ranging from chills to extreme shaking

▶ Hot stage, lasting 3 to 4 hours, characterized by a high fever (up to 107° F [41.7° C])

▶ Wet stage, lasting 2 to 4 hours and characterized by profuse sweating

The most severe form of malaria, which causes the most morbidity and mortality, is caused by *P. falciparum*. Severe malaria symptoms include seizures, delirium, and coma (cerebral malaria); pulmonary involvement (respiratory distress, pulmonary edema, nasal flaring, intercostal or subcostal chest retraction, use of accessory muscles, abnormally deep breathing); severe anemia; and renal failure (oliguria, anuria, and uremia).

DIAGNOSTIC TESTS

▶ Peripheral blood smears identify the parasites in RBCs. The immunochromatographic test *Para*Sight F, which detects monoclonal antibody to *P. falciparum*–specific histidine-rich protein 2, is an alternative sensitive and

What happens in malaria

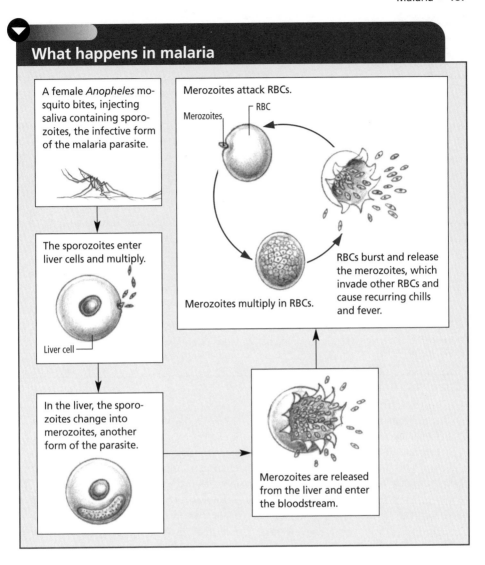

A female *Anopheles* mosquito bites, injecting saliva containing sporozoites, the infective form of the malaria parasite.

The sporozoites enter liver cells and multiply.

Liver cell

In the liver, the sporozoites change into merozoites, another form of the parasite.

Merozoites are released from the liver and enter the bloodstream.

Merozoites attack RBCs.

Merozoites
RBC

Merozoites multiply in RBCs.

RBCs burst and release the merozoites, which invade other RBCs and cause recurring chills and fever.

specific test for laboratories that are not equipped to identify parasites in RBCs. A rapid dipstick test (OptiMAL) that detects the lactate dehydrogenase (LDH) of the parasite can distinguish *P. falciparum* from other species. Thrombocytopenia, elevated LDH levels, and atypical lymphocytes in a patient are suggestive of malarial infection.

▶ Polymerase chain reaction and nucleic acid sequence-based amplification are more expensive but sensitive tests available for diagnosis.

TREATMENT

All forms of malaria except chloroquine-resistant *P. falciparum* are best treated with oral chloroquine (Aralen). Symptoms and parasitemia decrease within 24 hours after such therapy begins, and the patient usually recovers within 3 to 4 days. If the patient is comatose or vomiting frequently, chloroquine is given I.M.

ALERT Malaria caused by *P. falciparum*, which is resistant to chloroquine, requires treatment with quinine (Qualaquin),

Special considerations for antimalarial drugs

Chloroquine
• Perform baseline and periodic ophthalmologic examinations, and report blurred vision, increased sensitivity to light, and muscle weakness to the physician.
• Consult with the physician about altering therapy if muscle weakness appears in a patient on long-term therapy.
• Monitor the patient for tinnitus and other signs of ototoxicity, such as nerve deafness and vertigo.
• Caution the patient to avoid excessive exposure to the sun to prevent exacerbating drug-induced dermatoses.

Primaquine
• Give with meals or antacids.
• Halt administration if you observe a sudden fall in hemoglobin concentration or in RBC or leukocyte count or marked darkening of the urine, suggesting impending hemolytic reaction.

Pyrimethamine
• Administer with meals to minimize GI distress.
• Check blood counts (including platelets) twice per week. If signs of folic or folinic acid deficiency develop, reduce the dosage or discontinue use of medication while the patient receives parenteral folinic acid until blood counts become normal.

Quinine
• Use with caution in patients with cardiovascular conditions. Discontinue use of medication if you see any signs of idiosyncrasy or toxicity, such as headache, epigastric distress, diarrhea, rashes, or pruritus (in a mild reaction) or delirium, seizures, blindness, cardiovascular collapse, asthma, hemolytic anemia, or granulocytosis (in a severe reaction).
• Monitor blood pressure frequently while administering quinine I.V. infusion. Rapid administration causes marked hypotension.

doxycycline (Doryx), clindamycin (Cleocin), or pyrimethamine-sulfadoxine (Fansidar). Alternative therapies include atovaquone-proguanil (Malarone) and mefloquine.

The only drug that is currently effective against the hepatic stage of the disease is primaquine. This drug can induce hemolytic anemia, especially in patients with glucose-6-phosphate dehydrogenase deficiency. (See *Special considerations for antimalarial drugs.*)

For travelers going to an endemic area, prophylaxis may be required. (See *How to prevent malaria.*) Any traveler who develops an acute febrile illness should seek prompt medical attention, regardless of the prophylaxis taken.

NURSING CONSIDERATIONS

❯ Obtain a detailed patient history, noting any recent travel, foreign residence, blood transfusion, or drug addiction. Record symptom pattern, temperature, type of malaria, and any systemic signs. Report all cases of malaria to local or state public health authorities, who will then contact the Centers for Disease Control and Prevention.

❯ Assess the patient on admission and daily thereafter for fatigue, fever, orthostatic hypotension, disorientation, myalgia, and arthralgia. Enforce bed rest during periods of acute illness.

❯ Protect the patient from secondary bacterial infection by following proper handwashing and sterile techniques.

 SAFETY Protect yourself by wearing gloves when handling blood or body fluids.

❯ To reduce fever, administer antipyretics as ordered. Document onset, duration, and symptoms before and after febrile episodes.

❯ Fluid balance is fragile in patients with malaria, so keep a strict record of intake and output. Monitor I.V. fluids closely because fluid overload can lead to pulmonary edema and aggravate cerebral symptoms. Observe blood chemistry levels for hyponatremia and increased blood urea nitrogen, creatinine,

How to prevent malaria

Advise patients about the following actions that should be taken to help prevent malaria:
- Drain, fill, and eliminate mosquito breeding areas.
- Install screens in living and sleeping quarters in endemic areas.
- Use a residual insecticide on clothing and skin to prevent mosquito bites.
- Seek treatment for known cases.
- Question blood donors about a history of malaria or possible exposure to malaria. They *may* give blood if:
  - They haven't taken any antimalarial drugs and are asymptomatic after 6 months outside an endemic area
  - They were asymptomatic after treatment for malaria more than 3 years ago
  - They were asymptomatic after receiving malaria prophylaxis more than 3 years ago
- Seek prophylactic drug therapy before traveling to an endemic area. Agents include mefloquine, doxycycline, chloroquine, hydroxychloroquine, or malarone (a combination of atovaquone and proguanil). Prophylactic drug therapy is usually started 2 weeks before visiting the endemic area and continued for 6 weeks after leaving the area.

and bilirubin levels. Monitor urine output hourly, and maintain it at 40 to 60 ml/hour for an adult and at 15 to 30 ml/hour for a child. Immediately report any decrease in urine output or the onset of hematuria as a possible sign of renal failure; be prepared to perform peritoneal dialysis for uremia caused by renal failure.

▶ Slowly administer packed RBCs or whole blood while checking for crackles, tachycardia, and shortness of breath.

▶ If humidified oxygen is ordered, note the patient's response, particularly any changes in rate or character of respirations or any improvement in mucous membrane color.

▶ Watch for and immediately report signs of internal bleeding, such as tachycardia, hypotension, and pallor.

▶ Encourage frequent coughing and deep breathing, especially if the patient is on bed rest or has pulmonary complications. Record the amount and color of sputum.

▶ Watch for adverse effects of drug therapy, and take measures to relieve them.

▶ If the patient is comatose, make frequent, gentle changes in his or her position, and administer passive range-of-motion exercises every 3 to 4 hours. If the patient is unconscious or disoriented, use restraints as needed, and keep an airway available as appropriate.

▶ Provide emotional support and reassurance, especially in critically ill patients.

Patient teaching

▶ Explain the procedures and treatment to the patient and family; answer any questions clearly.

▶ Suggest that family members be tested for malaria.

▶ Emphasize the need for follow-up care to check the effectiveness of treatment and to manage residual problems.

▶ Teach the patient about possible complications, including signs and symptoms that should be reported to the practitioner immediately.

▶ Teach the patient about prescribed medications, including drug dosage, schedule of administration, and duration of therapy.

DROPLET PRECAUTIONS
CONTACT PRECAUTIONS

Marburg virus infection

Marburg virus causes severe hemorrhagic fever: In a 1967 outbreak in Marburg, Germany, mortality rates reached 23%. Hemorrhagic fevers caused by Ebola and Marburg are considered the most severe viral hemorrhagic fevers, with overall 25% to 100% mortality rates. Hemorrhage and widespread necrosis, varying from mild to massive, occur in many organs. Effusions may occur in serous cavities as well. The systems most commonly involved are the liver, lung, and lymphoid systems. Usually the lung shows varying degrees of interstitial pneumonitis, diffuse alveolar damage, and hemorrhage. Acute tubular necrosis and microvascular thrombosis may also be observed.

CAUSES

Marburg virus belongs to the Filoviridae family of viruses. The vector is unknown, but the infection is thought to be spread by direct contact with infected patients, their blood, or their secretions or excretions. Aerosol transmission is suspected. Animal reservoirs may be primates; in other types of hemorrhagic fevers, rats, mice, domestic livestock, and monkeys serve as intermediate hosts.

COMPLICATIONS

Complications of Marburg virus infection include myalgia and arthralgia, headache, fatigue, bulimia, amenorrhea, hearing loss, tinnitus, unilateral orchitis, and suppurative parotitis. Hemorrhagic fever commonly produces ocular pain, photophobia, increased lacrimation, and decreased visual acuity. Late complications include uveitis, transverse myelitis, and recurrent hepatitis.

ASSESSMENT FINDINGS

Initial symptoms begin after an incubation of 2 to 14 days and may include progressive fever (that may be biphasic), chills, malaise, generalized myalgia and arthralgia, headache, anorexia, cough, severe sore throat, epigastric pain, vomiting, and diarrhea. On about the fifth day of illness, a distinct morbilliform rash develops on the trunk and the patient may exhibit an expressionless ghostlike facies. Patients with progressive disease hemorrhage from mucous membranes, venipuncture sites, and body orifices, with disseminated intravascular coagulation (DIC) a feature of late disease.

Typical findings on examination may include conjunctival injection, facial and truncal flushing, petechiae, purpura, ecchymoses, icterus, epistaxis, GI and genitourinary bleeding, and lymphadenopathy. In severe hemorrhagic fever, hypotension and shock occur, as well as bradycardia, pneumonitis, pleural and pericardial effusions, hemorrhage, encephalopathy, seizures, coma, and death.

DIAGNOSTIC TESTS

▶ Enzyme-linked immunosorbent assays for virus-specific immunoglobulin (Ig) M and IgG are helpful in diagnosis.

 ALERT These serologic tests are useful because of their sensitivity; however, antibody may not be detected during the acute stages of Marburg virus infection. Polymerase chain reaction on serum may be done during the acute stages of infection with viral hemorrhagic fever as it is more sensitive.

▶ Direct examination of blood and tissue (such as by skin biopsy) identifies the viral antigen by enzyme immunoassay.
▶ Blood tests in viral hemorrhagic fevers often show leukopenia, leukocytosis, thrombocytopenia, hemoconcentration and, occasionally, DIC.
▶ Elevated hepatocellular enzyme levels and hypoalbuminemia are typically present.
▶ Proteinuria is a universal finding.

TREATMENT

Early diagnosis and supportive care can be lifesaving with special care given to fluid and electrolyte management. To date, antiviral agents, passive antibodies, and interferon have been unsuccessful in the treatment of Marburg virus infection. Supportive therapy should include meeting nutritional needs, supporting organ systems, and providing comfort.

NURSING CONSIDERATIONS

 SAFETY All body fluids and excretions (blood, saliva, urine, stool, sputum, and emesis) are considered infectious as they can harbor virions and should be handled with great care. Survivors of hemorrhagic fever can produce infectious virions for prolonged periods, so strict contact precautions must be observed. It is also recommended that the patient be placed in a private room away from traffic patterns throughout the course of illness. The patient's urine, stool, sputum, and blood, along with any objects that have come in contact with the patient or the patient's body fluids (such as laboratory equipment), should be disinfected with a 0.5% sodium hypochlorite solution.

▶ Administer antipyretics as ordered, and provide comfort measures.

▶ Because fluid balance is fragile in patients with viral hemorrhagic fever, keep a strict record of intake and output. Monitor I.V. fluids closely. Observe laboratory studies, and watch for evidence of overt or covert bleeding. Monitor urine output hourly, and report any decrease or the onset of hematuria as a possible sign of renal failure.

▶ Watch for and immediately report signs of internal bleeding, such as tachycardia, hypotension, or pallor.

▶ If oxygen is ordered, note the patient's response, particularly any changes in the rate or character of respirations, or any improvement in mucous membrane color.

▶ Encourage frequent coughing and deep breathing, especially if the patient is on bed rest or has pulmonary complications. Record the amount and color of sputum.

▶ Watch for adverse effects of drug therapy, and take measures to relieve them.

▶ If the patient is comatose, change his or her position gently and frequently, and administer passive range-of-motion exercises every 3 to 4 hours. If the patient is unconscious or disoriented, use restraints as needed, and keep an airway available as appropriate.

▶ Provide emotional support and reassurance, especially in critical illness.

Patient teaching

▶ Tell the patient that recovery often requires months and that weight gain and return of strength are slow.

▶ Tell the patient and family that those who were exposed to the patient should be watched closely for signs of early disease.

 PREVENTION Tell the patient and family that an important measure for preventing viral hemorrhagic fever is avoidance of insect bites from the vectors and exposure to sources of infection, such as specific reservoirs.

▶ Vaccines against these viruses are being tested in preliminary primate studies.

Melioidosis

Also known as Whitmore disease, melioidosis is caused by *Burkholderia pseudomallei* bacteria, which thrive in tropical climates. It is considered a potential biological warfare agent in the aerosolized form because it is highly infectious and resistant to routine antibiotics. Melioidosis can also result from wound penetration or ingestion of the bacteria. It commonly occurs in two forms: chronic melioidosis, which causes osteomyelitis and lung abscesses, and the rare acute melioidosis, which causes pneumonia, bacteremia, and prostration. Acute melioidosis is often fatal; however, most melioidosis infections are chronic and asymptomatic.

CAUSES

B. pseudomallei (formerly *Pseudomonas pseudomallei*) is a motile, aerobic, non-spore-forming, saprophytic, gram-negative bacillus. The organism is distributed widely in contaminated soil and water in tropical regions, especially in Southeast Asia where it is endemic, and is spread through direct contact with the contaminated source. Human cases have resulted from sexual contact and I.V. drug use. It has been observed in immigrants, military personnel, and travelers. The incubation period can vary from days to months to years; after an aerosol attack, the incubation period ranges from 10 to 14 days.

Bacteria that enter skin through a laceration or abrasion cause a local infection, ulceration, swollen lymph glands, and increased mucus production (when they enter through mucous membranes). Bacteria that enter the respiratory tract can cause pulmonary infections (pneumonia, pulmonary abscesses, and pleural effusions) and, possibly, cutaneous abscesses that may take months to appear. When bacteria enter the bloodstream, chronically ill patients (such as those with human immunodeficiency virus or diabetes) develop respiratory distress, headaches, fever, diarrhea, pus-filled lesions on the skin, and abscesses throughout the body.

The chronic form of melioidosis involves multiple abscesses that may affect the liver, spleen, skin, or muscles. Melioidosis can also become reactive many years after the primary infection.

COMPLICATIONS

Complications from melioidosis include septicemia, osteomyelitis, meningitis, and brain, liver, or splenic abscess. Prior to the use of antibiotics, untreated patients with septicemia had a mortality rate as high as 95%. Mortality remains higher than 50% for septicemic disease and reaches 20% for localized disease despite treatment; the overall mortality rate is 40%.

ASSESSMENT FINDINGS

Generalized symptoms of melioidosis include fever, rigors, night sweats, myalgia, anorexia, and headache. Depending on the route of exposure, symptoms may include chest pain, cough, photophobia, lacrimation, and diarrhea. Physical findings may include hepatomegaly or splenomegaly. When septicemia is present, flushing, cyanosis, and rigors occur and may be accompanied by confusion, dyspnea, abdominal pain, muscle tenderness, pharyngitis, diarrhea, and jaundice. A disseminated pustular eruption with regional lymphadenitis, cellulitis, or lymphangitis and severe urticaria may appear. Ecthyma gangrenosum–like lesions and cutaneous abscesses (that sometimes ulcerate) may develop. Although the initial foci in these severe cases begin with skin or lung infections, metastasis to the liver, spleen, kidney, brain stem, and/or parotid gland occurs, leading to acidosis, shock, and death within 48 hours of presentation.

DIAGNOSTIC TESTS

▶ Isolation of *B. pseudomallei* in a culture of exudate, blood, urine, skin lesions, or sputum confirms the diagnosis. Gram stain may reveal small, gram-negative bacilli.

ALERT Blood culture results may be negative (the median time for growth is 48 hours). In patients with septicemic melioidosis, blood culture results may be negative until just before death.

▶ Antibodies to the bacteria measured in the blood may be found after 7 to10 days.

▶ Complement fixation tests are more specific and are considered positive for melioidosis when a fourfold increase in the titer occurs.

▶ Blood work may reveal a mild leukocytosis with a left shift or leukopenia, anemia, hepatic impairment, renal insufficiency, and coagulopathy.

▶ Chest radiography may show diffuse nodular shadowing in up to 80% of patients.

▶ Plain radiography and magnetic resonance imaging of bone and musculoskeletal soft tissue may show findings consistent with disseminated melioidosis.

▶ Ultrasonography and computed tomography may reveal multiple, small, discrete abscesses in the liver and spleen suggestive of visceral melioidosis.

TREATMENT

Cases of melioidosis are reportable to the local health authorities. For localized disease, an extended course of oral amoxicillin-clavulanic acid (Augmentin), doxycycline (Doryx), or trimethoprim-sulfamethoxazole (Bactrim) may be used. For extrapulmonary disease, treatment with antibiotics may continue for as long as 12 months. Severe cases of melioidosis or septicemia may be treated initially with parenteral therapy for 2 weeks, followed by 6 months of treatment with ceftazidime (Fortaz) combined with trimethoprim-sulfamethoxazole. Alternative therapy in severe cases includes imipenem-cilastatin (Primaxin) or meropenem (Merrem) with or without trimethoprim-sulfamethoxazole. Abscesses should be also be drained surgically.

 ALERT Prolonged therapy is necessary for the prevention of relapse in patients with melioidosis. Relapse has been reported to occur in 23% of cases.

 SAFETY Standard precautions apply to patients with melioidosis. Person-to-person transmission is unlikely.

No vaccine is currently available for melioidosis.

NURSING CONSIDERATIONS

▶ Observe and record the character of wound exudate and sputum; provide wound care as indicated.

▶ Monitor the patient's vital signs and blood studies; watch for complications or progression of disease.

Patient teaching

▶ Reinforce the importance of completing the course of antibiotic therapy as prescribed. Review signs and symptoms to report to the health care provider.

▶ Immunocompromised patients should avoid contact with soil or standing water in areas where melioidosis is endemic. Wearing boots and gloves during agricultural work is advised.

Droplet Precautions

Meningitis

Meningitis is an inflammation of the meninges (dura mater, arachnoid, and pia mater). It can be acute, with symptoms occurring in hours to days, or chronic, with an onset and duration of weeks to months. Meningitis usually results from a viral or, less commonly, bacterial infection. Viral meningitis is usually mild and often clears on its own in 10 days or less. Bacterial meningitis requires prompt treatment with I.V. antibiotics.

Causes

Noninfectious causes of meningitis include medications (such as nonsteroidal antiinflammatory drugs and antibiotics) and carcinomatosis. Viruses cause most cases of aseptic meningitis. (See *Lymphocytic choriomeningitis.*)

Other infectious agents include bacterial, fungal, mycobacterial, and parasitic agents. *Neisseria meningitidis* is implicated in most epidemics. Transmission takes place through inhalation of infected droplets from a carrier, with the virus often localizing in the nasopharynx. After incubating about 3 to 4 days, the microorganisms spread through the bloodstream to the joints, skin, adrenal glands, lungs, and central nervous system. Resulting tissue damage may be due to the effects of bacterial endotoxins. In fulminating meningococcemia and meningococcal bacteremia, hemorrhage, thrombosis, and necrosis occur.

Complications

Complications of meningitis include visual impairment, optic neuritis, cranial nerve palsies, personality changes, paresis or paralysis, vasculitis, endocarditis or pericarditis, and respiratory failure. Other complications include disseminated intravascular coagulation, septic arthritis, pericarditis, endophthalmitis, neurologic deterioration, and death.

Assessment findings

Two-thirds of patients infected with meningitis present with fever, headache, neck stiffness, photophobia, nausea, vomiting, and signs of cerebral dysfunction (lethargy, confusion, coma).

 ALERT Atypical presentation may occur in elderly individuals (especially those with diabetes or renal or liver disease), those with neutropenia, and immunocompromised patients (transplant recipients and those with human immunodeficiency virus [HIV] and acquired immunodeficiency syndrome).

Signs of increased intracranial pressure include headache, vomiting and, rarely, papilledema. Signs of meningeal irritation include nuchal rigidity, positive Brudzinski's and Kernig's signs, exaggerated and symmetrical deep tendon reflexes, and opisthotonos. (See *Two signs of meningitis,* page 196.)

Other manifestations are irritability, sinus arrhythmias, and photophobia, diplopia, and other visual problems. The patient may also develop delirium, deep stupor, and coma.

Systemic findings can provide clues to the etiology of the organism. A morbilliform rash with pharyngitis and adenopathy may indicate a viral etiology (Epstein-Barr virus [EBV], cytomegalovirus [CMV], adenovirus, HIV). Macules and petechiae that rapidly evolve into purpura may indicate meningococcemia. Varicella-zoster virus often produces vesicular lesions in a dermatomal distribution, whereas genital vesicles suggest herpes simplex virus type 2. *Streptococcus pneumoniae* and *Haemophilus influenzae* may cause sinusitis or otitis. Rhinorrhea or otorrhea indicates a cerebrospinal fluid (CSF) leak, possibly from a basilar skull fracture, most commonly caused by *S. pneumoniae.* Systemic disease may produce hepatosplenomegaly and lymphadenopathy, possibly indicating a viral (EBV, CMV, HIV) or fungal (histoplasmosis) origin. A heart murmur occurs in infective endocarditis, and mumps meningitis can produce parotitis.

Lymphocytic choriomeningitis

Lymphocytic choriomeningitis (LCM) is a mild, biphasic, febrile illness lasting about 2 weeks. Infection occurs through inhalation of the LCM virus or arenavirus from infectious aerosolized particles of the host (rodents such as mice or hamsters) or its excreta (urine, feces, or saliva) 1 to 3 weeks before the onset of symptoms. It can also result from contact with food that has been contaminated with the virus or by contamination of mucous membranes, skin lesions, or cuts with infected body fluids. Handlers of infected animals or their excreta are at risk for this disease. Most cases occur in the northeast and eastern seaboard areas of the United States. LCM is more common during fall and winter.

The incubation period is 8 to 13 days after exposure. Early characteristics include fever, malaise, anorexia, weakness, muscle aches, retro-orbital headache, nausea, and vomiting. Sore throat, nonproductive cough, joint pain, chest pain, testicular pain, and parotid (salivary gland) pain may occur. Meningeal symptoms appear in 15 to 21 days, with signs and symptoms of meningitis (fever, increased headache, and stiff neck) or encephalitis (drowsiness, confusion, sensory disturbances, and motor abnormalities such as paralysis). Alopecia may also occur.

Complications include temporary or permanent neurologic damage, possible maternal transmission (pregnancy-related infection is associated with spontaneous abortion, congenital hydrocephalus, chorioretinitis, and mental retardation), myelitis, Guillain-Barré-type syndrome, orchitis or parotitis, myocarditis, psychosis, joint pain and arthritis, and prolonged convalescence with continuing dizziness, somnolence, and fatigue.

Diagnosis is made by detection of immunoglobulin M antibodies by enzyme-linked immunosorbent assay from serum or cerebrospinal fluid (CSF) (the preferred diagnostic test). Lumbar-puncture CSF is typically abnormal and reveals increased opening pressure, increased protein levels, and a lymphocytic pleocytosis, usually in the range of several hundred white blood cells. Treatment is generally supportive and includes bed rest, anti-inflammatory drugs, and analgesics. Ribavirin has been shown to be effective against LCM in vitro. Acute hydrocephalus may require surgical shunting to relieve increased intracranial pressure.

Prevention involves teaching rodent control measures, basic hygiene practices, use of a personal respirator, importance of adequate ventilation, and use of a liquid disinfectant, such as a diluted household bleach solution, to clean areas with rodent droppings.

DIAGNOSTIC TESTS

▶ Lumbar puncture shows typical CSF findings and establishes a diagnosis. It often indicates elevated CSF pressure, which varies depending on the causative agent.

▶ Cultures of the primary site of infection (blood, urine, nose and throat secretions) can identify the organism. CSF culture and sensitivity tests usually identify the infecting organism, unless it is viral in origin.

TREATMENT

Treatment of meningitis includes appropriate antimicrobial therapy (commonly penicillin, ceftriaxone (Rocephin), vancomycin, or chloramphenicol for bacterial infection) and supportive care. Treatment for viral meningitis is usually supportive; acyclovir (Zovirax) may be administered for herpes simplex virus infections; CMV infections may be treated with ganciclovir and foscarnet (Foscavir). Fungal infections are treated with amphotericin B (Abelcet) and fluconazole (Diflucan). The combination of rifampin, isoniazid, and pyrazinamide (Rifater) may be used in tubercular meningitis. Dexamethasone may be used as adjunctive therapy to increase penetration of the drug into the CSF. Mannitol may be used to decrease cerebral edema. Anticonvulsants,

Two signs of meningitis

BRUDZINSKI'S SIGN: Place the patient in a dorsal recumbent position, put your hands behind the neck, and bend it forward. Pain and resistance may indicate meningeal inflammation, neck injury, or arthritis. If the patient also flexes the hips and knees in response to this manipulation, chances are meningitis is present.

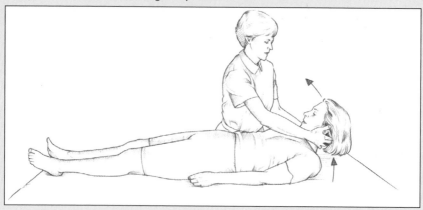

KERNIG'S SIGN: Place the patient in a supine position. Flex the leg at the hip and knee, and then straighten the knee. Pain or resistance points to meningitis.

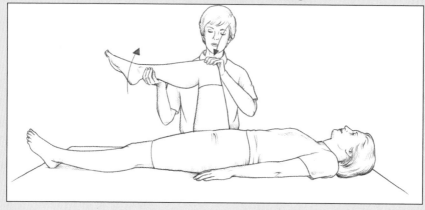

sedatives, antipyretics, and analgesics may also be indicated. Appropriate therapy is indicated for any coexisting conditions (endocarditis or pneumonia).

NURSING CONSIDERATIONS

▶ Give I.V. antibiotics as ordered to maintain blood and CSF drug levels; monitor renal and liver function as well as blood counts and therapeutic levels as indicated.

▶ Maintain a patent airway and provide oxygen as ordered; suction and turn the patient frequently.

▶ Monitor vital signs as well as intake and output; maintain I.V. therapy as ordered.

● Monitor neurologic status using the Glasgow Coma Scale, and implement seizure precautions (see *Glasgow Coma Scale*).

▶ Watch for complications, such as DIC, arthritis, endocarditis, and pneumonia.

▶ Report all cases of meningococcal disease to the state health department or the Centers for Disease Control and Prevention.

 SAFETY Droplet precautions are required in cases of meningitis caused by known or suspected *H. influenzae* type B or *Neisseria meningitidis* (meningococcal meningitis). Droplet precautions may be discontinued 24 hours after antibiotic therapy is initiated and the patient is responding.

Use standard precautions in cases of fungal meningitis and aseptic (nonbacterial or viral) bacterial gram-negative enteric meningitis in neonates and in cases of meningitis caused by *Listeria monocytogenes* and *S. pneumoniae*.

Patient teaching

▶ Teach the patient and family about the illness and expected recovery.

▶ Teach the patient about prescribed medications, including drug dosage, schedule of administration, and duration of therapy.

▶ Review with the patient symptoms that should be reported to the health care provider, signs of complications, medication dosage and adverse effects, and the need for follow-up.

 PREVENTION As a preventive measure, the meningococcal vaccine is recommended for children ages 11 to 18.

 SAFETY Prophylaxis for meningococcal meningitis is recommended for those in close contact with an infected patient, such as household contacts, day-care center employees who eat or sleep in the facility, individuals living together in military barracks or boarding schools, and medical personnel who perform mouth-to-mouth resuscitation.

Glasgow Coma Scale

To quickly assess a patient's level of consciousness and to uncover baseline changes, use the Glasgow Coma Scale. This assessment tool grades consciousness in relation to eye opening and motor and verbal responses. A decreased reaction score in one or more categories warns of an impending neurologic crisis. A patient scoring 7 or less is comatose and probably has severe neurologic damage.

Test	Patient's reaction	Score
Best eye opening response	Open spontaneously	4
	Open to verbal command	3
	Open to pain	2
	No response	1
Best motor response	Obeys verbal command	6
	Localizes painful stimuli	5
	Flexion-withdrawal	4
	Flexion-abnormal (decorticate rigidity)	3
	Extension (decerebrate rigidity)	2
	No response	1
Best verbal response	Oriented and converses	5
	Disoriented and converses	4
	Inappropriate words	3
	Incomprehensible sounds	2
	No response	1
Total		3 to 15

Meningoencephalitis, primary amebic

Primary amebic meningoencephalitis (PAM) is an acute, fulminant, and rapidly fatal infection involving the central nervous system. It is caused by the parasite *Naegleria fowleri*, a free-living ameboflagellate found in soil and fresh or brackish water (lakes, rivers, ponds). PAM develops with a rapid onset within several days of exposure and causes death within 4 to 5 days, often partly because of delayed diagnosis. Very few survivors have been reported (fewer than 12 of an estimated 200 cases).

The life cycle of *N. fowleri* has three stages: the trophozoite, a temporary flagellar stage known as ameboflagellate, and the cyst. The vegetative or feeding stage is the trophozoite stage of the ameba. This form is found in cerebrospinal fluid (CSF) or in tissue. In tissue, trophozoites ingest red and white blood cells, causing destruction. The ameboflagellate stage is a temporary form in which it neither feeds nor divides. This stage occurs when the trophozoites are exposed to a change in ionic concentration, such as in distilled water. It reverts back to the trophozoite stage within 24 hours. The resistant, protective form of the parasite is the cystic stage, which is never seen because the infection is so rapid and fatal that the patient typically dies before it occurs.

CAUSES

PAM can be contracted while swimming or diving in warm water contaminated with *N. fowleri*. In arid climates, PAM may be caused by inhalation of cysts. It enters the nose and invades the olfactory mucosa and bulbs. From there it tends to penetrate into cribriform plate, reaching the subarachnoid space and choroid plexus. It grows and multiplies in the CSF and the brain due to the glucose, protein, and oxygen supply in those regions. The CSF supports the growth and multiplication of the amebae. The organisms destroy the ependymal layer of the third, fourth, and lateral ventricles, producing acute ependymitis, but the nuclear membrane is left intact. (See *Normal circulation of CSF*.)

COMPLICATIONS

PAM is typically fatal, with the cause of death usually pulmonary edema or cardiorespiratory arrest within a week of the first symptoms. Persistent seizures have been reported in those who have otherwise recovered.

ASSESSMENT FINDINGS

History reveals exposure to fresh warm water, such as bathing in a pond or lake, 2 to 6 days prior to the onset of illness. Signs of PAM are similar to those of bacterial meningitis. The patient usually presents with symptoms of high fever, sudden onset of a frontal or bitemporal headache, nausea, and vomiting. The patient reports a stiff neck, photophobia (later sign), and alteration in taste (ageusia) or smell (parosmia). Neurologic exam reveals positive Kernig's and Brudzinski's signs, mental status changes, and signs of encephalitis and eventual herniation (cranial nerve palsies, seizures, coma). There is a rapid onset of coma and death.

DIAGNOSTIC TESTS

▶ *N. fowleri* trophozoites in nasal discharge, CSF, or brain biopsy samples provide diagnosis.

▶ Polymerase chain reaction also aids in diagnosis.

▶ Species-specific DNA probe can identify *N. fowleri* in environmental samples.

TREATMENT

Early diagnosis, treatment, and aggressive supportive care provide an increased chance of survival in patients with PAM. Amphotericin B (Abelcet) is an effective antifungal drug against *Naegleria* species and should be initiated promptly. The drug treatment of choice is amphotericin B combined with miconazole and rifampin. Ventriculostomy may be necessary in patients with signs of increased intracranial pressure and possible herniation.

Normal circulation of CSF

CSF is produced from blood in a capillary network (choroid plexus) in the brain's lateral ventricles. From the lateral ventricles, CSF flows through the interventricular foramen (foramen of Monro) to the third ventricle. From there, it flows through the aqueduct of Sylvius to the fourth ventricle and through the foramina of Luschka and Magendie to the cisterna of the subarachnoid space.

Then, the fluid passes under the base of the brain, upward over the brain's upper surfaces, and down around the spinal cord. Eventually, CSF reaches the arachnoid villi, where it's reabsorbed into venous blood at the venous sinuses.

Normally, the amount of fluid produced (about 500 ml/day) equals the amount absorbed. The average amount of CSF circulating at one time is 150 to 175 ml.

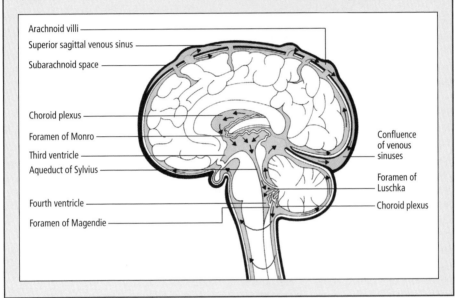

Arachnoid villi
Superior sagittal venous sinus
Subarachnoid space
Choroid plexus
Foramen of Monro
Third ventricle
Aqueduct of Sylvius
Fourth ventricle
Foramen of Magendie

Confluence of venous sinuses
Foramen of Luschka
Choroid plexus

NURSING CONSIDERATIONS

▶ Give antibiotics as ordered, and monitor renal and liver functioning as well as blood counts and therapeutic drug levels as indicated.
▶ Maintain a patent airway, and provide oxygen as ordered; suction and turn the patient frequently.
▶ Monitor vital signs as well as intake and output.
▶ Monitor neurologic status and report changes in trends.
▶ Provide comfort measures, and watch for complications.
▶ Provide emotional support for the patient and family.

Patient teaching
▶ Teach the patient and family about the illness and expected recovery.

 SAFETY Clusters of PAM cases have been associated with poorly chlorinated pools. Recommend that swimming pools be adequately chlorinated because *N. fowleri* trophozoites and cysts are susceptible to chlorine.

CONTACT PRECAUTIONS

Methicillin-resistant *Staphylococcus aureus* infection

Methicillin-resistant *S. aureus* (MRSA), a mutation of a very common bacterium, is spread easily by direct person-to-person contact. Once limited to large teaching hospitals and tertiary care centers, MRSA infection is now endemic in nursing homes, long-term care facilities, and community hospitals. It's also seen in patients who haven't been hospitalized, as community-acquired MRSA infections are increasing.

Those most at risk for MRSA infection include immunosuppressed patients, burn patients, intubated patients, and those with central venous catheters, surgical wounds, or dermatitis. Others at risk include people with prosthetic devices, such as heart valves, and postoperative wound infections. Other risk factors include prolonged hospital stays, extended therapy with multiple or broad-spectrum antibiotics, and close proximity to those colonized or infected with MRSA. Also at risk are patients with acute endocarditis, bacteremia, cervicitis, meningitis, pericarditis, and pneumonia. Community-acquired MRSA infections are becoming more common among athletes.

CAUSES

MRSA can persist on most environmental surfaces. In hospitals and other health care facilities, it's transmitted mainly by health care workers' hands. However, outbreaks have also been reported in sports such as wrestling and rugby as well as in other types of close contact. Other populations at risk include military recruits, children in day-care facilities, prison inmates, homosexual men, and veterinarians who have contact with farm animals, especially pigs. The most common route of transmission in the community is thought to be through an open wound, such as a superficial abrasion, or from contact with a carrier. Other methods of transmission include poor handwashing, poor personal hygiene (not showering after workouts), sharing personal items (razors, towels, clothing), or failure to properly clean and disinfect exercise and training equipment.

Many colonized individuals become silent or asymptomatic carriers. The most frequent site of colonization is the anterior nares (40% of adults and most children become transient nasal carriers). Less common sites are the groin, axilla, and gut. Typically, MRSA colonization is diagnosed by isolating bacteria from nasal secretions.

In individuals in whom the natural defense system breaks down, such as after an invasive procedure, trauma, or chemotherapy, the normally benign bacteria can invade tissue, proliferate, and cause infection. Up to 90% of *S. aureus* isolates or strains are resistant to penicillin, and about 50% of all *S. aureus* isolates are resistant to methicillin as well as nafcillin and oxacillin. Strains may also have developed resistance to cephalosporins, aminoglycosides, erythromycin (E-mycin), tetracycline, and clindamycin (Cleocin).

MRSA infection has become prevalent with the overuse of antibiotics. Over the years, this has given once-susceptible bacteria the chance to develop defenses against antibiotics. This new capability allows resistant strains to flourish when antibiotics kill their more-sensitive cousins.

COMPLICATIONS

Complications from MRSA include sepsis and death.

ASSESSMENT FINDINGS

Most community-acquired MRSA infections begin with symptoms of folliculitis or a similar soft-tissue or skin infection: small, red bumps that resemble pimples, boils, or spider bites. These can quickly turn into deep, painful abscesses. The bacteria can remain confined to the skin, or they can burrow deep into the body and cause life-threatening infections in joints, bones, surgical wounds, heart valves, lungs, and the blood-stream.

The initial clinical examination may reveal a limited area of redness, warmth, and swelling that is consistent with folliculitis. Occasionally, the patient may have swelling and pain in a joint. In more advanced cases, moderate to severe pain at the site of the infection may be reported; the pain may be due to soft-tissue necrosis. In severe infections, endocarditis, septicemia, necrotizing fasciitis, osteomyelitis, multisystem organ failure, or death due to overwhelming sepsis may occur. Severe cases may progress extremely rapidly.

DIAGNOSTIC TESTS

▶ MRSA can be cultured from the suspected site (such as a wound) as well as from blood, urine, or sputum.

TREATMENT

Trimethoprim-sulfamethoxazole (Bactrim), with or without rifampin, is used to treat MRSA infections. Other agents include doxycycline (Doryx), clindamycin (Cleocin), tetracycline, and minocycline (Arestin). To eradicate MRSA colonization in the nares, topical mupirocin (Bactroban) may be applied to the insides of the nostrils and an oral antibiotic may be used. Other treatments include surgical debridement of involved wounds and systemic supportive therapy.

NURSING CONSIDERATIONS

 SAFETY Good hand hygiene is the most effective way to prevent the spread of MRSA infection. People in contact with infected patients should wash their hands carefully before and after patient care. Use an antiseptic soap such as chlorhexidine, which has a residual antimicrobial effect on the skin.

◐ Contact precautions are appropriate for hospitalized patients, with a disinfected private room made available with dedicated equipment.

▶ Change gloves when contaminated or when moving from a potentially contaminated area of the body to a noncontaminated area in order to prevent transfer of microorganisms.

▶ Consider grouping infected patients together (also known as cohorting) and having the same nursing staff care for them.

▶ Don't lay equipment that has been used on the patient on the bed or bed stand. Be sure to wipe it with an appropriate disinfectant before leaving the room.

▶ Ensure judicious and careful use of antibiotics. Encourage physicians to limit the use of antibiotics.

Patient teaching

▶ Instruct the patient to take antibiotics for the full period prescribed, even if feeling better.

▶ Instruct the patient's family and friends to wear protective clothing when they visit, and show them how to dispose of it.

▶ Provide teaching and emotional support to the patient and family members.

 SAFETY Athletes should be instructed not to share personal hygiene products such as razors or towels. Medical and training staff should practice universal precautions, including proper disposal of bandages after dressing changes and routine cleaning of equipment (training tables, whirlpools, and exercise mats).

Molluscum contagiosum infection

M. contagiosum is a virus that causes a self-limiting skin disease resulting in lesions on affected areas. In adults it is considered a sexually transmitted disease. Patients who are severely immunocompromised may experience a longer disease course with more extensive and atypical lesions.

When infection occurs, the epidermal keratinocytes are targeted and viral replication occurs within the cytoplasm of the infected cell. This generates characteristic cytoplasmic inclusion bodies that appear most evident in the stratum granulosum and stratum corneum layers of the epidermis. Hyperproliferation of the epidermis also occurs because of a doubling in the epidermal basal layer.

CAUSES

Children may acquire *M. contagiosum* through skin-to-skin contact with another affected child, by sharing gymnasium equipment, or through public baths and swimming pools. Parents may report recent exposure to other children affected with *M. contagiosum* at school, camp, or public recreational facilities. The infection can also be transmitted by sexual contact with an affected partner. Individuals who are immunosuppressed may experience a more severe localized eruption. The infection usually resolves spontaneously by 18 months but can persist for as long as 5 years.

COMPLICATIONS

Complications of *M. contagiosum* include autoinoculation from trauma (shaving) or by manipulation of lesions by the patient. Cellulitis and secondary infections can also occur, resulting in abscess formation or necrotizing cellulitis.

ASSESSMENT FINDINGS

Skin lesions are about 0.04 to 0.08″ (1 to 2 mm) in diameter and appear as waxy, flesh-colored, dome-shaped, umbilicated papules with a smooth surface. In children, lesions usually are distributed on the trunk, arms, legs, and face, whereas in immunocompetent adults, lesions are found on the genitalia, lower abdomen, inner upper thighs, and/or buttocks. Lesions may be few in number or numerous, depending on the patient's immune state. Patients with human immunodeficiency virus have been known to have hundreds of systemic lesions, which are often larger than 0.8″ (2 cm) in diameter and confluent. Pruritus and perilesional eczematous reactions may also develop. The average duration of an untreated lesion is 6 to 9 months but may be as long as 5 years. *M. contagiosum* is rarely found in the oral mucosa or conjunctiva but may be located on the face.

DIAGNOSTIC TESTS

▸ Skin biopsy of the lesion confirms the diagnosis.
▸ Microscopic examination of cellular exudate in a squash preparation reveals intracytoplasmic *Molluscum* inclusion bodies (Henderson-Paterson bodies).

TREATMENT

The course of *M. contagiosum* usually is self-limited, and lesions generally heal without scarring. However, intervention may be indicated if lesions persist. Therapeutic modalities include topical application of various medications, radiation therapy, and/or surgery. Each technique might result in scarring or postinflammatory pigmentary changes.

ALERT Multiple treatment sessions are often necessary because of the recurrence of treated lesions and/or the appearance of new lesions by autoinoculation.

Topical medications are used first in treating active disease; acid and intralesional therapies are used when topical therapy fails.

Topical therapy may include imiquimod (Aldara) cream, which may be used in conjunction with the vesicant cantharidin. Tretinoin (Accutane) has reportedly been successful in the treatment of small *M. contagiosum* lesions. Tretinoin, cantharidin, and imiquimod may be self-administered by the patient. The physician may apply bichloracetic acid, trichloroacetic acid, salicylic acid, lactic acid, glycolic acid, or silver nitrate in the office. Topical podophyllotoxin cream has been effective in studies, and subcutaneous interferon alfa administered intralesionally may be useful in immunocompromised children.

Other techniques (curettage, cryosurgery, electrodesiccation, pulsed dye laser, and intense pulsed light) are effective in removing lesions but may result in scarring or postinflammatory pigment changes.

Nursing considerations

▶ Assist with treatments as indicated.
▶ Administer medications as ordered, and monitor for adverse effects.
▶ Provide skin care and comfort measures.

Patient teaching

▶ Teach the patient about the infection, including how it is transmitted, possible cause, and treatment.
▶ Teach the patient about prescribed medications, including drug dosage, schedule of administration, and duration of therapy.
▶ Tell the patient to apply ointments sparingly and only where directed; teach the patient about how to care for the affected area.
▶ If the patient is taking tretinoin, explain that it may cause photosensitivity. Warn patients of childbearing age that tretinoin is teratogenic and is known to cause extreme birth defects.

▶ Tell the patient that follow-up is recommended. Repeat examination is recommended 2 to 4 weeks after treatment as retreatment is often necessary; affected partners should also receive treatment.
▶ Teach the patient about possible complications, including signs and symptoms of infection, and highlight any complications that should be reported to the practitioner immediately.

 PREVENTION Tell the patient that good personal hygiene is important in preventing transmission of this disease. Because it is spread by close personal contact with infected people, tell the patient to avoid skin-to-skin contact with others. Transmission in children often results from swimming in pools and sharing baths, towels, gym equipment, and benches; and avoiding such practices reduces transmission. Tell the patient to avoid touching or scratching the lesions because the rash can spread by autoinoculation. Tell adults to avoid sexual contact with infected people as it is unclear whether condoms can prevent spread of the disease.
▶ Tell the patient that having multiple sexual partners and frequent unprotected sex increases the risk of infection.

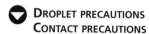

Monkeypox

Monkeypox is a rare viral disease that is identified mostly in the rainforest countries of Central and West Africa. The virus was originally discovered in laboratory monkeys and later recovered from an African squirrel, which was thought to be the natural host. It may also infect other rodents, such as rats and mice. The first human cases of monkeypox were reported in remote African locations in 1970. In June 2003, there was an outbreak in the United States involving people who had become ill following contact with infected prairie dogs.

Causes

The monkeypox virus, belonging to the orthopoxvirus group of viruses, causes monkeypox, which is related to variola and cowpox. People can contract monkeypox from an infected animal through a bite or by direct contact with the animal's blood, body fluids, or lesions. It may also be acquired by ingestion of the infected animal's inadequately cooked flesh. The infection is spread person to person via respiratory droplets during direct and prolonged face-to-face contact. Monkeypox is less infectious than smallpox, but it can also be spread through direct contact with an infected person's body fluids or with virus-contaminated objects, such as bedding or clothing.

Complications

Complications of monkeypox reported from African outbreaks include pitted scars, deforming scars, secondary bacterial infection, bronchopneumonia, respiratory distress, keratitis, corneal ulceration, blindness, septicemia, and encephalitis. Death may also occur.

Assessment findings

The signs and symptoms of monkeypox are similar to those of smallpox but milder. After an incubation period of about 12 days, the patient may report fever, headache, sore throat, cough, muscle aches, backache, swollen lymph nodes, and a general feeling of discomfort and exhaustion. Monkeypox, smallpox, and chickenpox are very similar, and the most reliable clinical sign that differentiates monkeypox from smallpox or chickenpox is the enlarged lymph nodes seen in monkeypox, especially the submental, submandibular, cervical, and inguinal nodes. A papular rash begins on the face or any other area of the body (even in areas that are usually covered) within 1 to 3 days after the onset of fever. The lesions go through several stages before crusting and falling off. Enanthema, which are lesions and inflammation of the pharyngeal, conjunctival, and genital mucosae, may develop. Exanthema lesions appearing in crops may occur within a particular body region and evolve synchronously over 14 to 21 days. The lesions do not have a strong centrifugal distribution and progress from macules to papules to vesicles and pustules. Umbilication, crusting, and desquamation follow. Most lesions are 0.2 to 0.6" (3 to 15 mm) in diameter and appear often on the face, trunk, extremities, and scalp. Lesions may also be seen on the palms of the hands and soles of the feet. Necrosis, petechiae, and ulceration may occur. Pruritus may be present, but pain may indicate a secondary bacterial infection. In children, the lesions may appear as erythematous papules that are 1 to 5 mm in diameter, suggestive of mosquito bite reactions. Subtle umbilication may be seen. The patient may develop deep pock scars as the lesions resolve. The duration of illness is 2 to 4 weeks.

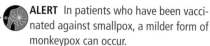

ALERT In patients who have been vaccinated against smallpox, a milder form of monkeypox can occur.

DIAGNOSTIC TESTS

▶ The virus may be isolated from vesicular fluid to aid in diagnosis and differentiation from other rash-producing viruses.
▶ Tissue may be obtained for DNA sequence-specific testing for the monkeypox virus.

TREATMENT

There is no specific treatment for monkeypox, but the smallpox vaccine appears to reduce the risk of contracting the disease.

 PREVENTION Persons who are investigating monkeypox outbreaks and caring for infected individuals or animals should receive a smallpox vaccination. Persons exposed to individuals or animals confirmed to have monkeypox should also receive vaccinations (up to 14 days after exposure).

Vaccinia immune globulin may be considered in some cases, such as in patients who are severely immunocompromised. There are no data available on the effectiveness of cidofovir (Vistide) in the treatment of monkeypox.

NURSING CONSIDERATIONS

▶ Notify the local health department immediately if you suspect monkeypox.

 SAFETY A combination of standard, contact, and droplet precautions should be applied in all health care settings where an infected person is being treated. Because of the risk of airborne transmission of monkeypox, droplet precautions should be applied whenever possible using an N-95 (or comparable) filtering disposable respirator that has been fit-tested. Surgical masks may be worn if a respirator is not available. Isolation continues until all lesions are crusted over or until the local or state health department advises that isolation is no longer necessary.

▶ Wash hands thoroughly after contact with an infected patient or contaminated objects.
▶ Place the patient in a private room. Use a negative-pressure room if available.
⊘ When transporting the patient, place a mask over his or her nose and mouth, and cover the exposed skin lesions with a sheet or gown. If the patient is to remain at home, he or she should maintain the same precautions.

Patient teaching

▶ Review the disorder and treatment with the patient and family; encourage follow-up treatment.
▶ Teach the patient about the infection, including how it is transmitted, possible cause, and treatment. Teach the patient and family proper handwashing technique.
▶ Teach the patient about the prescribed medications, including drug dosage, schedule of administration, duration of therapy, and possible adverse effects.
▶ Review signs and symptoms of complications to report to the health care provider.

 SAFETY Veterinarians, state and local public health authorities, and the Centers for Disease Control and Prevention provide guidelines for the importation of exotic animals as domestic pets. This action poses a health threat by introducing nonindigenous pathogens. Animals (or those in contact with them) that have signs of respiratory distress, mucocutaneous lesions, rhinorrhea, ocular discharge, and/or lymphadenopathy should be quarantined immediately. Tell patients and families that avoidance of contact, especially bites, scratches, and exposure to fluids and secretions, is essential.

Mononucleosis, infectious

Mononucleosis is an acute infectious disease caused by the Epstein-Barr virus (EBV), a member of the herpes group. It primarily affects young adults and children, but some cases are so mild that the infection is overlooked. Infectious mononucleosis characteristically produces fever, sore throat, and cervical lymphadenopathy. It may also cause hepatic dysfunction, increased lymphocyte and monocyte counts, and development and persistence of heterophile antibodies. The prognosis is excellent, and major complications are uncommon.

Circulating B cells spread the infection throughout the reticular endothelial system, which includes the liver, spleen, and peripheral lymph nodes. Infection of B lymphocytes produces a humoral and cellular response to the virus. The T-lymphocyte response is essential in controlling the infection because this response determines the clinical expression of viral infection. A rapid and efficient T-cell response results in control of the infection and lifelong suppression of EBV, whereas an ineffective T-cell response may lead to excessive and uncontrolled B-cell proliferation, resulting in B-lymphocyte malignancies.

CAUSES

EBV is transmitted through contact with body secretions, primarily oropharyngeal secretions, and infects the B cells in the oropharyngeal epithelium. The organism may also be shed from the uterine cervix, so genital transmission may occur in some cases. It can also be transmitted by blood transfusions and has been reported after cardiac surgery as part of the post-pump perfusion syndrome. Infectious mononucleosis is probably contagious during the period before symptoms develop until the fever subsides and oropharyngeal lesions disappear.

COMPLICATIONS

Complications from mononucleosis include splenic rupture, aseptic meningitis, encephalitis, hemolytic anemia, pericarditis, and Guillain-Barré syndrome.

ASSESSMENT FINDINGS

The symptoms of mononucleosis mimic those of many other infectious diseases, including hepatitis, rubella, and toxoplasmosis. Typically, after an incubation period of about 10 days in children and 30 to 50 days in adults, mononucleosis produces prodromal symptoms, such as headache, malaise, and fatigue. After 3 to 5 days, patients typically develop a triad of symptoms: sore throat, cervical lymphadenopathy, and temperature fluctuations, with an evening peak of 101° to 102° F (38.3° to 38.9° C). Splenomegaly, hepatomegaly, stomatitis, exudative tonsillitis, or pharyngitis may also develop.

ALERT Exudative pharyngitis that occurs in patients with mononucleosis is commonly confused with group A streptococcal pharyngitis. About 30% of patients with EBV infectious mononucleosis have group A streptococcal infection of the oropharynx. A throat culture or rapid test may be falsely positive for group A streptococci (streptococcal pharyngitis) in a patient with mononucleosis. In addition, non-exudative pharyngitis (with or without tonsillar enlargement) is common and resembles viral pharyngitis.

Sometimes, a maculopapular rash that resembles rubella develops early in the illness; jaundice occurs in about 5% of patients. Major complications are rare but may include splenic rupture, aseptic meningitis, encephalitis, hemolytic anemia, idiopathic thrombocytopenic purpura, and Guillain-Barré syndrome. Symptoms usually subside about 6 to 10 days after the onset of infection but may persist for weeks.

DIAGNOSTIC TESTS

▶ The monospot test is positive in infectious mononucleosis.

▶ Laboratory tests may reveal a leukocyte count that increases to 10,000 to 20,000/µl during the second and third weeks of illness. Lymphocytes and monocytes account for 50% to 70% of the total leukocyte count; 10% of the lymphocytes are atypical. Heterophile antibodies (agglutinins for sheep red blood cells) in serum drawn during the acute illness at 3- to 4-week intervals may rise to four times the normal number. Liver function studies are abnormal.

▶ Indirect immunofluorescence shows antibodies to EBV and cellular antigens. Such testing is usually more definitive than testing heterophile antibodies.

TREATMENT

Infectious mononucleosis resists prevention and antimicrobial treatment. Therapy is essentially supportive: relief of symptoms, bed rest during the acute febrile period, and acetaminophen (Tylenol) or ibuprofen (Motrin) for headache and sore throat. Sore throat can also be ameliorated with warm salt-water gargles. If severe throat inflammation causes airway obstruction, steroids can be used to relieve swelling. Splenic rupture, marked by sudden abdominal pain, requires splenectomy. About 20% of patients will also have streptococcal pharyngotonsillitis and should receive antibiotic therapy.

NURSING CONSIDERATIONS

▶ Administer medications as ordered; provide warm saline gargles for symptomatic relief of sore throat; provide adequate fluids and nutrition.

▶ Plan care to provide frequent rest periods; provide comfort measures and diversional therapy.

▶ Monitor vital signs and laboratory studies, and watch for signs of complications.

Patient teaching

▶ Teach the patient and family about the illness and expected recovery. Review symptoms that should be reported to the health care provider, signs of complications, and the need for follow-up.

▶ Teach the patient about prescribed medications, including the drug dosage, schedule of administration, and duration of therapy.

▶ Explain that convalescence may take several weeks, usually until the patient's leukocyte count returns to normal.

▶ During the acute illness, stress the need for bed rest. Warn the patient to avoid excessive activity, which could lead to splenic rupture. If the patient is a student, explain that undertaking less demanding school assignments and seeing friends are fine, but he or she should avoid long, difficult projects until after recovery.

▶ To minimize throat discomfort, encourage the patient to drink milkshakes, fruit juices, and broths and to eat cool, bland foods. Suggest gargling with saline mouthwash and taking aspirin as needed.

 PREVENTION Patients should avoid exposing other people to their affected body secretions because virus remains viable for months after the initial infection.

DROPLET PRECAUTIONS

Mumps

Mumps, also known as infectious or epidemic parotitis, is an acute viral disease caused by a paramyxovirus. It causes painful enlargement of the salivary or parotid glands. It may also infect the testes, the central nervous system (CNS), and the pancreas. The prognosis for complete recovery is good, although mumps sometimes causes complications.

CAUSES

The mumps paramyxovirus is found in the saliva of an infected person and is transmitted either by respiratory droplets or by direct contact. The virus is present in the saliva 7 days before to 9 days after the onset of parotid gland swelling and in the urine for as long as 2 weeks after swelling begins; the 48-hour period immediately preceding the onset of swelling is probably the time of highest communicability. The incubation period ranges from 14 to 29 days (the average is 18 days). One attack of mumps (even if unilateral) almost always confers lifelong immunity.

Mumps is most prevalent in children between ages 6 and 8. Infants younger than age 1 seldom get this disease because of the passive immunity received from maternal antibodies. Peak incidence occurs during late winter and early spring.

After the virus enters the respiratory system, it replicates locally and then disseminates to target tissue, such as the CNS and salivary glands (particularly the parotid glands). A secondary phase of viremia commences when replication of the virus occurs at the target organs. The virus can travel through the bloodstream to the kidneys, potentially impairing renal function. Cell necrosis and inflammation occur with mononuclear cell infiltration. The salivary glands show edema and desquamation of ductal lining, and focal hemorrhage and destruction of epithelium may occur, leading to ductal plugging.

COMPLICATIONS

Meningoencephalitis is the most frequent complication of mumps and affects 10% of patients. Signs and symptoms of meningoencephalitis include fever, meningeal irritation (nuchal rigidity, headache, and irritability), vomiting, drowsiness, and a cerebrospinal fluid lymphocyte count ranging from 500 to 2,000/μl. Recovery is usually complete, but complications can occur.

Other complications of mumps may include hearing loss, orchitis, oophoritis, pancreatitis, transient myelitis, polyneuritis, myocarditis, nephritis, arthritis, thyroiditis, thrombocytopenic purpura, mastitis, and pneumonia. Epididymo-orchitis, the abrupt onset of testicular swelling and tenderness, scrotal erythema, lower abdominal pain, nausea, vomiting, fever, and chills, occurs in about 25% of postpubertal males and may cause sterility.

ASSESSMENT FINDINGS

The clinical features of mumps vary widely. Diagnosis is usually made after the characteristic signs and symptoms develop, especially parotid gland enlargement with a history of exposure to mumps. Mumps usually begins with prodromal symptoms that last for 24 hours and include myalgia, anorexia, malaise, headache, and low-grade fever followed by an earache that's aggravated by chewing, parotid gland tenderness and swelling, a temperature of 101° to 104° F (38.3° to 40° C), and pain when chewing or when drinking sour or acidic liquids. One or more of the other salivary glands may become swollen simultaneously with the swelling of the parotid gland or several days later. (See *Parotid inflammation in mumps.*)

DIAGNOSTIC TESTS

▶ Mumps virus can be isolated in a cell culture from throat washings, urine, or spinal fluid.

▶ Complement fixation, neutralization, hemagglutination inhibition, and enzyme immunoassay are serologic tests that can confirm infection or vaccination.

Parotid inflammation in mumps

The mumps virus (paramyxovirus) attacks the parotid glands—the main salivary glands. Inflammation causes characteristic swelling and discomfort associated with eating, drinking, swallowing, and talking.

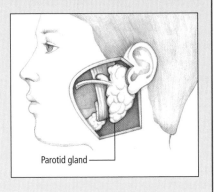

Parotid gland

▶ Blood work shows an elevated serum amylase level in patients with mumps parotitis and pancreatitis; the serum lipase level is elevated in pancreatitis. A complete blood count may show elevated lymphocytes. Elevated serum C-reactive protein may occur in mumps orchitis.

TREATMENT

Treatment includes analgesics for pain, antipyretics for fever, and adequate fluid intake to prevent dehydration from fever and anorexia. If the patient can't swallow, consider I.V. fluid replacement. Warm salt-water gargles, soft foods, and extra fluids may also help relieve symptoms.

NURSING CONSIDERATIONS

▶ Stress the need for bed rest during the febrile period. Give analgesics and apply warm or cool compresses to the neck to relieve pain. Give antipyretics and tepid sponge baths for fever.
▶ During the acute phase, observe the patient closely for signs of CNS involvement,

such as altered level of consciousness and nuchal rigidity.
▶ Report all cases of mumps to the state health department or the Centers for Disease Control and Prevention.

 SAFETY Because the mumps virus is present in the saliva throughout the course of the disease, follow droplet precautions until symptoms subside. After the onset of swelling, susceptible health care workers should not provide care if immune caregivers are available.

Patient teaching

▶ To prevent dehydration, encourage the patient to drink fluids. To minimize pain and anorexia, advise the patient to avoid spicy, irritating foods and foods that require a lot of chewing. Offer a soft, bland diet.
▶ List the complications the patient should watch for and report to the physician.

PREVENTION Emphasize the importance of routine immunization with live attenuated mumps virus (paramyxovirus) at age 12 to 15 months. The vaccine is usually given in a combination that includes measles, mumps, and rubella (MMR). A second dose of MMR vaccine is recommended at age 4 to 6 years; if this dose is missed, it should be given before age 12. Immunization within 24 hours of exposure may prevent or attenuate the disease. Immunity against mumps lasts at least 12 years.

 SAFETY Droplet precautions continue until 9 days after the onset of parotid swelling, and affected children should be excluded from school and day-care centers for that 9-day period. If outbreaks occur in a school or day-care center, recommend that all children and staff be vaccinated, as appropriate (pregnant women and severely immunocompromised people should not receive the vaccination; alternatives may include immune globulin). If vaccination is withheld for medical, religious, or other reasons, the individuals should be excluded from school or day care until at least 26 days after the onset of parotitis in the last person affected in the school.

Mycobacterium avium complex

M. avium complex consists of two species, *M. avium* and *M. intracellulare.* They together are referred to as *M. avium-intracellulare. M. avium* complex causes lung disease in healthy individuals and disseminated infection in immunocompromised hosts. Patients with underlying lung disease or immunosuppression may develop progressive disease. *M. avium* complex is the most common cause of infection in patients with acquired immunodeficiency syndrome (AIDS).

CAUSES

M. avium complex has been isolated from fresh water and salt water worldwide. Common environmental sources include aerosolized water, piped hot water systems (including household and hospital water supplies), bathrooms, house dust, soil, birds, farm animals, and cigarette components such as tobacco, filters, and paper. It has also been associated with hot tubs. *M. avium* complex is transmitted by inhalation through the respiratory tract and also by ingestion through the GI tract. *M. avium* complex invades the mucosal epithelium, infecting macrophages, and is eventually carried to local lymph nodes by the lymphatic system. In immunocompromised hosts, the infection can spread to the liver, spleen, bone marrow, and other sites. Pulmonary disease is the most common manifestation, as well as lymphadenitis in children and cervical adenitis in adults.

COMPLICATIONS

Complications in patients with AIDS include anemia, weight loss, and death. Those with lung disease may also develop respiratory insufficiency.

ASSESSMENT FINDINGS

M. avium complex infection usually presents as pulmonary infection in immunocompetent hosts, disseminated infection in those with advanced AIDS, or lymphadenitis in children. Physical findings depend on the form of infection and the health of the patient.

Immunocompetent hosts that develop pulmonary infection may have a cough, sputum production, weight loss, fever, lethargy, and night sweats, with an insidious onset of symptoms that last for weeks to months. Lung crackles and rhonchi can be heard on auscultation; tachypnea, dullness on chest percussion, and/or bronchial breath sounds may also be present.

In those with advanced AIDS (CD4 counts of less than 50 cells/μl), fever is common, as are sweating, weight loss, fatigue, diarrhea, shortness of breath, and right upper quadrant abdominal pain. Generalized wasting, skin pallor, tender hepatosplenomegaly, and lymphadenopathy are often present. Other manifestations include mastitis, pyomyositis, cutaneous abscess, brain abscess, and GI mycobacteriosis.

Lymphadenitis of unilateral cervical lymph nodes often occurs in children ages 1 to 4. Affected nodes most often include the submandibular and submaxillary, although preauricular, postauricular, and submental nodes may be affected. Rarely, axillary, epitrochlear, or inguinal nodes are affected. The nodes are rubbery to firm on palpation and may group together as the disease progresses. The skin over the area may appear shiny, thin, and erythematous. The lymph nodes usually enlarge and then resolve spontaneously; however, caseation may occur with nodes rupturing through the skin, forming sinus tracts with chronic discharge.

With skin and soft-tissue infections, osteomyelitis, peritonitis (in patients with cirrhosis), bursitis, septic arthritis, and tenosynovitis may occur. Affected joints will be painful and swollen.

DIAGNOSTIC TESTS

▶ Sputum acid-fast bacillus (AFB) stains are positive for *M. avium* complex in most patients with pulmonary infection. Mycobacterial cultures grow in about 1 to 2 weeks.

 ALERT To obtain the best specimen for AFB staining and culture, sputum should be obtained early in the morning on three different days.

▶ Enzyme immunoassay is useful in serodiagnosis, detecting serum immunoglobulin A antibody to *M. avium* complex–specific glycopeptidolipid core antigen.

▶ Chest radiography and computed tomography may show nodules.

▶ Biopsy specimens of nodes, bronchoscopy, or transbronchial specimens are positive for *M. avium* complex. In children, needle aspiration of the node may be performed.

▶ Blood cultures are usually positive later in the course of infection. Elevated transaminase and alkaline phosphatase levels occur in disseminated disease. Complete blood count shows anemia and occasionally pancytopenia due to bone marrow suppression secondary to the infection.

▶ Lymph node, bone marrow, or liver biopsy can confirm a diagnosis of disseminated infection in patients with AIDS.

TREATMENT

In addition to supportive therapy for oxygenation, hydration, and nutrition, antimycobacterial agents are used. Clarithromycin (Biaxin), azithromycin (Zithromax), rifabutin (Mycobutin), ethambutol (Myambutol), levofloxacin (Levaquin), and amikacin are preferred therapies; newer fluoroquinolones, linezolid (Zyvox), and ketolides may also be effective. Aerosolized amikacin is an effective adjunct therapy. Treatment of infection in immunocompetent patients and those with disseminated disease involves a combination of agents.

Lymphadenitis in children is treated with surgical excision of the affected lymph nodes. The surgical cure rate is less than 90%, and although antibiotics are generally not required, they may be beneficial in patients with extensive lymphadenitis or in those with a poor surgical response.

Prophylaxis in patients with AIDS who have low CD4 cell counts consists of clarithromycin, azithromycin, or rifabutin. Prophylaxis dramatically reduces the incidence of disease in patients with AIDS.

NURSING CONSIDERATIONS

▶ Administer medications as ordered, and monitor for adverse effects.

▶ Administer blood transfusions, if ordered, and monitor blood counts.

▶ Monitor respiratory rate, breath sounds, and oxygenation status; encourage deep breathing and coughing; suction as indicated.

Patient teaching

 PREVENTION It is recommended that patients with AIDS and CD4 cell counts less than 50 cells/μl should receive a prophylactic antibiotic to prevent infection with *M. avium* complex. Clarithromycin or azithromycin is usually used; alternatively, rifabutin can be used.

Those who have received treatment for *M. avium* complex should remain on the treatment regimen until their CD4 count increases to more than 100 cells/μl.

▶ Teach the patient about prescribed medications, including drug dosage, schedule of administration, adverse effects, and duration of therapy.

▶ Tell the patient how to recognize signs of anemia and other complications, and encourage follow-up with health care providers.

Mycotoxicosis

Diseases caused by mycotoxins are called mycotoxicoses. Trichothecene mycotoxins are low-molecular-weight compounds produced by more than 350 species of fungi and are pathogenic to animals and humans. The T-2 mycotoxin is the most extensively studied of the trichothecenes and is the only mycotoxin known to have been used as a biological weapon. Mycotoxins such as trichothecene are potential biological weapon agents because they can be absorbed through intact skin and cause systemic toxicity. Mycotoxins can be delivered by food or water sources as well as via droplets, aerosols, or smoke from dispersal systems and exploding munitions.

CAUSES

Mycotoxicoses occur when mycotoxins enter the body, usually by ingestion. Different mycotoxins cause different diseases. Trichothecene mycotoxins are very cytotoxic and potentially immunosuppressive. Mycotoxins can be absorbed by topical, oral, and inhalational routes and can act as a dermal irritant and blistering agent. Local or systemic toxicity can result from any route of exposure (dermal, oral, or inhalational), depending on the mycotoxin.

COMPLICATIONS

Complications may include vascular collapse, desquamation and necrosis of dermal layers, severe dizziness, ataxia, and prostration.

ASSESSMENT FINDINGS

Patients with cutaneous symptoms may report seeing clouds of a yellow-colored smoke or aerosol, but blue and green aerosols have also been reported. Yellow droplets may be present on clothing, and affected individuals may experience immediate pain and burning on exposed skin surfaces and in the eyes.

Redness, rash, and blistering may be present; other symptoms of mycotoxin exposure may include vomiting, diarrhea, dyspnea, and bleeding. With virulent toxins such as trichothecene, some symptoms may appear within seconds of exposure while others develop over hours, days, or longer.

With systemic exposure, trichothecene mycotoxicoses produce more severe symptoms such as mild ataxia. Ocular exposure causes tearing, pain, conjunctivitis, and blurred vision. Nasal mucosa exposure results in sinus irritation, pain, rhinorrhea, sneezing, and potentially epistaxis. Oral and oropharyngeal exposure produces pain and blood-tinged saliva and sputum. Pulmonary symptoms include cough, dyspnea, and wheezing. Other symptoms include tachycardia, nausea, vomiting, anorexia, watery diarrhea, and abdominal cramping.

Chronic exposure to trichothecene toxin can produce the clinical syndrome of alimentary toxic aleukia, which is similar to radiation sickness. Weeks after exposure, bone marrow suppression with significant leukopenia, granulocytopenia, and thrombocytopenia occur with severe coagulopathy. Petechial hemorrhages and ulcerated and necrotic lesions can result in significant bleeding from the esophagus and GI tract. Edema accompanying the mucosal injury may threaten the airway.

DIAGNOSTIC TESTS

‣ Spectrometric evaluation of nasal, throat, or respiratory secretions helps diagnose trichothecene mycotoxin exposure. Toxin can be detected in the postexposure phase in serum, urine, and/or tissue samples.
‣ Enzyme-linked immunosorbent assay and antibody assays for mycotoxin exposure are available.
‣ Serial absolute lymphocyte counts can help detect early bone marrow suppression.
‣ A coagulation panel identifies those at risk for developing severe coagulopathy.

TREATMENT

The trichothecene toxin decontamination procedure, which includes removing the patient's clothing and scrubbing the skin surfaces with soap and water within 6 hours of exposure, can remove 80% to 98% of the toxin and prevent adverse reactions.

 SAFETY Trichothecene toxin is a potent dermally active toxin that can be transmissible if not properly decontaminated. Standard precautions should be used prior to approaching the patient. In addition, clothing from the patient should be contained to avoid contamination of the health care environment.

Patients who have ingested trichothecene toxin may be given activated charcoal. In those with severe neutropenia, filgrastim (Neupogen) may be given. Supportive measures are otherwise instituted for airway compromise, impaired hemodynamic status, and GI symptoms. Eye exposure calls for irrigation of the area with copious amounts of water.

NURSING CONSIDERATIONS

❯ Assist with decontamination as appropriate.
❯ Monitor respiratory status. Provide support for airway, breathing, and circulation per facility protocol as indicated.
❯ If the patient requires mechanical ventilation, monitor oxygenation status and provide suction as indicated; turn the patient every 2 hours, and provide respiratory treatments as ordered.
❯ Monitor cardiovascular status, vital signs, and intake and output; maintain fluid status.
❯ Maintain I.V. therapy as ordered; monitor laboratory results.
❯ Contact the local poison control center for additional guidance; depending on the situation, specific guidelines may need to be followed concerning weapons of mass destruction. Consultation with the Federal Bureau of Investigation and the Department of Homeland Security is required in any situation in which biological weapon exposure is suspected.

Patient teaching

❯ Teach the patient about the prescribed medication, including drug dosage, schedule of administration, adverse effects, and duration of therapy.
❯ Teach the patient about possible complications, including signs and symptoms to report to the practitioner. Review the disease course and treatment regimen; if wound care is required, have the patient perform return demonstrations.

Myocarditis

Myocarditis is focal or diffuse inflammation of the cardiac muscle (myocardium). It may be acute or chronic and can occur at any age. In many cases, myocarditis fails to produce specific cardiovascular symptoms or electrocardiographic abnormalities, and recovery is usually spontaneous and without residual defects. Occasionally, myocarditis is complicated by heart failure; in rare cases, it leads to cardiomyopathy.

CAUSES

Myocarditis can result from a wide variety of infectious organisms, autoimmune disorders, exogenous agents, and genetic and environmental factors. Viral infections are the most common cause of myocarditis in the United States and Western Europe. The more common viruses include coxsackievirus A and B strains and, possibly, poliomyelitis, influenza, rubeola, rubella, and adenoviruses and echoviruses. Bacterial infections that may cause myocarditis include diphtheria, tuberculosis, typhoid fever, tetanus, and staphylococcal, pneumococcal, and gonococcal infections. Helminthic infections, such as trichinosis and parasitic infections, especially trypanosomiasis (Chagas disease) in infants and immunosuppressed adults, can be the cause, as can toxoplasmosis. Other causes include hypersensitive immune reactions such as acute rheumatic fever, systemic immune diseases, postcardiotomy syndrome, radiation therapy, and certain drugs and chemicals. Venemous bites or stings that may result in myocarditis include those of the scorpion, snake, black widow spider, and wasp.

COMPLICATIONS

Complications from myocarditis include arrhythmias, thromboembolism, chronic valvulitis (when disease results from rheumatic fever), and recurrence of disease.

Occasionally left-sided heart failure can occur, and cardiomyopathy is rare.

ASSESSMENT FINDINGS

Myocarditis usually causes nonspecific symptoms, such as fatigue, dyspnea, palpitations, and fever that reflect the accompanying systemic infection. Occasionally, it may produce mild, continuous pressure or soreness in the chest. The patient history commonly reveals recent febrile upper respiratory tract infection, viral pharyngitis, or tonsillitis. Physical examination shows supraventricular and ventricular arrhythmias, S_3 and S_4 gallops, a faint S_1, possibly a murmur of mitral insufficiency (from papillary muscle dysfunction) and, if pericarditis is present, a pericardial friction rub. Although myocarditis is usually self-limiting, it may induce myofibril degeneration that results in right- and left-sided heart failure, with cardiomegaly, jugular vein distention, dyspnea, persistent fever with resting or exertional tachycardia disproportionate to the degree of fever, and supraventricular and ventricular arrhythmias. Sometimes myocarditis recurs or produces chronic valvulitis (when it results from rheumatic fever), cardiomyopathy, arrhythmias, and thromboembolism.

DIAGNOSIS

▸ Cardiac enzymes may show elevated creatine kinase-MB, aspartate aminotransferase, and lactate dehydrogenase levels. An increased white blood cell count and erythrocyte sedimentation rate as well as elevated antibody titers (such as antistreptolysin-O titer in rheumatic fever) may be present.
▸ Although endomyocardial biopsy confirms the diagnosis, the procedure is rarely performed because it is invasive and costly. A negative biopsy doesn't exclude the diagnosis, and a repeat biopsy may be needed.
▸ Electrocardiography typically shows diffuse ST-segment and T-wave abnormalities as in pericarditis, conduction defects (prolonged PR interval), and other supraventricular arrhythmias.

▶ Echocardiography demonstrates some degree of left ventricular dysfunction, and radionuclide scanning may identify inflammatory and necrotic changes characteristic of myocarditis.

▶ Serum and viral antibody titers may identify viral causation; stool and throat cultures may identify bacteria.

TREATMENT

Treatment includes antibiotics for bacterial infection, modified bed rest to decrease heart workload, and careful management of complications. Inotropic support of cardiac function may be needed. Heart failure requires restriction of activity to minimize myocardial oxygen consumption, supplemental oxygen therapy, sodium restriction, diuretics to decrease fluid retention, and cardiac glycosides to increase myocardial contractility. However, cardiac glycosides should be administered cautiously because some patients with myocarditis may show a paradoxical sensitivity to even small doses. Arrhythmias necessitate prompt but cautious administration of antiarrhythmics because these drugs depress myocardial contractility. Thromboembolism requires anticoagulation therapy. Treatment with corticosteroids or other immunosuppressants may be used to reduce inflammation, but they haven't been shown to change the progression of myocarditis infections.

Surgical treatment may include placement of left ventricular assistive devices and extracorporeal membrane oxygenation for support of cardiogenic shock. Cardiac transplantation has been beneficial for giant cell myocarditis.

NURSING CONSIDERATIONS

▶ Assess cardiovascular status frequently, watching for signs of heart failure and arrhythmias.

▶ Observe for signs of adverse effects of medications; if the patient is receiving cardiac glycosides, monitor for digoxin toxicity and for factors that may potentiate toxicity (electrolyte imbalance or hypoxia).

▶ Stress the importance of bed rest, and assist with care as needed.

Patient teaching

▶ During recovery, recommend that the patient resume normal activities slowly and avoid competitive sports.

▶ Instruct the patient to obtain prompt treatment of causative disorders.

▶ Instruct the patient to practice good hygiene, including thorough handwashing, and to thoroughly wash and cook food.

 PREVENTION Encourage the patient and family to obtain appropriate vaccinations. Vaccinations ultimately can reduce the incidence of myocarditis caused by measles, rubella, mumps, poliomyelitis, and influenza. Research is ongoing for the development of vaccines for other cardiotropic viruses in order to prevent viral myocarditis.

Necrotizing fasciitis

Most commonly referred to as flesh-eating bacteria, necrotizing fasciitis is a progressive, rapidly spreading inflammatory infection located in the deep fascia that destroys fascia and fat with secondary necrosis of subcutaneous tissue. It is also referred to as hemolytic streptococcal gangrene, acute dermal gangrene, suppurative fasciitis, and synergistic necrotizing cellulitis. The mortality rate is very high but drops significantly with early intervention and treatment. Treating patients aggressively with surgery, antibiotics, and hyperbaric oxygen therapy can significantly reduce mortality.

CAUSES

Necrotizing fasciitis is most commonly caused by the pathogenic bacteria *Streptococcus pyogenes*, also known as group A *Streptococcus*, of which there are more than 80 types in existence. The bacteria enter the body through a wound, such as a pinprick, needle puncture, bruise, blister, or abrasion, or through a traumatic injury or surgical incision. They can also enter through a breach in a mucous membrane barrier. Other aerobic and anaerobic pathogens, including *Staphylococcus aureus*, *Bacteroides*, *Clostridium*, *Peptostreptococcus*, Enterobacteriaceae, coliforms, *Proteus*, *Pseudomonas*, and *Klebsiella*, may also be present. These pathogens can proliferate in an environment of tissue hypoxia caused by trauma, recent surgery, or medical compromise. The end product of this invasion is necrosis of the surrounding tissue, which accelerates the disease process by creating an even more favorable environment for the organisms.

COMPLICATIONS

Complications include renal failure, septic shock with cardiovascular collapse, scarring with cosmetic deformities, myositis, and myonecrosis.

ASSESSMENT FINDINGS

Pain that is out of proportion to the size of the wound or injury is usually the first symptom of necrotizing fasciitis. The infective process begins with a mild area of erythema at the site, changing in color from red to purple to blue, with the formation of fluid-filled blisters and bullae within 48 hours. By days 4 and 5, multiple patches of this erythema form, producing large areas of gangrenous skin. By days 7 to 10, dead skin begins to separate at the margins of the erythema, revealing extensive necrosis of the subcutaneous tissue. Other clinical symptoms include fever and hypovolemia. In later stages, hypotension, respiratory insufficiency, and overwhelming sepsis requiring supportive care ensue. In the most severe cases, necrosis advances rapidly until several large areas of the body are involved and the patient becomes less alert, delirious, or even unresponsive.

DIAGNOSTIC TESTS

▶ Cultures of microorganisms obtained from the periphery of the spreading infection or biopsy of deeper tissue obtained during surgical debridement detect the organism. Gram stain and culture of biopsied tissue are useful in establishing the type(s) of invasive organisms present and the effective treatment against them.
▶ Radiographic studies show the presence of subcutaneous gases, and computed tomography can locate necrosis. In combination with clinical assessment, magnetic resonance imaging determines areas of necrosis and the need for surgical debridement.
▶ A complete blood count would show an elevated white blood cell count, an elevated blood urea nitrogen, and a decreased serum sodium level.

TREATMENT

Prompt and aggressive exploration and debridement of suspected necrotizing fasciitis are mandatory for early, definitive diagnosis and to improve prognosis. Ninety percent of patients who present with clinical signs and symptoms will need immediate surgical debridement, fasciotomy, or amputation.

Penicillin, clindamycin (Cleocin), metronidazole (Flagyl), ceftriaxone (Rocephin), gentamicin, chloramphenicol (Amphicol), and ampicillin, alone or in combination, are effective in treating the organisms involved with necrotizing fasciitis. Recommendations for specific drugs change as new antibiotics are developed and new resistance emerges.

Hyperbaric oxygen therapy may be used to improve the tissue defense against infection as well as to prevent the necrosis from spreading by increasing the normal oxygen saturation of infected wounds by 1,000-fold, causing a bactericidal effect. It is typically started after the first surgical debridement and continues for a total of 10 to 15 sessions.

NURSING CONSIDERATIONS

▶ Administer antibiotic therapy immediately.
▶ Assess the patient's pain level, mental status, wound status, and vital signs to recognize the progression of the wound changes or the development of new signs and symptoms. Changes must be reported immediately.
▶ Provide supportive care, such as endotracheal intubation, cardiac monitoring, fluid replacement, and supplemental oxygen as indicated.
▶ Institute strict sterile technique, good hand hygiene, and barriers between health care providers and patients to prevent contamination.

 SAFETY Health care workers with sore throats should see their physician to determine whether they have a streptococcal infection. If infection is present, they shouldn't return to work until 24 hours after the initiation of antibiotic therapy.

 ALERT Watch for signs and symptoms of toxic shock syndrome, which is associated with any streptococcal soft-tissue infection, and the development of shock, acute respiratory distress syndrome, renal impairment, or bacteremia, any of which can lead to sudden death.

Patient teaching

▶ Patients at risk for necrotizing fasciitis include elderly people and those with human immunodeficiency virus infection or a history of alcohol abuse or varicella infection. Patients with chronic illnesses (cancer, diabetes, cardiopulmonary disease, and kidney disease requiring hemodialysis) and those using steroids are more susceptible due to their debilitated immune response. Teach patients how to prevent this disorder by receiving prompt treatment for injuries and illnesses and maintaining optimum health with proper nutrition, exercise, and adequate rest.
▶ Review signs and symptoms of complications that should be reported to the health care provider.
▶ Explain the disorder and its treatment to the patient; review the medications prescribed, including the dosage schedule and adverse effects.

Nocardiosis

Nocardiosis is an acute, subacute, or chronic bacterial infection caused by weakly gram-positive bacilli of the genus *Nocardia*—usually *Nocardia asteroides*. It can occur in cutaneous, lymphocutaneous, and subcutaneous forms following local traumatic inoculation. Dissemination from these sites is more likely in immunocompromised hosts. Pleuropulmonary nocardiosis is thought to arise from inhalation exposure. Disseminated nocardiosis is spread first through the bloodstream, usually from a pulmonary focus, and then to the central nervous system (CNS) or skin. Most persons with disseminated disease are immunocompromised or receiving immunosuppressive therapy.

CAUSES

Nocardia are aerobic bacilli with branching filaments that resemble fungi. Normally found in soil, these opportunistic pathogens cause occasional sporadic disease in humans and animals throughout the world. Their incubation period is unknown but is probably several weeks. The usual mode of transmission is inhalation of organisms suspended in dust. Transmission by direct inoculation through puncture wounds or abrasions is less common.

COMPLICATIONS

Complications include meningitis, seizures, and cardiac arrhythmias. Other potential complications include tracheitis, bronchitis, pericarditis, endocarditis, peritonitis, mediastinitis, septic arthritis, and keratoconjunctivitis.

ASSESSMENT FINDINGS

The physical findings in patients with nocardiosis will vary depending on the site of infection and extent of dissemination. Nocardiosis originating as a pulmonary infection produces a cough with thick, tenacious,

purulent, mucopurulent, and possibly blood-tinged sputum. It may also cause a fever as high as 105° F (40.6° C), chills, night sweats, anorexia, malaise, and weight loss. This infection may lead to pleurisy, intrapleural effusions, and empyema.

If the infection spreads through the blood to the brain, abscesses form, causing confusion, disorientation, dizziness, headache, nausea, and seizures. Rupture of a brain abscess can cause purulent meningitis. Extrapulmonary, hematogenous spread may cause endocarditis or lesions in the kidneys, liver, subcutaneous tissue, and bone.

Cutaneous nocardiosis may present as a cutaneous, lymphocutaneous, or subcutaneous infection. Cutaneous nocardiosis manifests with symptoms of cellulitis or nontender erythematous nodules at the site of traumatic inoculation. These nodules may drain purulent material. Lymphocutaneous nocardiosis is evident by lesions with ascending regional lymphadenopathy, which may also drain purulent material. In tropical areas of the world, mycetoma of the extremities may occur as a chronic, swollen, purulence-draining, subcutaneous infection.

DIAGNOSTIC FINDINGS

▶ The diagnosis of nocardiosis is established with culture of the causative organism from the infection site (respiratory secretions, skin biopsy samples, and aspirates from abscesses).

 ALERT The microbiology laboratory should always be notified when nocardiosis is suspected as nocardiae are very slow growing, especially when sputum is the specimen. *Nocardia* species can usually be isolated in 3 to 5 days, some up to 7 days.

▶ There are no characteristic chest radiography or computed tomography findings, but these imaging methods may show irregular nodules (which may cavitate), pulmonary infiltrates, lung abscess formation, and pleural effusion.

▶ In brain infection with meningitis, lumbar puncture shows nonspecific changes such as increased opening pressure. Cerebrospinal fluid (CSF) shows increased white blood cell and protein levels and decreased glucose levels compared with serum glucose.

TREATMENT

Sulfonamides are the preferred antimicrobial therapy for nocardiosis, especially sulfadiazine because of its CNS and CSF penetration. An alternative to sulfadiazine is trimethoprim-sulfamethoxazole (Bactrim); others include carbapenem, meropenem (Merrem), third-generation cephalosporins (cefotaxime [Claforan] or ceftriaxone [Rocephin]), and amikacin, either alone or in combination. Meropenem with amikacin is often preferred. Oral therapy with minocycline (Arestin) and amoxicillin-clavulanic acid (Augmentin) is prescribed for mild cases or given after I.V. antibiotic therapy for continued treatment. Antimicrobial therapy for pulmonary or disseminated nocardiosis is continued for 6 to 12 months, including at least 1 month of treatment after resolution of clinical signs. Treatment also includes surgical drainage of abscesses and excision of necrotic tissue. The acute phase requires complete bed rest; as the patient improves, activity can increase.

 SAFETY Because it isn't transmitted from person to person, nocardiosis requires only standard precautions.

NURSING CONSIDERATIONS

▶ Provide adequate nourishment through total parenteral nutrition, nasogastric tube feedings, or a balanced diet.

▶ Give the patient tepid sponge baths and antipyretics, as ordered, to reduce fever.

▶ Monitor for allergic reactions to antibiotics.

▶ High-dose sulfonamide therapy (especially sulfadiazine) predisposes the patient to crystalluria and oliguria, so assess him or her frequently, force fluids, and alkalinize the urine with sodium bicarbonate, as ordered, to prevent these complications.

▶ In patients with pulmonary infection, administer chest physiotherapy. Auscultate the lungs daily, checking for increased crackles or consolidation. Note and record the amount, color, and thickness of sputum.

▶ In brain infection, regularly assess neurologic function. Watch for signs of increased intracranial pressure, such as a decreased level of consciousness and respiratory abnormalities.

▶ In long-term hospitalization, turn the patient often and assist with range-of-motion exercises.

▶ Provide support and encouragement to help the patient and family cope with this long-term illness.

Patient teaching

▶ Before the patient is discharged, stress the need to comply with treatment and follow a regular medication schedule to maintain therapeutic blood levels. Explain the importance of frequent follow-up examinations.

▶ Educate the patient about the prescribed medications, including drug dosage and adverse effects. Stress the importance of continuing to take medications even after symptoms subside.

▶ Review symptoms of complications to report to the health care provider.

CONTACT PRECAUTIONS

Norwalk virus infection

Norwalk virus, among a group called noroviruses, is a single-stranded RNA virus of the Caliciviridae family that causes acute gastroenteritis lasting 24 to 48 hours. Recurrent infections may occur throughout life because of the diversity of strains and the lack of long-term immunity. The virus is shed in vomitus and feces, and contamination can occur through an infected water supply, undercooked foods, or improper handwashing by an infected food preparer. Secondary transmission commonly occurs among close contacts of the infected person. Cruise ships are particularly vulnerable because of crowding and the difficulty in performing decontamination during short periods ashore.

CAUSES

Norwalk virus is highly contagious and transmitted via the fecal-oral route and through aerosolized particles during vomiting. The most common routes of infection include person-to-person contact and contaminated food or water supplies. Foods often involved include salad, cake frosting, clams, oysters, and meats. The virus can survive freezing as well as heating temperatures of up to 140° F (60° C). The infection causes damage to microvilli in the small intestine, producing malabsorption; vomiting occurs as a result of changes in gastric motility and delayed gastric emptying.

COMPLICATIONS

Complications from Norwalk virus infection include dehydration and, rarely, death. Severe dehydration can cause electrolyte abnormalities (hyponatremia, hypokalemia, hypochloremia, and metabolic alkalosis), hypovolemic shock, and cardiovascular collapse. Norwalk virus infection can exacerbate inflammatory bowel disease and has also caused encephalopathy in pediatric patients.

ASSESSMENT FINDINGS

Symptoms develop 24 to 48 hours after ingestion of contaminated food or water or contact with an infected individual. Each gastroenteritis episode is short-lived, lasting about 1 to 2 days. Signs and symptoms typically include nausea and profuse, nonbloody, nonbilious vomiting as well as watery diarrhea, abdominal cramps, headache, low-grade fever, and myalgia. Tachycardia and possibly hypotension may occur if the patient is dehydrated. Physical examination of the abdomen usually reveals the absence of tenderness and peritoneal signs.

DIAGNOSTIC TESTS

▶ Stool specimens can detect isolates for Norwalk virus, although isolated cases of infection usually don't require laboratory testing. Stool culture will be negative for infectious bacteria and hemoglobin, and fecal leukocytes will be absent. Because studies are very costly, stool evaluation is not recommended unless strong public health indications exist.

 SAFETY Two or more people living in different households who shared a common meal or three or more people living in the same household who are symptomatic is considered an epidemic and the cause of gastroenteritis should be investigated. Epidemics can occur from a common source. In an epidemic setting, the health department may evaluate infected stool with polymerase chain reaction (PCR) for noroviruses.

▶ PCR or electron microscopy can detect the virus; newer diagnostics such as microarrays are currently under investigation.
▶ Serum electrolytes, blood urea nitrogen, and creatinine show values associated with dehydration in severe cases of gastroenteritis.
▶ Radioimmunoassay and enzyme-linked immunosorbent assay techniques have been developed to detect the virus and the viral antigen.

TREATMENT

The disease is usually self-limiting and lasts about 24 to 48 hours. The patient is usually treated with outpatient therapy, which includes oral rehydration with electrolyte replacement fluids and rest. If the patient is severely dehydrated, I.V. hydration is necessary as well as electrolyte monitoring and replacement. Antidiarrheal agents may be used sparingly but should be avoided in children.

NURSING CONSIDERATIONS

 PREVENTION Secondary spread of infection can be prevented through appropriate handwashing and disposal of infectious materials. In an inpatient setting, contact precautions will help limit spread. Notify the health department so it can investigate outbreak centers and prevent further transmission. Notify the state or local health department of all suspected Norwalk virus outbreaks (two or more people who shared a common meal or three or more people living in the same household who are symptomatic) so that potential outbreak centers can be investigated and further transmission limited.

▶ Plan your care to allow uninterrupted rest periods for the patient.

▶ If the patient is nauseated, advise him or her to avoid quick movements.

▶ If the patient can tolerate oral fluid intake, replace lost fluids and electrolytes with broth, ginger ale, and lemonade, as tolerated. Warn the patient to avoid milk and milk products, which may provoke recurrence.

▶ Monitor fluid status carefully; assess vital signs, daily weight, and intake and output; watch for signs of dehydration and electrolyte imbalance.

▶ Administer I.V. fluids and electrolytes as ordered.

▶ To ease anal irritation, clean the area carefully, apply a repellent cream such as petroleum jelly, and provide warm sitz baths and witch hazel compresses.

Patient teaching

▶ Teach the patient about gastroenteritis, including the symptoms, causes, and treatment.

▶ Instruct the patient to drink unsweetened fruit juice, tea, bouillon, or other clear broths and to eat bland, soft foods, such as cooked cereal, rice, and applesauce. Tell the patient to avoid foods that are spicy, greasy, or high in roughage (whole-grain products, raw fruits or vegetables) as they can precipitate recurrent diarrhea.

 PREVENTION Advise patients who expect to travel, especially to developing nations, to pay close attention to what they eat and drink. Review proper hygiene measures, including proper handwashing technique, to prevent recurrence. Instruct patients to cook foods, especially pork, thoroughly; to refrigerate perishable foods, such as milk, mayonnaise, potato salad, and cream-filled pastry; to always wash hands with warm water and soap before handling food, especially after using the bathroom; to clean utensils thoroughly; and to eliminate flies and roaches in the home.

▶ Disease transmission may be decreased with education regarding handwashing for food preparers, day-care employees, resort/cruise guests, and family or close contacts of infected individuals.

Opisthorchiasis

Opisthorchis sinensis, also known as *Clonorchis sinensis,* is a trematode, or fluke, that causes infection in the liver. It is most commonly called the Chinese liver fluke. *O. viverrini* is a Southeast Asian liver fluke, and *O. felineus* is a cat liver fluke. Trematode infections occur worldwide and cause various clinical infections in humans. The parasites are known for their conspicuous suckers, which are the organs of attachment. Flukes are generally classified as blood flukes, liver flukes, lung flukes, or intestinal flukes, depending on where in the body they manifest themselves. Fluke infection in the United States is extremely rare; it is seen mostly in travelers and emigrants from endemic areas.

Liver flukes have a complex life cycle that involves a definitive host and two intermediate aquatic hosts. Humans are infected when they eat the encysted metacercariae in undercooked, raw, or pickled fish or vegetables. After digestion of the cyst in the duodenum, the larvae enter the biliary duct and lay eggs, which are passed into the stool. The eggs enter freshwater areas, forming miracidium and infecting aquatic snails, which are the intermediate host.

CAUSES

Liver flukes are found predominantly in China, Japan, Korea, and Vietnam. The definitive hosts include grazing herbivores, such as sheep and cattle, as well as dogs, cats, rabbits, and humans. Eggs passed in the feces are deposited in the environment and hatch in freshwater areas within 10 days, longer if temperatures are cool. They are known to survive in cold water for several years. The embryos develop into miracidia, which swim to and penetrate the soft tissue of snails. The miracidia undergo several developmental stages (sporocysts, rediae, cercariae) within the snail and are then released and penetrate freshwater fish (second intermediate host). There they encyst as metacercariae in the

muscles or under the scales of the fish. People become infected by ingesting undercooked fish or raw or undercooked vegetables containing metacercariae. After ingestion, the metacercariae excyst in the duodenum and ascend through the ampulla of Vater into the biliary ducts, where they attach and develop into adults, laying eggs after 3 to 4 weeks. Adult flukes reside in the biliary and pancreatic ducts, where they attach to the mucosa.

COMPLICATIONS

Complications include bacterial infections, anemia, malnutrition, and hepatomegaly. In rare cases, cholangitis, cholecystitis, biliary obstruction, and cholangiocarcinoma may develop.

ASSESSMENT FINDINGS

Most patients with opisthorchiasis are asymptomatic; the presence and severity of symptoms depend on the quantity of liver flukes in the individual as well as the specific location of infection. Those with fewer than 100 flukes usually experience no symptoms other than general malaise, dyspepsia, abdominal pain, diarrhea, or constipation. As flukes invade the liver and biliary passages, more severe infections may present with fever, acute pain, hepatomegaly, splenomegaly, progressive ascites, edema, jaundice, tachycardia, weight loss, and eosinophilia. No correlation has been found between the severity of disease and fecal liver fluke egg output; the flukes block the gallbladder and bile ducts, so eggs may no longer appear in the feces.

DIAGNOSTIC TESTS

▶ Diagnosis is based on microscopic identification of eggs in stool specimens. The presence of fewer than 100 eggs per gram of feces is considered a mild infection, and more than 30,000 eggs per gram of feces indicate severe infection. If eggs are not detected in the stool, duodenal drainage aspiration may detect them.

▶ Indirect evidence of opisthorchiasis in the bile ducts can be obtained with radiography, ultrasonography, computed tomography, and magnetic resonance imaging.

▶ Serologic tests that can aid in diagnosis include indirect hemagglutination, indirect immunofluorescence, and enzyme-linked immunosorbent assay.

▶ Blood work showing high bilirubin, alkaline phosphatase, and serum transaminase levels coupled with low serum albumin levels indicates liver involvement. Eosinophilia may be present in patients with acute symptomatic infection.

TREATMENT

Praziquantel (Biltricide) is the drug of choice to treat opisthorchiasis. Surgical management may be needed for complications of trematode infection. Anemia may be treated with iron supplements and vitamins.

NURSING CONSIDERATIONS

▶ Although isolation is unnecessary, properly dispose of stool and soiled linen and carefully wash your hands after patient contact.

▶ If the patient is receiving nasogastric (NG) suction, be sure to provide mouth care.

▶ Maintain NG tube patency, and check for secretion returns every 4 hours.

▶ Question family members and other contacts about symptoms.

▶ Weigh the patient daily, and monitor intake and output. Replace fluids as needed.

▶ Provide a nutritionally adequate diet, and administer nutritional supplements as prescribed.

▶ Administer anthelmintic drug therapy as ordered. Monitor NG tube aspirate to ensure drug absorption.

▶ Tell the patient to swallow praziquantel tablets whole with some liquid during meals. Instruct him or her to avoid keeping the tablet in the mouth because it has bitter taste that can produce nausea or vomiting.

Patient teaching

▶ Inform patients about the danger of eating raw or undercooked vegetables and fish.

 SAFETY To prevent ingestion of infective forms of *Opisthorchis* and avoid infection, advise thorough cooking of fish and other types of seafood (such as crab and crayfish) as well as aquatic vegetables, fruits, and plants. Thorough washing of raw vegetables and aquatic fruits can help prevent infection. Advise immunocompromised patients to avoid consumption of contaminated water, water plants, fruits, fish, crab, and raw liver.

▶ Tell the patient that freezing fish intended for raw consumption kills parasites, unlike brining and pickling.

▶ Explain to the patient that encysted metacercariae can be killed by washing water-grown vegetables in 6% vinegar or potassium permanganate for 5 to 10 minutes. In endogenous areas, this may be more successful than attempts to halt the consumption of raw vegetables.

▶ Advise the patient that molluscicidals can prevent transmission of trematodes.

▶ Tell the patient to take medication as prescribed, and stress the importance of finishing medication as ordered.

Osteomyelitis

Osteomyelitis is a pyogenic bone infection that may be chronic or acute. The disease commonly results from a combination of traumatic injury and acute infection originating elsewhere in the body. Osteomyelitis usually remains a local infection, but it can spread through the bone to the marrow, cortex, and periosteum. Acute osteomyelitis is typically caused by hematogenous spread that most commonly affects rapidly growing children, particularly boys. Multiple draining sinus tracts and metastatic lesions characterize the rarer chronic osteomyelitis, which is more prevalent in adults.

In children, the most common disease sites include the lower end of the femur and the upper end of the tibia, humerus, and radius. In adults, the disease commonly localizes in the pelvis and vertebrae and usually results from contamination related to surgery or trauma. The prognosis for a patient with acute osteomyelitis is good if he or she receives prompt treatment. The prognosis for patients with chronic osteomyelitis is poor.

CAUSES

Infection causes osteomyelitis. Bacterial pyogens are the most common agents, but the disease may also result from fungi or viruses. The most common pyogenic organisms are *Staphylococcus aureus*, *Streptococcus pyogenes*, *Pseudomonas aeruginosa*, *Haemophilus influenzae*, and *Enterobacter* species. Typically, these organisms find a site of local infection and spread through the blood directly to bone. As the organisms grow and produce pus within the bone, pressure builds within the rigid medullary cavity and forces the pus through the haversian canals. A subperiosteal abscess forms, depriving the bone of its blood supply and eventually causing necrosis. In turn, necrosis stimulates the periosteum to create new bone (involucrum). The old, dead bone (sequestrum) detaches and works its way out through either an abscess or the sinuses. By the time the body processes sequestrum, osteomyelitis is chronic.

COMPLICATIONS

Osteomyelitis may lead to chronic infection, skeletal deformities, joint deformities, disturbed bone growth (in children), differing leg lengths, and impaired mobility.

ASSESSMENT FINDINGS

The patient's history may reveal a previous injury, surgery, or primary infection. The patient may complain of a sudden, severe pain in the affected bone and related chills, nausea, and malaise. He or she may describe the pain as unrelieved by rest and worse with motion and may refuse to use the affected area. The patient may also have tachycardia, fever, swelling, restricted movement, and tenderness and warmth over the infection site.

The chronic and acute forms of osteomyelitis usually have similar clinical features, but chronic infection can persist intermittently for years, flaring up spontaneously after minor trauma. Sometimes the only sign of chronic infection is persistent pus drainage from an old pocket in a sinus tract.

DIAGNOSTIC TESTS

▶ Blood work will reveal leukocytosis and an increased erythrocyte sedimentation rate if the patient has osteomyelitis. Blood culture can be used to identify the pathogen.
▶ Radiography may show bone involvement only after the disease has been active for some time, usually 2 to 3 weeks.
▶ Bone scans can be used to detect early infection. Computed tomography and magnetic resonance imaging may be necessary to determine the extent of infection.

TREATMENT

To decrease internal bone pressure and prevent infarction, treatment for acute osteomyelitis begins even before the diagnosis is confirmed. After drawing samples for blood culture, high doses of I.V. antibiotics are typically administered; usually, a penicillinase-resistant agent, such as nafcillin or oxacillin (Bactocill), is administered for at least 4 to 6 weeks. The infected site may be drained surgically to relieve pressure and remove sequestrum. The infected bone is usually immobilized with a cast or traction or by complete bed rest. The patient receives analgesics and I.V. fluids as needed.

If an abscess forms, treatment includes incision and drainage followed by culture of the drainage. Anti-infective therapy may include systemic antibiotics; intracavitary instillation of antibiotics through closed-system continuous irrigation with low intermittent suction; limited irrigation with a blood drainage system equipped with suction such as a Hemovac; or local application of packed, wet, antibiotic-soaked dressings.

Some patients may receive hyperbaric oxygen therapy to increase the activity of naturally occurring white blood cells. Additional measures include using free tissue transfers and local muscle flaps to fill in dead space and increase blood supply.

Chronic osteomyelitis may also require surgery: sequestrectomy to remove dead bone and saucerization to promote drainage and decrease pressure. The typical patient reports severe pain and requires prolonged hospitalization. Unrelieved chronic osteomyelitis in an arm or a leg may require amputation.

NURSING CONSIDERATIONS

▶ Use sterile technique when changing dressings and irrigating wounds.
▶ Assess vital signs, wound appearance, and new pain (which may indicate secondary infection) daily.
▶ Carefully monitor drainage and suctioning equipment. Monitor the amount of solution instilled and drained.
▶ Support the affected limb with firm pillows. Keep it level with the body; don't let it sag.
▶ Provide thorough skin care. Turn the patient gently every 2 hours, and watch for signs of developing pressure ulcers.

▶ Provide complete cast care. Support the cast with firm pillows. Check circulation and drainage. Assess increasing drainage, and report as appropriate. Monitor vital signs for excessive blood loss.
▶ Assess the patient's pain pattern. Give analgesics as needed, and monitor the response.

Patient teaching

▶ Explain tests and treatments, including preoperative and postoperative procedures.
▶ Review prescribed medications. Discuss possible adverse reactions to drug administration, and instruct the patient about which adverse reactions to report to the physician. Emphasize importance of taking antibiotics as ordered, even if feeling better.
▶ Before discharge, teach the patient how to protect and clean the wound site and, most importantly, how to recognize signs of recurring infection (elevated temperature, redness, localized heat, and swelling).

Otitis externa

Otitis externa, also known as external otitis and swimmer's ear, is inflammation of the skin of the external ear canal and auricle. The condition is most common in the summer and may be acute or chronic. With treatment, acute otitis externa usually subsides within 7 days. It may become chronic, however, and tends to recur.

CAUSES

Otitis externa usually results from bacteria (such as *Pseudomonas aeruginosa*, *Staphylococcus aureus*, group A streptococci), fungi (*Aspergillus*), yeast (*Candida*), or dermatologic conditions (seborrhea or psoriasis). Trauma to the middle ear, such as cleaning too vigorously with cotton-tipped swabs, can also cause otitis externa.

COMPLICATIONS

Without effective treatment, otitis externa can lead to otitis media and hearing loss. In patients with severe otitis externa, cellulitis, abscesses, discoloration, disfigurement of the pinna, lymphadenopathy, osteitis, septicemia, and stenosis may develop. Malignant otitis externa, most common in patients with type 1 diabetes mellitus and among the elderly, may develop as a result of a fulminant *Pseudomonas* infection.

ASSESSMENT FINDINGS

Acute otitis externa characteristically produces moderate to severe pain that's exacerbated by manipulating the auricle or tragus, clenching the teeth, opening the mouth, or chewing. Its other clinical effects may include fever, foul-smelling discharge, crusting in the external ear, regional cellulitis, partial hearing loss, and itching. It's usually difficult to view the tympanic membrane because of pain in the external canal. Hearing acuity is normal unless complete occlusion has occurred.

Fungal otitis externa may be asymptomatic, although *Aspergillus niger* produces a black or gray, blotting, paperlike growth in the ear canal. In chronic otitis externa, pruritus replaces pain, and scratching may lead to scaling and skin thickening. Aural discharge may also be seen.

Otoscopy reveals a swollen external ear canal (sometimes to the point of complete closure), periauricular lymphadenopathy (tender nodes anterior to the tragus, posterior to the ear, or in the upper neck) and, occasionally, regional cellulitis. In fungal otitis externa, removal of the growth reveals thick, red epithelium. Pain on palpation of the tragus or auricle distinguishes acute otitis externa from acute otitis media. In chronic otitis externa, physical examination reveals thick, red epithelium in the ear canal. Severe chronic otitis externa may reflect underlying diabetes mellitus, hypothyroidism, or nephritis.

DIAGNOSTIC TESTS

▸ Microscopic examination or culture and sensitivity testing identifies the causative organism and determines the course of antibiotic treatment.

TREATMENT

To relieve the pain of otitis externa, treatment includes heat therapy to the periauricular region (heat lamp; hot, damp compresses; or a heating pad), aspirin, or acetaminophen (Tylenol) plus codeine. Instillation of antibiotic eardrops (with or without hydrocortisone) follows cleaning of the ear and removal of debris. However, a corticosteroid helps reduce the inflammatory response. If fever persists or regional cellulitis or tender postauricular adenopathy develops, a systemic antibiotic is necessary. If the ear canal is too edematous for the instillation of eardrops, an ear wick may be used for the first few days.

NURSING CONSIDERATIONS

▸ Monitor vital signs, particularly temperature. Watch for and record the type and amount of aural drainage.

PREVENTION

Preventing otitis externa

Any patient who has experienced otitis externa should be taught to prevent a recurrence by avoiding irritants, such as hair-care products and earrings, and by avoiding cotton-tipped applicators or other objects when cleaning the ears. Encourage the patient to keep water out of the ears when showering or shampooing by using lamb's wool earplugs coated with petroleum jelly. Also, parents of young children should be told that modeling clay makes a tight seal to prevent water from getting into the external ear canal.

In addition, when the patient goes swimming he or she should keep the head above water or wear earplugs. Following swimming, the patient should instill one or two drops of a mixture that is one-half 70% alcohol and one-half white vinegar to toughen the skin of the external ear canal.

▶ Remove debris, gently clean the ear canal, and instill antibiotic drops as ordered. To instill eardrops in an adult, grasp the helix and pull upward and backward to straighten the canal. To instill eardrops in a child, pull the earlobe downward and backward. To ensure that the drops reach the epithelium, insert a wisp of cotton moistened with eardrops.

▶ If the patient has chronic otitis externa, clean the ear thoroughly. Use wet soaks intermittently on oozing or infected skin.

▶ If the patient has a chronic fungal infection, clean the ear canal well and then apply an exfoliative ointment.

Patient teaching

▶ Instruct the patient about proper hand-washing technique, and stress the need for daily ear cleaning.

▶ Teach the patient and family how to properly instill eardrops, ointment, and ear wash.

▶ Tell the patient to notify the physician if an allergic reaction to the antibiotic drops or ointment develops; this may be indicated by increased swelling and discomfort of the area and worsening of other symptoms.

▶ Answer the patient's questions, and encourage him or her to discuss concerns about hearing loss. Reassure the patient that hearing loss from an external ear infection is temporary.

▶ If the patient has difficulty understanding procedures because of hearing loss, offer clear, concise explanations of treatments and procedures, including written information. Face the patient when speaking; enunciate words clearly, slowly, and in a normal tone; and allow adequate time for the patient to grasp what you have said. Provide a pencil and paper to aid communication, and alert the staff regarding communication challenges.

▶ Caution the patient to take the prescribed antibiotic on time, to finish the prescription, and to report any adverse reactions.

▶ Urge prompt treatment for otitis externa to prevent perforation of the tympanic membrane. (See *Preventing otitis externa*.)

Otitis media

Otitis media is inflammation of the middle ear that may be suppurative or secretory, acute or chronic, persistent, or unresponsive. With prompt treatment, the prognosis for acute otitis media is excellent; however, prolonged accumulation of fluid can cause chronic otitis media and perforation of the tympanic membrane. Patient risk factors for otitis media include age, anatomic anomalies, gastroesophageal reflux, the presence of adenoids, and genetic predisposition. Environmental risk factors include upper airway infections or allergies, seasonality (the incidence is higher in fall and winter), day-care center attendance, bottle-feeding, exposure to passive smoking, and use of pacifiers. Common pathogens associated with otitis media include *Streptococcus pneumoniae*, *Haemophilus influenzae*, *Moraxella catarrhalis*, *Staphylococcus aureus*, group A *Streptococcus*, and mixed anaerobes.

CAUSES

Otitis media results from disruption of eustachian tube patency. In the suppurative form, bacterial infection is usually the cause; other causes include respiratory tract infection, allergic reaction, nasotracheal intubation, or positional changes that allow flora to reflux through the eustachian tube and colonize the middle ear. Chronic suppurative otitis media results from inadequate treatment for acute otitis episodes, infection by resistant bacteria or, rarely, tuberculosis. Obstruction of the eustachian tube causes a buildup of negative pressure and eustachian tube dysfunction. Barotrauma from rapid aircraft descent in a person with an upper respiratory tract infection or during rapid underwater ascent in scuba diving may produce barotitis media. Chronic secretory otitis media may result from mechanical obstruction (adenoidal tissue overgrowth or tumors), edema (allergic rhinitis or chronic sinus infection), or inadequate treatment for acute suppurative otitis media.

COMPLICATIONS

Complications include spontaneous rupture of the tympanic membrane, mastoiditis, meningitis, cholesteatomas (cystlike masses in the middle ear), septicemia, abscesses, vertigo, lymphadenopathy, sigmoid sinus or jugular vein thrombosis, suppurative labyrinthitis, facial paralysis, otitis externa, tympanosclerosis, and permanent hearing loss.

ASSESSMENT FINDINGS

Many patients are asymptomatic. Clinical features of acute suppurative otitis media include severe, deep, throbbing pain; signs of upper respiratory tract infection; mild to very high fever; hearing loss; tinnitus; dizziness; nausea; and vomiting. Bulging of the tympanic membrane with erythema may occur; purulent drainage may be present from tympanic membrane rupture. Pain may stop suddenly when the membrane ruptures. Acute secretory otitis media produces a severe conductive hearing loss, a sensation of fullness in the ear, and popping, crackling, or clicking sounds on swallowing or with jaw movement. Accumulation of fluid may cause the patient to hear an echo when speaking and to have a vague feeling of top-heaviness. In chronic otitis media, thickening and scarring of the tympanic membrane occur with decreased or absent tympanic membrane mobility.

DIAGNOSTIC TESTS

▶ Otoscopic or neuroscopic examination is used to diagnose the disorder, remove debris, and perform minor surgery. Pneumatoscopy shows decreased tympanic membrane mobility.

ALERT This procedure is painful when the tympanic membrane is obviously bulging and erythematous.

▶ Culture and sensitivity testing of exudate is used to identify the causative organism.

▶ Radiographic studies or computed tomography depict mastoid involvement.

PREVENTION

Preventing otitis media

To help prevent a recurrence of otitis media, instruct the patient or parents how to recognize upper respiratory infections, and encourage early treatment. Encourage the patient or parents to consider a pneumococcal vaccine to prevent infections that can cause respiratory and aural infections.

Tell parents to wash children's toys and promote frequent handwashing. For infants, tell parents to avoid the use of pacifiers and encourage breast-feeding for at least the first 6 months of the child's life. (It has been shown that breast milk contains antibodies that protect infants from ear infections.) If the child is bottle-fed, instruct the parents not to feed the infant in a supine position and to refrain from putting the infant to bed with a bottle, which can cause reflux of nasopharyngeal flora. Also, teach the parent to keep the child away from secondhand smoke.

To promote eustachian tube patency, instruct the patient to perform Valsalva's maneuver several times a day, especially during airplane travel. Outline possible adverse reactions to the prescribed medications, emphasizing those that require immediate medical attention.

▶ Tympanometry and audiometry measure how well the tympanic membrane functions in order to detect hearing loss and evaluate the condition of the middle ear.

▶ Biopsy is used to rule out malignancy and identify tissue.

TREATMENT

Antibiotics are given in infants younger than 6 months or in older children if the diagnosis is certain or is severe. Alternatively, the patient may be observed for 48 to 72 hours and given analgesics (ibuprofen [Motrin] and acetaminophen [Tylenol]). Infants with frequent recurrences may be prescribed antibiotic prophylaxis.

ALERT Patients with persistent pain or fever should be reexamined within 48 hours. If the child fails to improve, antibiotic therapy should be initiated. If the patient fails to improve with antibiotic therapy, an alternate antibiotic should be initiated and compliance emphasized.

To reduce middle ear fluid accumulation, an osteopathic manipulation technique (Galbreath technique) may help open eustachian tubes and is similar to having the child blow up a balloon. Other treatments include decongestant therapy, myringotomy, and aspiration of middle ear fluid followed by insertion of a polyethylene tube. Treatment for chronic otitis media includes elimination of eustachian tube obstruction and surgery.

NURSING CONSIDERATIONS

▶ Provide comfort measures; administer pain medication and antibiotics as ordered; and apply heat to help relieve pain.

▶ After myringotomy, sterile cotton may be placed loosely in the external ear to absorb drainage; it should be changed when damp. Watch for headache, fever, severe pain, or disorientation.

▶ After tympanoplasty, reinforce dressings, observe for excessive bleeding, and administer analgesics. Warn against nose blowing or getting the ear wet when bathing.

Patient teaching

▶ Parents should be aware that analgesics, not antibiotics, relieve the ear pain of acute otitis media. Stress the importance of taking antibiotics as prescribed, even if feeling better.

 PREVENTION Eliminating the child's exposure to tobacco smoke helps prevent recurrence. Regular exercises to increase upper airway pressure and to force inflation of the middle ear may be useful (Galbreath technique or blowing up balloons).

▶ Provide guidelines to patients and parents regarding how to prevent recurrence. (See *Preventing otitis media.*)

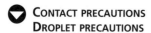

Parainfluenza

Parainfluenza refers to any of a group of respiratory illnesses caused by paramyxoviruses, a subgroup of the myxoviruses. Affecting both the upper and lower respiratory tracts, these self-limiting diseases resemble influenza but are milder and seldom fatal. They primarily affect young children.

CAUSES

Parainfluenza is transmitted by direct contact or by inhalation of contaminated airborne droplets. Paramyxoviruses occur in five serotypes—1, 2, 3, 4a, and 4b—that are linked to several diseases: croup (types 1, 2, and 3), bronchiolitis (types 1 and 3 particularly, but all may cause it), tracheobronchitis (type 3); pharyngitis (types 1, 2, 3, and 4a and 4b), bronchitis (types 1 and 3), and pneumonia (types 1 and 3). Parainfluenza type 3 ranks second to respiratory syncytial viruses as the most common cause of lower respiratory tract infections in children. Types 4a and 4b rarely cause symptomatic infections in humans.

Parainfluenza is rare among adults but widespread among children, especially boys. By age 8, most children demonstrate antibodies to parainfluenza types 1 and 3. Most adults have antibodies to all five types as a result of childhood infections and subsequent multiple exposures. Incidence rises in the winter and spring.

Parainfluenza infection in the respiratory tract leads to the secretion of high levels of inflammatory cytokines, with a peak duration of secretion 7 to 10 days after initial exposure. Increasing levels of certain chemokines are detected in the nasal secretions of pediatric patients. These chemokines are responsible for pathologic changes in the respiratory tract and the clinical manifestations of this condition. The features include airway inflammation, necrosis and sloughing of respiratory epithelium, edema, excessive mucus production, and interstitial infiltration of lung. Edema of the mucus layer causes swelling (vocal cords, larynx, trachea, and bronchi), which can lead to airflow obstruction and subsequent stridor.

COMPLICATIONS

Complications of parainfluenza include croup, bronchiolitis, and pneumonia.

ASSESSMENT FINDINGS

After a short incubation period (usually 3 to 6 days), signs and symptoms emerge that are similar to those of other respiratory diseases: sudden fever, nasal discharge, reddened throat (with little or no exudate), chills, and muscle pain. Bacterial complications are uncommon, but in infants and very young children parainfluenza may lead to croup or laryngotracheobronchitis. Re-infection is usually less severe and affects only the upper respiratory tract.

DIAGNOSTIC TESTS

▶ A swab of nasal secretions is useful for rapid viral testing. Virus isolation and serum antibody titers differentiate parainfluenza from other types of respiratory illness but is rarely done.

TREATMENT

Depending on the severity of symptoms, parainfluenza may require bed rest, antipyretics, analgesics, and antitussives or no treatment at all. Complications, such as croup and pneumonia, require appropriate treatment. No vaccine is effective against parainfluenza. Corticosteroids should be administered along with nebulization to treat respiratory symptoms and reduce airway edema.

NURSING CONSIDERATIONS

▶ Throughout the illness, monitor respiratory status and temperature, and ensure adequate fluid intake and rest.
▶ Monitor cough and breath sounds, hoarseness, severity of retractions, inspiratory stridor, cyanosis, respiratory rate and character

(especially prolonged and labored respirations), restlessness, fever, and heart rate.

▶ Keep the child as quiet as possible but avoid sedation, which may depress respiration. If the patient is an infant, position him or her in an infant seat or prop the baby up with a pillow; place an older child in Fowler's position. A cool vaporizer air may soothe air passages.

▶ Control the child's energy output and oxygen demand by providing age-appropriate diversional activities to keep him or her occupied quietly.

⬤ Use contact and droplet precautions with patients suspected of having respiratory syncytial virus or parainfluenza infections. Wash your hands carefully before leaving the room to avoid transmitting germs to other patients, particularly infants.

▶ Control fever with sponge baths and antipyretics. Keep a hypothermia blanket on hand if the patient's temperature rises above 102° F (38.9° C). Watch for seizures in infants and young children with high fevers. Give I.V. antibiotics as ordered.

▶ Relieve sore throat with soothing, water-based ices, such as fruit sorbet and ice pops. Avoid thicker, milk-based fluids if the patient has thick mucus or swallowing difficulties. Apply petroleum jelly or another ointment around the nose and lips to decrease irritation from nasal discharge and mouth breathing.

▶ Institute measures to prevent the patient from crying, which increases respiratory distress. As necessary, adapt treatment to conserve the patient's energy and to include parents, who can provide reassurance.

 ALERT Watch for signs of complete airway obstruction, such as increased heart and respiratory rates, use of respiratory accessory muscles in breathing, nasal flaring, and increased restlessness.

Patient teaching

▶ If the child is hospitalized, advise the parents that he or she may be placed in a cool-mist tent (with or without oxygen) to provide high humidity.

▶ Tell the parents that bed rest is essential to conserve energy and limit oxygen needs. To ease the child's breathing, advise the parents to use pillows to prop him or her into a sitting or semi-sitting (semi-Fowler's) position. Advise them that keeping the child quiet and comfortable reduces oxygen needs. Holding the child as often as possible will provide soothing and comfort.

▶ Urge parents to ensure adequate hydration by giving fluid electrolyte replacement, and instruct them to avoid thicker, milk-based fluids. To relieve sore throat, suggest fruit sorbet or ice pops. Instruct the parents to withhold solid food until the child can breathe and swallow more easily. Inform them that the child may have little or no appetite until he or she feels better.

▶ Warn parents not to give aspirin to reduce fever because of its link to Reye syndrome in children.

▶ Suggest using a cool-mist humidifier (vaporizer) in the home or the use of warm moist air from the shower to ease breathing.

CONTACT PRECAUTIONS

Paratyphoid fever

Transmitted by the fecal-oral route, typhoid and paratyphoid fever are bacterial infections of the intestinal tract and bloodstream. Affected patients usually experience mild fever, malaise, anorexia, headache, constipation, or diarrhea 1 to 3 weeks after exposure. Symptoms in paratyphoid fever are similar to those of typhoid fever but are generally milder. Most patients recover completely, although intestinal complications can result in death. With early treatment, the mortality rate is less than 1%. Paratyphoid fever is preventable through clean water, proper hygiene, and good sanitation practices. Contaminated water is one of the pathways of transmission of the disease.

CAUSES

Typhoid and paratyphoid fevers are caused by the bacteria *Salmonella typhi* and *Salmonella paratyphi*, respectively. The bacteria are passed in the feces and urine of infected people. People become infected after eating food or drinking beverages that have been contaminated by an infected person or by drinking water that has been contaminated by sewage containing the bacteria. Once the bacteria enter the body, they multiply, spreading from the intestines to the bloodstream. After recovery, a small number of carriers continue to harbor the bacteria and can be a source of infection for others. Transmission of paratyphoid in less-industrialized countries may be due to contaminated food or water, such as by shellfish taken from sewage-contaminated beds. In areas with chlorinated water where water quality is high, transmission is more likely to occur through food contaminated by infected food handlers.

COMPLICATIONS

Complications may include intestinal perforation or hemorrhage, abscesses, thrombophlebitis, cerebral thrombosis, pneumonia, osteomyelitis, myocarditis, and acute circulatory failure.

ASSESSMENT FINDINGS

Paratyphoid fever has three stages: early stage, toxic stage, and recovery. The incubation period is 1 to 2 weeks but is often shorter in children. Symptom onset may be gradual in adults but is often sudden in children. A patient in the early stage may present with high fever. Those in the toxic stage have abdominal pain and intestinal symptoms, such as loss of appetite, vomiting, constipation, or diarrhea. The pain may resemble that of appendicitis. There is also a long period of recovery from fever (defervescence). In adults, these three phases may occur over 4 to 6 weeks; in children, they are shorter and occur over 10 days to 2 weeks.

Intestinal perforation or hemorrhage may occur during the toxic stage. In addition, the patient typically develops an enlarged spleen and about 30% develop rose spots on the front of the chest during the first week of illness. The rose spots change into small hemorrhages that may be difficult to see in blacks or Native Americans. The diagnosis is usually made on the basis of a history of recent travel and culturing the paratyphoid organism.

DIAGNOSTIC TESTS

▶ Diagnosis depends on the isolation of the organism in a culture, particularly blood or feces. *S. paratyphi* is also easily cultured from samples of urine or bone marrow.

TREATMENT

Paratyphoid fever is treated with a 2- to 3-week course of antibiotics, usually trimethoprim-sulfamethoxazole (Bactrim), amoxicillin (Amoxil), or ampicillin. In resistant strains, third-generation cephalosporins may be used, such as ceftriaxone (Rocephin), cefotaxime (Claforan), cefixime (Suprax), or chloramphenicol. Other treatments include bed rest and fluid and electrolyte replacement. The administration of camphorated tincture of opium, kaolin with pectin, diphenoxylate, codeine, or small doses of morphine may be necessary to relieve diarrhea and control cramps in patients who must remain active. Patients with intestinal perforation or hemorrhage may need surgery. Patients with severe infections may require fluid replacement or blood transfusions.

 PREVENTION Vaccination against paratyphoid fever is recommended when traveling to countries with high rates of enteric fever. It is not routinely recommended except for those who will have prolonged exposure to potentially contaminated food and water in high-risk areas.

NURSING CONSIDERATIONS

▶ Plan your care to allow uninterrupted rest periods for the patient. Rest usually helps to relieve the patient's symptoms, increase resistance, and conserve strength. Provide comfort measures.

▶ Monitor fluid status carefully. Take vital signs at least every 4 hours, weigh the patient daily, monitor for fluid and electrolyte balance, and record intake and output.

▶ Watch for signs of dehydration, such as dry skin and mucous membranes, fever, and sunken eyes. If dehydration occurs, administer oral and I.V. fluids as ordered.

◗ Wash your hands thoroughly after giving care to avoid spreading infection, and use contact precautions when caring for these patients.

▶ To ease anal irritation caused by diarrhea, clean the area carefully and apply a repellent cream such as petroleum jelly. Warm sitz baths and application of witch hazel compresses can also soothe irritation.

 SAFETY Use contact precautions if the patient is incontinent or diapered; otherwise, standard precautions are appropriate. Remember to always wash your hands thoroughly before and after any contact with the patient and advise other personnel to do the same, and ensure proper disposal of soiled linens.

Patient teaching

▶ Teach the patient about the disease, including symptoms, causes, and prescribed treatments.

▶ Carefully review the proper use of prescribed medications with the patient, including the desired effects of the drugs and their possible adverse effects.

▶ Tell the patient to report any signs of complications, such as dehydration, bleeding, or recurrence of symptoms.

 PREVENTION Public health interventions include education regarding personal hygiene, handwashing after toilet use and before food preparation, and using a safe water supply as well as installation of proper sanitation systems. Individuals who are disease carriers should be excluded from food handling.

▶ Travelers in countries with high rates of paratyphoid fever should be careful to wash their hands before eating and to avoid meat, egg, or poultry dishes unless the food has been thoroughly cooked.

Pasteurellosis

Pasteurella multocida is a small, gram-negative, nonmotile, non-spore-forming coccobacillus that often exists in the upper respiratory tract of many livestock, poultry, and domestic pet species, especially cats and dogs. Infection in humans is usually associated with an animal bite, scratch, or lick, but infection without animal contact may occur as well. Wound infections associated with animal bites require broad-spectrum antimicrobials targeted at both aerobic and anaerobic gram-negative bacteria. Bite injuries can be aggressive, with symptoms appearing within 24 hours. The wounds can develop progressive soft-tissue inflammation resembling group A beta-hemolytic *Streptococcus pyogenes* infections.

CAUSES

P. multocida infection usually results from being bitten, licked, or scratched by an infected pet or by sharing food or plates with infected pets. However, the infection may be idiopathic, with no history of pet exposure. Immunosuppression may increase the incidence of the disease.

COMPLICATIONS

Complications of pasteurellosis include deep tissue injury such as tenosynovitis, septic arthritis, and osteomyelitis. Severe, disseminating infections, such as endocarditis and meningitis, may (rarely) develop.

ASSESSMENT FINDINGS

The patient may have a positive history of occupational or recreational exposure to animals. Physical findings relate to the infection site. Local infection may show erythema, warmth, pain and tenderness, purulent discharge, lymphadenitis, joint swelling, and decreased range of motion. Respiratory infection may show sinus tenderness, hoarseness, pharyngeal erythema, rales and rhonchi

upon chest auscultation, dullness to percussion, and changes in vocal fremitus. If the central nervous system is involved, neurologic deficits may occur, as well as signs of meningeal irritation (nuchal rigidity, Brudzinski's sign, Kernig's sign). Abdominal signs include tenderness, guarding and rebound, hepatosplenomegaly, and costovertebral angle tenderness. Ocular symptoms may include corneal ulcer, conjunctival injection, and decreased visual acuity. Cardiovascular symptoms may include hypotension, tachycardia, new cardiac murmur, or embolic phenomenon. Lymph nodes may show regional adenopathy.

DIAGNOSTIC TESTS

❱ Gram stain of purulent material or other fluid specimens (blood, sputum, and cerebrospinal fluid) may show small, gram-negative, nonmotile, non-spore-forming pleomorphic coccobacilli. Wright, Giemsa, and Wayson stains enhance bipolar staining.
❱ Computed tomography and magnetic resonance imaging can evaluate tenosynovitis, septic arthritis, osteomyelitis, and meningeal signs.
❱ Lumbar puncture is performed if meningitis is suspected; arthrocentesis is performed if septic arthritis is suspected.
❱ Echocardiography evaluates suspected endocarditis.
❱ Abdominal paracentesis assesses ascites in spontaneous bacterial peritonitis, especially in those who have significant liver disease with a history of pet exposure.

TREATMENT

Animal bite wounds require wound care with an antiseptic solution coupled with removable of nonviable tissue. Soaking has not been proven to be of any benefit, although copious irrigation with a small-gauge catheter on a syringe removes debris and decreases the concentration of bacteria in a contaminated wound. Surgical care may require debridement and closure depending on the extent of the wound. The wound may need to be sharply debrided initially to remove nonviable tissue and reduce the risk of infection as well as to allow easier suturing by providing a more even edge. Minor injuries are sutured if the person is at low risk for infection, and suturing is considered for those at risk if they are treated within 8 to 10 hours of injury. Otherwise, the wound is left open until the risk of infection is reduced by cleansing, debridement, and prophylactic antibiotics.

Tetanus prophylaxis, rabies prophylaxis, and antimicrobial treatment should be instituted. Most *Pasteurella* isolates are susceptible to amoxicillin (Amoxil), amoxicillin-clavulanic acid (Augmentin), minocycline (Arestin), fluoroquinolones (ciprofloxacin [Cipro], ofloxacin, levofloxacin [Levaquin], moxifloxacin), and trimethoprim-sulfamethoxazole (Bactrim). Infections that are more severe may require parenteral antibiotics, such as ampicillin-sulbactam (Unasyn), ticarcillin-clavulanate (Timentin), piperacillin-tazobactam (Zosyn), cefoxitin, and carbapenems (imipenem-cilastatin [Primaxin], meropenem [Merrem], ertapenem [Invanz]) because they provide gram-positive, gram-negative, and anaerobic coverage.

NURSING CONSIDERATIONS

▶ Institute antibiotic therapy as ordered, and monitor for response.

▶ Assess the patient's pain level, mental status, wound status, and vital signs frequently and carefully in order to recognize the progression of wound changes or the development of new signs and symptoms. Changes must be reported and documented immediately.

▶ The need for supportive care, such as endotracheal intubation, cardiac monitoring, fluid replacement, and supplemental oxygen should be assessed and provided as warranted. Neurologic assessments should be performed and any changes reported.

▶ Care of postoperative patients and patients with trauma wounds requires strict sterile technique, good hand hygiene, and barriers between health care providers and patients to prevent contamination.

▶ Assess immunization status; provide tetanus prophylaxis as indicated.

▶ Assess the need for rabies vaccinations, and institute as ordered and as indicated.

▶ Encourage the patient to verbalize feelings about his or her appearance. Recognize the importance of body image.

▶ Assist with general hygiene and comfort measures as needed.

▶ Administer an analgesic and an antibiotic, as ordered, and monitor the patient's response.

Patient teaching

▶ Explain tests and treatments, including preoperative and postoperative procedures.

▶ Review prescribed medications and adverse reactions; instruct the patient to report adverse effects to the physician.

▶ Instruct the patient to complete the entire course of the prescribed antibiotic, even if the wound appears to have healed. Advise the patient to notify the physician about any adverse reactions to systemic antibiotic therapy.

▶ Before discharge, teach the patient how to protect and clean the wound site and how to recognize signs of infection (elevated temperature, redness, localized heat, and swelling). Discuss the importance of follow-up appointments.

CONTACT PRECAUTIONS

Pediculosis

Any human infestation of lice is known as pediculosis. Pediculosis can occur anywhere on the body. In the most common type, pediculosis capitis, lice feed on the scalp and, rarely, on the skin under the eyebrows, eyelashes, and beard. In pediculosis corporis, lice live next to the skin in clothing seams. In pediculosis pubis, lice are found primarily in pubic hairs but may extend to the eyebrows, eyelashes, and axillary or body hair. All types of lice feed on human blood and lay eggs (nits) on body hairs or clothing fibers. After the nits hatch, the lice must feed within 24 hours or they die; lice mature within 2 to 3 weeks after hatching. When a louse bites, it injects a toxin into the skin that produces mild irritation and a purpuric spot.

CAUSES

Pediculosis capitis (head lice) is caused by *Pediculus humanus capitis*, while *Pediculus humanus corporis* causes pediculosis corporis (body lice). *Phthirus pubis* causes pediculosis pubis (crab lice).

Pediculosis capitis commonly affects children, spreading through shared clothing and personal articles or by being in close proximity (playrooms or institutions). Pediculosis corporis is associated with close, crowded living situations (crowded buses and trains) and prolonged wearing of the same clothing; it spreads through shared clothing and bedsheets. Pediculosis pubis is associated with crowded living conditions and is transmitted through sexual intercourse or by contact with clothing, bedsheets, or towels harboring lice.

COMPLICATIONS

Excoriation and secondary bacterial infections from scratching are common complications of pediculosis. Left untreated, pediculosis may result in dry, hyperpigmented, thickly encrusted, scaly skin with residual scarring. Lice may carry *Staphylococcus*

aureus and group A *Streptococcus pyogenes* on their surface and transmit pathogens to others. *P. humanus corporis* is a known vector of three major bacterial diseases (relapsing fever, typhus, and trench fever), all of which have caused epidemics.

ASSESSMENT FINDINGS

In a patient with pediculosis capitis, inspection notes excoriation (with severe itching), pruritic papules or wheals from bite marks, hair that is matted and may have exudates under the matting (in severe cases), and posterior auricular and cervical lymphadenopathy. Hair shafts display oval, gray-white nits that can't be removed easily. A patient with pediculosis corporis may have excoriated red papules on the axilla, groin, and trunk and small, gray-blue spots (maculae ceruleae) on the thighs or upper body. Nits are found on clothing, especially in the seams. Inspection of a patient with pediculosis pubis reveals skin irritation from scratching, maculae ceruleae, and inguinal and axillary lymphadenopathy. The nits are attached to pubic hairs.

DIAGNOSTIC TESTS

▶ Wood's light examination achieves fluorescence of the adult lice. Microscopic examination shows nits visible on the hair shaft.

 ALERT A patient with pediculosis pubis should also receive testing and a thorough examination for concomitant sexually transmitted infections and human immunodeficiency virus if he or she is considered to be at risk for these conditions.

TREATMENT

For pediculosis capitis and pediculosis pubis, a topical insecticide such as permethrin (Elimite) or pyrethrin (Rid Mousse) is the initial treatment of choice. The lotion is rubbed into the hair and rinsed after 10 minutes. Often a single treatment is sufficient. A fine-tooth comb dipped in vinegar helps remove nits, and washing hair with ordinary shampoo removes crusts. Oral anthelminthics (ivermectin [Stromectol], levamisole, albendazole [Albenza]) are effective against head lice infestation. To prevent re-infestation, clothes and bed linens must be washed in hot water, ironed, or dry cleaned. Storing clothes or linens for more than 30 days or placing them in dry heat of 140° F (60° C) kills lice (especially on items such as stuffed animals).

In heavy infestation with *P. humanus corporis*, treatment of the body with a pediculicide shampoo or lotion may be beneficial, especially if the patient also has head or pubic lice infestation. Oral ivermectin may also be necessary. Clothing and bed linens should be treated. Lindane (Kwell) should only be used in patients who cannot tolerate other therapies, or in those where other therapies have failed.

Nursing considerations

◐ Contact precautions should be maintained until treatment is complete to prevent spreading the infection.

▶ Have the patient's fingernails cut short to prevent skin breaks and secondary bacterial infections caused by scratching.

▶ Be alert for possible adverse reactions to treatment with an antiparasitic, including sensitivity reactions and, in some cases, central nervous system (CNS) toxicity.

▶ To prevent self-infestation, avoid direct contact with the patient's hair, clothing, and bedsheets. Use gloves, a gown, and a protective head covering when administering delousing treatment.

▶ After each treatment, inspect the patient for remaining lice and eggs.

▶ Administer antibiotics as ordered.

▶ Be aware of the stigma that is attached to the presence of lice. Provide emotional support to the patient and family.

 SAFETY Ask the patient with pediculosis pubis to notify sexual contacts so that they can be examined and treated. If the infestation occurs in a school-age child, notify the school. To prevent the spread to other hospitalized patients, examine all high-risk patients on admission, especially elderly patients from nursing homes, people living in crowded conditions, and homeless people.

Patient teaching

▶ Teach the patient and family how to inspect for and identify lice, eggs, and related lesions. Teach them how to decontaminate infestation sources, and stress the importance of not borrowing personal articles.

 PREVENTION To prevent the spread of body lice or prevent re-infestation, educate the patient about the need for personal hygiene and the importance of laundering clothing, bed linens, and towels.

▶ Instruct the patient and family about the use of the creams, lotions, powders, and shampoos that eliminate lice. Teach them how to remove nits from the hair and eyelashes.

▶ Instruct the patient in the proper application of lindane, which can be absorbed by the skin and cause CNS complications. Tell the patient to be alert for possible adverse reactions and to notify the physician if these occur.

Pelvic inflammatory disease

Pelvic inflammatory disease (PID) is an umbrella term that refers to any acute, subacute, recurrent, or chronic infection of the oviducts and ovaries, with adjacent tissue involvement. It involves inflammation of the cervix (cervicitis), uterus (endometritis), fallopian tubes (salpingitis), and ovaries (oophoritis); inflammation can extend to the connective tissue lying between the broad ligaments (parametritis). In some cases, PID can result from overgrowth of common bacterial species found in the cervical mucus. Early diagnosis and treatment help prevent damage to the reproductive system. Untreated PID can be fatal.

CAUSES

PID occurs when microorganisms ascend to the upper female genital tract from the vagina and cervix. The condition can result from infection with aerobic or anaerobic microorganisms. The microorganisms *Neisseria gonorrhoeae* and *Chlamydia trachomatis* are the most common causes because they most readily penetrate the bacteriostatic barrier of cervical mucus. Common bacteria found in cervical mucus include staphylococci, streptococci, diphtheroids, chlamydiae, and coliforms, including *Pseudomonas* and *Escherichia coli*. Uterine infection can result from any one or several of these microorganisms or may follow the multiplication of normally nonpathogenic bacteria in an altered endometrial environment. Bacterial multiplication is most common during parturition because the endometrium is atrophic, quiescent, and not stimulated by estrogen.

Those at risk for PID include people with any sexually transmitted infection or multiple sex partners. Conditions or procedures, such as conization or cauterization of the cervix, that alter or destroy cervical mucus, can allow bacteria to ascend into the uterine cavity. Any procedure that risks transfer of contaminated cervical mucus into the endometrial cavity by an instrument (such as a biopsy curette or an irrigation catheter) poses an increased risk of PID, as do tubal insufflation, abortion, or recent intrauterine device insertion. Infectious foci within the body, such as drainage from a chronically infected fallopian tube, a pelvic abscess, a ruptured appendix, or diverticulitis of the sigmoid colon increase the risk of PID, as do infection during or after pregnancy, cigarette smoking, multiparity, douching, and intercourse during menses.

COMPLICATIONS

Possible complications of PID may include potentially fatal septicemia from a ruptured pelvic abscess, pulmonary emboli, infertility, and shock.

ASSESSMENT FINDINGS

The most common symptom in the patient with PID is that is pain described as dull, aching, and constant. It begins a few days after the onset of the last menstrual period and tends to be accentuated by motion, exercise, or coitus. It usually lasts about 7 days. Other signs include abnormal mucopurulent vaginal discharge, irregular vaginal bleeding, fever, and malaise. Vaginal examination may reveal pain during movement of the cervix or palpation of the adnexa; lower abdominal tenderness may be noted on palpation.

DIAGNOSTIC TESTS

▶ Gram stain of secretions from the endocervix or cul-de-sac indicates the causative agent. Culture and sensitivity testing aids selection of the appropriate antibiotic.
▶ Blood work reveals an elevated C-reactive protein level, erythrocyte sedimentation rate, and white blood cell count.
▶ Ultrasonography, computed tomography, and magnetic resonance imaging may help to identify and locate an adnexal or uterine mass.

TREATMENT

To prevent progression of PID, antibiotic therapy should begin immediately after culture specimens are obtained. Therapy can be reevaluated as soon as laboratory results are available (usually after 24 to 48 hours). Infection may become chronic if it is treated inadequately. If the patient is hospitalized, cefoxitin plus doxycycline (Doryx) or clindamycin (Cleocin) plus gentamicin may be administered I.V. initially for the first 24 hours, followed by doxycycline (Doryx) given orally. If the patient is treated as an outpatient, ceftriaxone (Rocephin) or cefoxitin may be given I.M. in conjunction with oral doxycycline (Doryx) or probenecid (Probalan), with or without metronidazole (Flagyl). Supplemental treatment for patients with PID may include bed rest, an analgesic, and I.V. fluids as needed.

Development of a pelvic abscess necessitates adequate drainage. A ruptured pelvic abscess is a life-threatening condition. If this complication develops, the patient may need a total abdominal hysterectomy with bilateral salpingo-oophorectomy.

NURSING CONSIDERATIONS

▶ After establishing that the patient has no drug allergies, administer an antibiotic and an analgesic as ordered.
▶ Monitor vital signs for fever and fluid intake and output for signs of dehydration. Watch for abdominal rigidity and distention, which are possible signs of developing peritonitis.
▶ Provide frequent perineal care if vaginal drainage occurs.
◗ Use meticulous handwashing technique; institute wound and skin precautions if necessary.
▶ Encourage the patient to discuss her feelings. Offer emotional support as well, and help her develop effective coping strategies.

Patient teaching

▶ Teach the patient about her infection, including how it is transmitted, causes, and treatment.
▶ Teach the patient about prescribed medications, including drug dosage, schedule of administration, and duration of therapy as well as the signs of adverse effects to report. Discuss the importance of taking the medications as prescribed and to finish the dosage.
▶ Teach the patient about possible complications of PID, including signs and symptoms of recurrence or re-infection, and which signs to report to the practitioner immediately.
▶ To prevent recurrence, encourage compliance with treatment and explain the disease and its severity.
▶ Stress the need for the patient's sexual partner to be examined and, if necessary, treated for infection.
▶ Discuss the use of condoms to prevent the spread of sexually transmitted infections.
▶ Because PID may cause dyspareunia, advise the patient to check with her physician before resuming sexual activity.

 PREVENTION To prevent infection after minor gynecologic procedures, such as dilation and curettage, tell the patient to immediately report fever, increased vaginal discharge, or pain. After such procedures, instruct the patient to avoid douching or having intercourse for at least 7 days.

Pharyngitis

The most common throat disorder, pharyngitis is an acute or chronic inflammation of the pharynx. It's widespread among adults who live or work in dusty or dry environments, use their voices excessively, habitually use tobacco or alcohol, or suffer from chronic sinusitis, persistent cough, or allergies. Uncomplicated pharyngitis usually subsides in 3 to 10 days. Beta-hemolytic streptococci, which cause 15% to 20% of acute pharyngitis cases, may precede the common cold or other communicable diseases. Chronic pharyngitis commonly is an extension of nasopharyngeal obstruction or inflammation. Viral pharyngitis accounts for about 70% of acute pharyngitis cases.

CAUSES

Pharyngitis is usually caused by a virus, including rhinovirus, adenovirus, Epstein-Barr virus, herpes simplex virus, influenza virus, parainfluenza virus, coronavirus, enterovirus, respiratory syncytial virus, cytomegalovirus, and human immunodeficiency virus. The most common bacterial cause is group A beta-hemolytic streptococci. Other common causes include *Mycoplasma* and *Chlamydia*. The organisms may invade the pharyngeal mucosa directly, causing a local inflammatory response. In up to 30% of cases, no organism is identified.

COMPLICATIONS

Complications of pharyngitis include otitis media, sinusitis, mastoiditis, rheumatic fever, and nephritis.

ASSESSMENT FINDINGS

Pharyngitis produces a sore throat and slight difficulty swallowing. Swallowing saliva is usually more painful than swallowing food. Pharyngitis may also cause the sensation of a lump in the throat as well as a constant, aggravating urge to swallow. Associated

features may include mild fever, headache, muscle and joint pain, coryza, and rhinorrhea. Uncomplicated pharyngitis usually subsides in 3 to 10 days. More than 90% of cases of sore throat and fever in children are of viral origin, and associated symptoms usually include a runny nose and nonproductive cough. Physical examination of the pharynx reveals generalized redness and inflammation of the posterior wall along with red, edematous mucous membranes studded with white or yellow follicles. Exudate is usually confined to the lymphoid areas of the throat, sparing the tonsillar pillars. Bacterial pharyngitis usually produces a large amount of exudate.

DIAGNOSTIC TESTS

▶ A throat culture may be performed to identify bacterial organisms that may be the cause of inflammation.
▶ Serology testing may be conducted and titers drawn to help identify the contributing organism, but these tests are not very helpful in diagnosing acute pharyngitis.
▶ Computed tomography is helpful in identifying the location of abscesses.
▶ A white blood cell (WBC) count is used to determine atypical lymphocytes; an elevated total WBC count is present in pharyngitis.

TREATMENT

Treatment for acute viral pharyngitis is usually symptomatic and consists mainly of rest, warm saline gargles, throat lozenges containing a mild anesthetic, plenty of fluids, and analgesics as needed. If the patient can't swallow fluids, I.V. hydration may be required. More severe cases may necessitate antiviral therapy. In severe cases of herpes simplex pharyngitis and for immunocompromised patients, acyclovir (Zorivax), famciclovir (Famvir), and valacyclovir are considerations.

Suspected bacterial pharyngitis requires rigorous treatment with penicillin or another broad-spectrum antibiotic because *Streptococcus* is the chief infecting organism. Antibiotic therapy should continue for 48 hours until culture results are ready. If the culture (or a rapid strep test) is positive for group A beta-hemolytic streptococci, or if bacterial infection is suspected despite negative culture results, penicillin therapy should be continued for 10 days. This is to prevent the sequelae of acute rheumatic fever.

Chronic pharyngitis requires the same supportive measures as acute pharyngitis but with greater emphasis on eliminating the underlying cause, such as an allergen. Preventive measures include adequate humidification and avoiding excessive exposure to air conditioning. In addition, the patient should be urged to stop smoking.

NURSING CONSIDERATIONS

▶ Administer analgesics and warm saline gargles as ordered and as appropriate.
▶ Encourage the patient to drink plenty of fluids. Scrupulously monitor intake and output, and watch for signs of dehydration (cracked lips, dry mucous membranes, low urine output, poor skin turgor).
▶ Provide meticulous mouth care to prevent dry lips and oral pyoderma, and maintain a restful environment.
▶ Obtain throat cultures, and administer antibiotics as needed. If the patient has acute bacterial pharyngitis, emphasize the importance of completing the full course of antibiotic therapy.
▶ Maintain a restful environment, especially if the patient is febrile, to conserve energy.

▶ Encourage a soft, light diet with plenty of liquids to combat the commonly experienced anorexia. An antiemetic can be given before eating if ordered.
▶ Examine the skin twice a day for possible drug sensitivity rashes or for rashes indicating a communicable disease.
▶ Administer an analgesic as ordered.

Patient teaching

▶ If the patient has acute bacterial pharyngitis, emphasize the importance of completing the full course of antibiotic therapy. Tell the patient to call the physician if he or she experiences any adverse reactions.
▶ Teach the patient with chronic pharyngitis how to minimize sources of throat irritation in the environment, such as by using a bedside humidifier.
▶ Teach the patient about the infection, including how it is transmitted, possible cause, and treatment. Review signs and symptoms of complications to report to the health care provider.
▶ Refer the patient to a self-help group to stop smoking if appropriate.

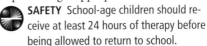 **SAFETY** School-age children should receive at least 24 hours of therapy before being allowed to return to school.

▶ Teach the patient to avoid using irritants, such as alcohol, which may exacerbate symptoms.

DROPLET PRECAUTIONS

Plague

Plague, also known as black death, is an acute infection caused by the gram-negative, non-motile, nonsporulating bacillus *Yersinia pestis*. Bubonic plague, the most common form, causes the characteristic swollen, and sometimes suppurating, lymph glands (buboes) that give this infection its name. Mortality is about 75% in untreated bubonic plague but is reduced to 5% with treatment. In pneumonic plague, mortality rates are in excess of 90% in untreated cases. Other types of plague include septicemic, meningeal, and pharyngeal.

CAUSES

Plague is usually transmitted to humans through the bite of a flea from an infected rodent host, such as a rat or prairie dog. Occasionally, transmission occurs from handling infected animals or their tissue; the infection is rarely transmitted from person to person. Respiratory droplets (coughing) are highly contagious in pneumonic plague, and transmission can occur after inhalation of *Y. pestis* in a laboratory.

COMPLICATIONS

Complications from plague include acute respiratory distress syndrome, chronic lymphedema from lymphatic scarring, disseminated intravascular coagulation, septic shock, and secondary infection of the buboes by *Staphylococcus* and *Pseudomonas* species.

ASSESSMENT FINDINGS

In bubonic plague, the incubation period is 2 to 8 days. The milder form begins with malaise and fever in addition to pain, swelling, and tenderness in regional lymph nodes. Lymph node damage (usually axillary or inguinal) produces painful, inflamed, and possibly suppurative buboes. Hemorrhagic areas become necrotic in the skin and appear dark ("black death"). This infection can

progress extremely rapidly within hours. Bubonic plague may also begin dramatically, with a sudden high fever of 103° to 106° F (39.4° to 41.1° C), chills, myalgia, headache, prostration, restlessness, disorientation, delirium, toxemia, and a staggering gait. Occasionally, abdominal pain, nausea, vomiting, and constipation followed by diarrhea (frequently bloody), skin mottling, petechiae, and circulatory collapse occur.

In pneumonic plague, the incubation period of 2 to 3 days is followed by high fever, chills, severe headache, tachycardia, tachypnea, dyspnea, and a productive cough (mucoid sputum at first, later frothy pink or red sputum). Pneumonic plague can quickly cause severe prostration, respiratory distress and, usually, death.

Septicemic plague usually develops without overt lymph node enlargement. The patient shows toxicity, hyperpyrexia, seizures, prostration, shock, and disseminated intravascular coagulation (DIC). Septicemic plague causes widespread nonspecific tissue damage (peritoneal or pleural effusions, pericarditis, and meningitis). With meningeal plague the patient has a fever, headache, nuchal rigidity, and buboes, especially axillary. Pharyngeal plague results from ingestion of the plague bacilli and produces symptoms of sore throat, fever, painful cervical lymph nodes, and pharyngeal erythema.

DIAGNOSTIC TESTS

▶ Blood culture results are often positive for *Y. pestis* in bubonic and septicemic plague; *Y. pestis* may be observed on a peripheral blood smear and in lymph node aspirates; in pharyngeal plague, *Y. pestis* is cultured from throat swabs and gram stain of sputum.
▶ Cerebrospinal fluid samples show pleocytosis with a predominance of polymorphonuclear leukocytes in meningeal plague; Gram stain may show gram-negative bacilli, and a limulus test detects endotoxin.
▶ Chest radiography detects patchy infiltrates, consolidation, or a persistent cavity with pneumonic plague.

TREATMENT

Treatment consists of large doses of strepto-mycin, the drug proven most effective against *Y. pestis*, with the alternative of doxy-cycline (Doryx). Chloramphenicol is the preferred drug in meningeal plague or for hypotensive patients with any type of plague. Supportive management aims to control fever, shock, and seizures and to maintain fluid balance through I.V. therapy, epineph-rine, and dopamine. Hemodynamic moni-toring and ventilatory support may be re-quired. As complications develop (toxemia, shock, DIC), they will need to be addressed. Enlarging or fluctuant buboes may require incision and drainage.

 PREVENTION Prophylactic antibiotics (doxycycline, trimethoprim-sulfamethoxa-zole [Bactrim]) should be administered to individuals who are exposed to bites of potentially infected rodent fleas during a plague outbreak, to those who have han-dled an animal known to be infected, or to those who have had close exposure to a person thought to have pneumonic plague.

NURSING CONSIDERATIONS

 SAFETY Practice strict droplet precautions for 48 to 72 hours after starting antibiotic therapy with all patients who have a sus-pected diagnosis of plague who have pneumonia symptoms. Cases of plague should be reported to the local health de-partment and the World Health Organiza-tion. Laboratory personnel should be alerted to the possibility of plague to pre-vent aerosolization of fluids.

◆ Carefully dispose of feces, sputum, and soiled dressings and linens. If the patient has pneumonic plague, wear a mask and follow droplet precautions. For more information, consult your infection control officer.

❱ Monitor vital signs, intake and output, and respiratory and hemodynamic status; pro-vide ventilator support and I.V. fluids as in-dicated; suction as indicated.

Patient teaching

 PREVENTION To help prevent plague, dis-courage contact with wild animals (espe-cially sick or dead animals), and support programs aimed at reducing insect and ro-dent populations. Recommend immuniza-tion with plague vaccine to travelers to, or residents of, endemic areas, and to scien-tists and laboratory personnel who rou-tinely work with the plague bacterium even though the effect is transient.

❱ Recommend removing food sources and nesting places used by rodents and having homes, workplaces and recreation areas made more "rodent-proof." Professionals should apply chemicals to kill fleas and rodents.

❱ Recommend that trained professionals fu-migate cargo areas of ships and docks.

❱ Instruct patients and family to report sick or dead animals to the local health depart-ment or law enforcement officials and to wear gloves when handling potentially in-fected animals.

❱ Educate patients regarding personal pro-tective measures, such as wearing protective clothing and applying insect repellents to clothing and skin to prevent flea bites.

❱ Tell the patient to restrain pets in endemic areas and regularly treat them to control fleas.

Pneumonia

Pneumonia is an acute infection of the lung parenchyma that often impairs gas exchange. Many types of organisms can cause pneumonia, including viral, bacterial, fungal, protozoal, mycobacterial, mycoplasmal, or rickettsial organisms. The infection may also be described by location: bronchopneumonia, lobular pneumonia, or lobar pneumonia.

Pneumonia is also classified into three types—primary, secondary, or aspiration pneumonia. Primary pneumonia results directly from inhalation or aspiration of a pathogen, such as bacteria or a virus; it includes pneumococcal and viral pneumonia. Secondary pneumonia may follow initial lung damage from a noxious chemical or other insult (super-infection) or may result from hematogenous spread of bacteria from a distant area. Aspiration pneumonia results from inhalation of foreign matter, such as vomitus or food particles, into the bronchi. Aspiration pneumonia is more likely to occur in elderly or debilitated patients, those receiving nasogastric tube feedings, and those with an impaired gag reflex, poor oral hygiene, or a decreased level of consciousness.

CAUSES

Pneumonia can be classified in several ways. Depending on the microbiologic etiology, pneumonia can be bacterial, viral, fungal, protozoan, mycobacterial, mycoplasmal, or rickettsial in origin. (See *Diagnosing and treating the types of pneumonia*, pages 246–249.)

In bacterial pneumonia, an infection initially triggers alveolar inflammation and edema. Capillaries become engorged with blood, causing stasis. As the alveolocapillary membrane breaks down, alveoli fill with blood and exudate, resulting in atelectasis. In severe bacterial infections, the lungs assume a heavy, liverlike appearance, as in acute respiratory distress syndrome (ARDS).

Viral infection typically causes diffuse pneumonia and first attacks bronchiolar epithelial cells, causing interstitial inflammation and desquamation. It then spreads to the alveoli, which fill with blood and fluid. In advanced infection, a hyaline membrane may form. As with bacterial infection, severe viral infection may clinically resemble ARDS.

In aspiration pneumonia, aspiration of gastric juices or hydrocarbons triggers similar inflammatory changes and also inactivates surfactant over a large area. Decreased surfactant leads to alveolar collapse. Acidic gastric juices may directly damage the airways and alveoli. Particles with the aspirated gastric juices may obstruct the airways and reduce airflow, thereby leading to secondary bacterial pneumonia.

Certain predisposing factors increase the risk of pneumonia. They include chronic illness and debilitation, cancer (particularly lung cancer), abdominal and thoracic surgery, atelectasis, common colds or other viral respiratory infections, chronic respiratory diseases, influenza, smoking, malnutrition, alcoholism, sickle cell disease, tracheostomy, exposure to noxious gases, aspiration, and immunosuppressive therapy.

COMPLICATIONS

Complications from pneumonia may include septic shock, hypoxemia, respiratory failure, empyema, lung abscess, bacteremia, endocarditis, pericarditis, and meningitis.

ASSESSMENT FINDINGS

The main symptoms of pneumonia are coughing, sputum production, pleuritic chest pain, shaking chills, shortness of breath, fever, and rapid, shallow breathing. Physical signs vary widely, ranging from diffuse, fine crackles to signs of localized or extensive consolidation and pleural effusion. There may also be associated symptoms of headache, sweating, loss of appetite, excess fatigue, and confusion (in older patients).

Diagnostic tests

▶ Chest radiography shows infiltrates with characteristics specific to the type of pneumonia present.

▶ Sputum stain demonstrates acute inflammatory cells; Gram stain and sputum culture may identify the organism. Tracheobronchial secretions or brushings or washings obtained via bronchoscopy may be used for smear and culture.

▶ Positive blood cultures in the patient with pulmonary infiltrates strongly suggest pneumonia produced by the organisms isolated from the blood cultures.

▶ Pleural effusions, if present, should be tapped and fluid analyzed for evidence of infection in the pleural space.

Treatment

Antimicrobial therapy varies with the causative agent and should be reevaluated early in the course of treatment. Supportive measures include humidified oxygen therapy for hypoxemia, mechanical ventilation for respiratory failure, a high-calorie diet and adequate fluid intake, bed rest, and an analgesic to relieve pleuritic chest pain. Patients with severe pneumonia who are on mechanical ventilation may require positive end-expiratory pressure to facilitate adequate oxygenation.

Nursing considerations

▶ Maintain a patent airway and adequate oxygenation. Monitor pulse oximetry and arterial blood gas levels. Administer oxygen as ordered.

▶ Teach the patient how to cough, breathe deeply, and clear secretions. In severe pneumonia that requires endotracheal intubation or tracheostomy (with or without mechanical ventilation), suction as needed to remove secretions.

 SAFETY In order to control the spread of infection, dispose of secretions properly. Tell the patient to sneeze and cough into a disposable tissue; tape a lined bag to the side of the bed for used tissues.

▶ Administer antimicrobials as ordered and pain medication as needed; record the patient's response.

▶ Monitor vital signs as well as intake and output; administer antipyretics for fever and I.V. fluids and electrolyte replacement as ordered.

▶ Maintain adequate nutrition to offset the hypermetabolic state; supplement oral feedings with nasogastric tube feedings or parenteral nutrition.

 PREVENTION To prevent aspiration pneumonia during nasogastric tube feedings, elevate the patient's head, check the tube's position, and administer the formula slowly. To prevent vomiting, don't give large volumes at one time. Keep the patient's head elevated for at least 30 minutes after the feeding. Check for residual formula at 4- to 6-hour intervals.

Patient teaching

▶ Review the patient's medication. Stress the need to take the entire course of medication, even if feeling better, to prevent a relapse.

▶ Teach the patient procedures to clear lung secretions, such as deep-breathing and coughing exercises, chest physiotherapy to mobilize secretions, and home oxygen therapy.

▶ Urge the patient to avoid irritants that stimulate secretions, such as cigarette smoke, dust, and significant environmental pollution.

 PREVENTION Advise the patient to avoid using antibiotics indiscriminately during minor viral infections because this may result in upper airway colonization with antibiotic-resistant bacteria. If the patient then develops pneumonia, the organisms producing the pneumonia may require treatment with more toxic antibiotics. Encourage pneumococcal (Pneumovax) vaccination and annual influenza vaccination for high-risk patients, such as those with chronic obstructive pulmonary disease, chronic heart disease, or sickle cell disease.

Diagnosing and treating the types of pneumonia

Type	Signs and symptoms
Aspiration	
Results from vomiting and aspiration of gastric or oropharyngeal contents into trachea and lungs	• Noncardiogenic pulmonary edema that may follow damage to respiratory epithelium from contact with stomach acid • Crackles, dyspnea, cyanosis, hypotension, and tachycardia • May be subacute with cavity formation; lung abscess may occur if foreign body is present
Bacterial	
Klebsiella	• Fever and recurrent chills; cough producing rusty, bloody, viscous sputum (currant jelly); cyanosis of lips and nail beds due to hypoxemia; and shallow, grunting respirations • Common in patients with chronic alcoholism, pulmonary disease, diabetes, or those at risk for aspiration
Staphylococcus	• Temperature of 102° to 104° F (38.9° to 40° C), recurrent shaking chills, bloody sputum, dyspnea, tachypnea, and hypoxemia • Should be suspected with viral illness, such as influenza or measles, and in patients with cystic fibrosis
Streptococcus (pneumoniae)	• Sudden onset of shaking chills and a sustained temperature of 102° to 104° F (38.9° to 40° C); commonly preceded by upper respiratory tract infection
Protozoan	
Pneumocystis carinii (jiroveci)	• Occurs in immunocompromised persons • Dyspnea and nonproductive cough • Anorexia, weight loss, and fatigue • Low-grade fever
Viral	
Adenovirus (insidious onset; generally affects young adults)	• Sore throat, fever, cough, chills, malaise, small amounts of mucoid sputum, retrosternal chest pain, anorexia, rhinitis, adenopathy, scattered crackles, and rhonchi

Diagnosis	Treatment
• *Chest radiography:* locates areas of infiltrates, which suggest diagnosis	• *Antimicrobial therapy:* penicillin G or clindamycin • *Supportive:* oxygen therapy, suctioning, coughing, deep breathing, and adequate hydration
• *Chest radiography:* typically, but not always, consolidation in the upper lobe that causes bulging of fissures • *White blood cell (WBC) count:* elevated • *Sputum culture and Gram stain:* may show gram-negative *Klebsiella*	• *Antimicrobial therapy:* an aminoglycoside and a cephalosporin
• *Chest radiography:* multiple abscesses and infiltrates; high incidence of empyema • *WBC count:* elevated • *Sputum culture and Gram stain:* may show gram-positive staphylococci	• *Antimicrobial therapy:* nafcillin or oxacillin for 14 days if staphylococci are penicillinase producing • *Supportive:* chest tube drainage of empyema
• *Chest radiography:* areas of consolidation, commonly lobar • *WBC count:* elevated • *Sputum culture:* may show gram-positive *S. pneumoniae;* this organism not always recovered	• *Antimicrobial therapy:* penicillin G (or erythromycin, if patient is allergic to penicillin) for 7 to 10 days beginning after obtaining culture specimen but without waiting for results (Resistance to penicillin is becoming much more common and, in the patient with risk factors for resistance [extreme age, daycare attendance, or immunosuppression], treatment with vancomycin, imipenem, or levofloxacin should be considered.)
• *Fiber-optic bronchoscopy:* obtains specimens for histologic studies • *Chest radiography:* nonspecific infiltrates, nodular lesions, or spontaneous pneumothorax	• *Antimicrobial therapy:* co-trimoxazole or pentamidine by I.V. administration or inhalation (prophylactic pentamidine may be used for high-risk patients) • *Supportive:* oxygen, improved nutrition, and mechanical ventilation
• *Chest radiography:* patchy distribution of pneumonia, more severe than indicated by physical examination • *WBC count:* normal to slightly elevated	• Treat symptoms only • Mortality low; usually clears with no residual effects

(continued)

Diagnosing and treating the types of pneumonia *(continued)*

Type	Signs and symptoms
Viral (continued)	
Chickenpox (varicella) (uncommon in children, but present in 30% of adults with varicella)	• Cough, dyspnea, cyanosis, tachypnea, pleuritic chest pain, hemoptysis, and rhonchi 1 to 6 days after onset of rash
Cytomegalovirus	• Difficult to distinguish from other nonbacterial pneumonias • Fever, cough, shaking chills, dyspnea, cyanosis, weakness, and diffuse crackles • Occurs in neonates as devastating multisystemic infection; in normal adults, resembles mononucleosis; in immunocompromised hosts, varies from clinically inapparent to devastating infection
Influenza (prognosis poor even with treatment; 30% mortality)	• Cough (initially nonproductive; later, purulent sputum), marked cyanosis, dyspnea, high fever, chills, substernal pain and discomfort, moist crackles, frontal headache, and myalgia • Death results from cardiopulmonary collapse
Measles (rubeola)	• Fever, dyspnea, cough, small amounts of sputum, coryza, rash, and cervical adenopathy
Respiratory syncytial virus (most prevalent in infants and children)	• Listlessness, irritability, tachypnea with retraction of intercostal muscles, wheezing, slight sputum production, fine moist crackles, fever, severe malaise, and cough

Diagnosis	Treatment
• *Chest radiography:* shows more extensive pneumonia than indicated by physical examination and bilateral, patchy, diffuse, nodular infiltrates • *Sputum analysis:* predominant mononuclear cells and characteristic intranuclear inclusion bodies, with characteristic skin rash, confirm diagnosis	• *Supportive:* adequate hydration, and oxygen therapy in critically ill patients • Therapy with I.V. acyclovir
• *Chest radiography:* in early stages, variable patchy infiltrates; later, bilateral, nodular, and more predominant in lower lobes • *Percutaneous aspiration of lung tissue, transbronchial biopsy, or open lung biopsy:* microscopic examination shows typical intranuclear and cytoplasmic inclusions; the virus can be cultured from lung tissue	• Generally, benign and self-limiting in mononucleosis-like form • *Supportive:* adequate hydration and nutrition, oxygen therapy, and bed rest • In immunosuppressed patients, disease is more severe and may be fatal; ganciclovir or foscarnet treatment warranted
• *Chest radiography:* diffuse bilateral bronchopneumonia radiating from hilus • *WBC count:* normal to slightly elevated • *Sputum smears:* no specific organisms	• *Supportive:* for respiratory failure, endotracheal intubation and ventilator assistance; for fever, hypothermia blanket or antipyretics; and for influenza A, amantadine or rimantadine
• *Chest radiography:* reticular infiltrates, sometimes with hilar lymph node enlargement • *Lung tissue specimen:* characteristic giant cells	• *Supportive:* bed rest, adequate hydration, and antimicrobials; assisted ventilation if necessary
• *Chest radiography:* patchy bilateral consolidation • *WBC count:* normal to slightly elevated	• *Supportive:* humidified air, oxygen, antimicrobials (commonly given until viral etiology confirmed), and aerosolized ribavirin • Usually complete recovery

Poliomyelitis

Poliomyelitis, also called polio or infantile paralysis, is an acute communicable disease caused by the poliovirus, an enterovirus. It ranges in severity from inapparent infection to fatal paralytic illness. Minor outbreaks still occur, usually among nonimmunized groups, with the disease occurring during the summer and fall. If the central nervous system (CNS) is spared, the prognosis is excellent. However, CNS infection can cause paralysis and death.

CAUSES

The poliovirus is transmitted from person to person by direct contact with infected oropharyngeal secretions or feces; the incubation period is 5 to 35 days. The virus enters through the alimentary tract, multiplies in the oropharynx and lower intestinal tract, and spreads to regional lymph nodes and the blood.

COMPLICATIONS

Complications from poliomyelitis include respiratory failure, pulmonary edema, pulmonary embolism, urinary tract infection, urolithiasis, atelectasis, pneumonia, cor pulmonale, soft-tissue and skeletal deformities, paralytic shock, and hypertension.

ASSESSMENT FINDINGS

Inapparent (subclinical) infections constitute 95% of all poliovirus infections. Abortive or inapparent poliomyelitis (minor illness) accounts for 4% to 8% of all cases and causes slight fever, malaise, headache, sore throat, inflamed pharynx, and vomiting. The patient usually recovers within 72 hours. Most cases of abortive poliomyelitis go unnoticed.

Major poliomyelitis involves the CNS and takes two forms: nonparalytic and paralytic. Children commonly show a biphasic course in which the onset of major illness occurs after recovery from the minor illness stage. Nonparalytic poliomyelitis produces moderate fever, headache, vomiting, lethargy, irritability, and pains in the neck, back, arms, legs, and abdomen. It also causes muscle tenderness, weakness, and spasms in the extensors of the neck, back, hamstring, and other muscles during range-of-motion exercises. Nonparalytic polio usually lasts about a week, with meningeal irritation persisting 2 weeks. Paralytic poliomyelitis develops within 5 to 7 days of the onset of fever with symptoms similar to those of nonparalytic poliomyelitis: asymmetrical weakness of various muscles, loss of superficial and deep reflexes, paresthesia, positive Kernig's and Brudzinski's signs, hypersensitivity to touch, urine retention, constipation, and abdominal distention. The extent of paralysis depends on the level of the spinal cord lesions (cervical, thoracic, or lumbar).

In both nonparalytic and paralytic forms of poliomyelitis, the patient will show tripod (arms extended behind for support when sitting up), Hoyne sign (head falls back when supine and shoulders are elevated), and an inability to raise the legs a full 90 degrees from a supine position. When the disease affects the medulla of the brain (bulbar paralytic poliomyelitis), the nerves of the respiratory tract are affected, leading to respiratory paralysis and weakness of the muscles supplied by the cranial nerves (particularly IX and X) and producing symptoms of encephalitis. Other signs include facial weakness, diplopia, dysphasia, difficulty chewing, inability to swallow or expel saliva, regurgitation of food through the nasal passages, dyspnea, and abnormal respiratory rate, depth, and rhythm, which may lead to respiratory arrest, fatal pulmonary edema, and shock.

DIAGNOSIS

▶ Cultures from throat washings early in the disease, from stools throughout the disease, and from cerebrospinal fluid (CSF) cultures in CNS infection detect the polio virus.
▶ Convalescent serum antibody titers four times greater than acute titers support the diagnosis.

▶ CSF pressure and protein levels may be slightly increased and the white blood cell count elevated initially. Thereafter, mononuclear cells constitute most of the diminished number of cells.

▶ Electromyographic findings in early poliomyelitis show a reduction in the recruitment pattern and a diminished interference pattern due to acute motor axon fiber involvement. Fibrillations develop in 2 to 4 weeks, and fasciculations also may be observed. Motor unit action potentials are affected, but motor nerve conduction velocities remain within normal limits. Compound muscle action potential is reduced in direct proportion to the number of motor axons that are affected. Sensory nerve conduction studies are normal.

TREATMENT

Treatment is supportive and includes analgesics to ease headache, back pain, and leg spasms; morphine is contraindicated because of the danger of additional respiratory suppression. Moist heat applications may also reduce muscle spasm and pain. Bed rest is necessary only until extreme discomfort subsides; in paralytic polio, this may take a long time. Paralytic polio also requires long-term rehabilitation, including physical therapy, braces, corrective shoes and, in some cases, orthopedic surgery.

NURSING CONSIDERATIONS

▶ Observe the patient for paralysis and other neurologic damage. Maintain a patent airway; prepare and assist with tracheotomy and mechanical ventilation as indicated.

 ALERT Check blood pressure frequently, especially in patients with bulbar poliomyelitis, which can cause hypertension or shock because of its effect on the brain stem.

▶ Provide an adequate, well-balanced diet and prevent pressure ulcers by good skin care and frequent repositioning.

 SAFETY To control the spread of poliomyelitis, wash your hands thoroughly after contact with the patient and instruct patients to do the same. Warn any facility worker who hasn't been vaccinated to avoid contact with the patient. Only those who have been vaccinated against poliomyelitis should have direct contact with the patient.

▶ Report all cases of poliomyelitis to the appropriate local public health department.

Patient teaching

▶ Inform ambulatory patients about the need for careful handwashing.

▶ Instruct the patient or caregivers about measures needed to manage symptoms and prevent complications.

PREVENTION Encourage parents to have children vaccinated against polio. Reassure them that the risk of vaccine-related disease is small. Inactivated poliovirus vaccine is administered in four doses at ages 2 months, 4 months, 6 to 18 months, and 4 to 6 years.

Powassan viral disease

The Powassan (POW) virus is a rare, tick-borne encephalitis virus related to the flavivirus. This disease had its earliest origins in the town of Powassan, Ontario. The virus is transmitted by *Ixodes cookei* ticks among small mammals in eastern Canada and the United States, where it has been responsible for 20 known cases. Other ticks may transmit the virus in a wider geographic area. POW virus can be transmitted within less than 15 minutes of tick attachment. It usually occurs in May through December after outdoor exposure. POW encephalitis is common and is usually severe, leaving the patient with neurologic deficits or causing death.

CAUSES

POW virus has been isolated from four species of tick in North America—*I. cookei*, *Ixodes marxi*, *Ixodes spinipalpus*, and *Dermacentor andersoni*—with *I. cookei* the most commonly involved. It is transmitted among several species of small wild mammals but is most often associated with the woodchuck. Infection rates can also be high in red and gray squirrels, Eastern chipmunks, porcupines, deer mice, voles, snowshoe hares, striped skunks, and raccoons. The virus can survive through winter in dormant ticks at various stages in their life cycle and be transmitted to mammals in the spring when the tick becomes active again. Studies in the former U.S.S.R. detected POW virus in mosquitoes and antibodies to the virus in a variety of bird species. Whether this is important in maintenance of the virus or for transmission to people is not known.

COMPLICATIONS

Complications of POW encephalitis include secondary bacterial infections of the respiratory and urinary tracts, neuronal injury and defects, impairment of intelligence, and psychiatric disturbances. Extrapyramidal features (especially dystonia and occasionally parkinsonism), weakness, seizure disorders, and death may occur.

ASSESSMENT FINDINGS

The incubation period is 7 to 14 days and onset is sudden, with headache, fever, disorientation, and convulsions. Prodromal symptoms include sore throat, sleepiness, headache, and disorientation. Encephalitis is characterized by vomiting, prolonged fever or fever of variable length, respiratory distress, and lethargy. Seizures are common, and patients may then become semicomatose with some paralysis, hypotonia, spasticity, or ophthalmoplegia.

DIAGNOSTIC TESTS

▶ Serology helps identify the POW virus antibody. Diagnosis may be facilitated by serologic assays, such as immunoglobulin (Ig) M-capture enzyme-linked immunosorbent assay (ELISA) and Ig ELISA. Early in infection, IgM antibody is more specific, whereas later IgG is more reactive. Nucleic acid detection tests for flavivirus can also be helpful.
▶ Brain biopsy may identify the virus and may be considered when a lumbar puncture is precluded or when the diagnosis is uncertain.

TREATMENT

There is no specific therapy for POW encephalitis. Supportive treatment includes appropriately managing the airway and hemodynamic status, maintaining fluid and electrolyte balance, treating fever, providing nutrition, and preventing complications of bed rest (bedsores, secondary pulmonary infection). Increased intracranial pressure should be managed in the intensive care setting with head elevation, gentle diuresis, mannitol, and hyperventilation. Seizures may be treated with anticonvulsants, such as phenytoin or other medications, and treatment for status epilepticus. There is no vaccine available for POW encephalitis.

Nursing considerations

▶ During the acute phase of the illness, assess neurologic function often. Observe the level of consciousness and signs of increased intracranial pressure (increasing restlessness, plucking at the bedcovers, vomiting, seizures, and changes in pupil size, motor function, and vital signs). Also watch for cranial nerve involvement (ptosis, strabismus, and diplopia), abnormal sleep patterns, and behavior changes.

▶ Maintain adequate fluid intake to prevent dehydration, but avoid fluid overload, which may increase cerebral edema. Measure and record intake and output accurately.

▶ Carefully position the patient to prevent joint stiffness and neck pain, and turn the patient often. Assist with range-of-motion exercises.

▶ Maintain adequate nutrition. Give the patient small, frequent meals, or supplement these meals with nasogastric tube or parenteral feedings.

◗ Maintain a quiet environment. Darkening the room may decrease headache. If the patient naps during the day and is restless at night, plan daytime activities to minimize napping and promote night-time sleep. If the patient has seizures, take precautions to protect the patient from injury.

▶ If the patient is delirious or confused, attempt to reorient him or her often. Providing a calendar or a clock in the patient's room may be helpful.

Patient teaching

▶ Teach the patient and family about the disease and its effects. Explain the diagnostic tests and treatment measures. Be sure to explain procedures to the patient even if he or she is comatose.

▶ Explain to the patient and family that behavior changes caused by encephalitis usually disappear, but permanent problems sometimes occur. If a neurologic deficit is severe

> ## Preventing POW viral disease
>
> *Ixodes cookei* is the tick that is primarily responsible for spreading POW viral disease, which usually causes encephalitis. In addition to protecting the skin from tick bites, reducing the incidence of the disease includes using environmental controls to minimize contact with small and medium-size mammals, such as the woodchuck, which are considered to be the primary vectors of POW virus.
>
> • Keep areas adjacent to the home clear of brush, weeds, trash, and other elements that could support small and medium-size mammals.
>
> • When removing rodent nests, avoid direct contact with nesting materials.
>
> • Use sealed plastic bags for disposal of infected animals to prevent direct contact with ticks.
>
> If a tick is found on the skin, prompt removal may help decrease the risk of transmission of a tickborne virus.

and appears permanent, refer the patient to a rehabilitation program as soon as the acute phase has passed.

 PREVENTION Explain that the best means of prevention is protection from tick bites. This includes using insect repellents, wearing light-colored clothing with long sleeves and pants tucked into socks or boots, avoiding or clearing brushy areas, and removing ticks before they attach or as soon after attachment as possible. Checking family pets can also prevent ticks from entering the home.

▶ Review with the patient preventive measures that can reduce the incidence of POW viral disease. (See *Preventing POW viral disease.*)

Prostatitis

Prostatitis, which is inflammation of the prostate gland, occurs in several forms. Acute prostatitis most often results from gram-negative bacteria and is easily recognized and treated. It is the most common cause of recurrent urinary tract infection (UTI) and more difficult to recognize. There are four forms of prostatitis: acute bacterial prostatitis, chronic bacterial prostatitis, chronic prostatitis/chronic pelvic pain syndrome, and asymptomatic inflammatory prostatitis.

CAUSES

Bacterial prostatitis often results from gram-negative Enterobacteriaceae (*Escherichia coli, Proteus mirabilis, Klebsiella* species, *Enterobacter* species, *Pseudomonas aeruginosa*, and *Serratia marcescens*). Anaerobic bacteria and gram-positive bacteria other than enterococci rarely cause acute bacterial prostatitis. *Staphylococcus aureus* infection can occur due to prolonged catheterization in hospital settings. Other organisms include *Neisseria gonorrhoeae, Mycobacterium tuberculosis, Salmonella* species, *Clostridium* species, and parasitic or mycotic organisms. Infection spreads from infected urine by reflux into the prostate gland, by the hematogenous route, from ascending urethral infection, or by invasion of rectal bacteria via the lymphatic vessels. Infection may also result from urethral procedures performed with instruments, such as cystoscopy and catheterization, or sexual intercourse. Chronic prostatitis usually results from bacterial invasion from the urethra, whereas granulomatous prostatitis occurs secondary to spread of *M. tuberculosis*. Nonbacterial prostatitis produces symptoms of prostatitis without bacterial infection.

COMPLICATIONS

UTI is the most common complication of prostatitis. An untreated infection can progress to prostatic abscess, acute urine retention from prostatic edema, pyelonephritis, and epididymitis.

ASSESSMENT FINDINGS

The patient with acute prostatitis may report sudden fever, chills, low back pain, myalgia, perineal fullness, perineal pain, arthralgia, frequent urination, urinary urgency, dysuria, nocturia, and transient erectile dysfunction. Some degree of urinary obstruction can occur, and the urine may appear cloudy. On palpation, the bladder may feel distended, swollen, firm, warm, and tender. Patients with chronic bacterial prostatitis may be asymptomatic or have milder symptoms of the acute version. Other symptoms include hemospermia, persistent urethral discharge, and painful ejaculation. The prostate may feel soft, and crepitation may be evident if prostatic calculi are present. Digital examination in granulomatous prostatitis may reveal a stony, hard induration of the prostate, and there is often a history of pulmonary or GI tuberculosis or receiving intravesical therapy for superficial bladder cancer. With nonbacterial prostatitis, the patient usually complains of dysuria, mild perineal or low back pain, and frequent nocturia.

DIAGNOSTIC TESTS

▶ A urine culture usually can be used to identify the causative infectious organism.
▶ Characteristic rectal examination findings suggest prostatitis (especially in the acute phase). The urine specimen should include midstream urine both before and after prostate massage.
▶ Blood cultures may be positive occasionally.
▶ Urodynamic evaluation may reveal detrusor hyperreflexia and pelvic floor myalgia from chronic spasms.
▶ Transrectal ultrasonography and computed tomography of the pelvis are useful in diagnosing and draining prostatic abscesses.

TREATMENT

Systemic antibiotic therapy, guided by sensitivity studies, is the treatment of choice for acute prostatitis. Agents that are effective against gram-negative bacteria include fluoroquinolones, trimethoprim-sulfamethoxazole (Bactrim), and ampicillin with gentamicin. Alpha-blocker therapy should also be considered. Alpha blockade with terazosin (Hytrin) may improve outflow obstruction and diminish intraprostatic urinary reflux. If drug therapy is unsuccessful, treatment may include transurethral resection of the prostate to remove all infected tissue.

For chronic bacterial prostatitis, trimethoprim-sulfamethoxazole fluoroquinolone antibiotics (ciprofloxacin [Cipro] or ofloxacin) or gatifloxacin-moxifloxacin is given for a 4- to 6-week course. Treatment for granulomatous prostatitis consists of antitubercular drug combinations. For nonbacterial prostatitis, a 2-week trial of an antibiotic such as trimethoprim-sulfamethoxazole, levofloxacin (Levaquin), or ciprofloxacin may help lead to the diagnosis; if the patient improves, treatment continues for a 4- to 6-week course.

Supportive therapy includes bed rest, adequate hydration, and administration of analgesics, antipyretics, and stool softeners as necessary. If symptoms are present in chronic prostatitis, treatment may consist of sitz baths and regular ejaculation to promote drainage of prostatic secretions. Anticholinergics, analgesics, and herbal supplements such as saw palmetto may help relieve the symptoms of nonbacterial prostatitis.

NURSING CONSIDERATIONS

▶ Administer analgesics for pain as ordered; ensure bed rest and adequate hydration.
▶ Provide stool softeners and sitz baths as ordered. Avoid rectal examination because it can precipitate bleeding.

▶ If transurethral resection of the prostate is performed, monitor postoperatively for signs of hypovolemia (decreased blood pressure, increased pulse rate, and pale, clammy skin). Provide catheter care and bladder irrigation as ordered; check the catheter every 15 minutes for the first 2 to 3 hours after surgery for patency, urine color and consistency, and excessive urethral meatus bleeding.

ALERT Watch for septic shock, the most serious complication of prostatic surgery. Immediately report severe chills, sudden fever, tachycardia, hypotension, or other signs of shock. Watch for pulmonary embolism, heart failure, and acute renal failure.

Patient teaching

▶ Teach the patient about his infection, including possible causes and treatment. Provide preoperative and postoperative education if the patient requires surgery.
▶ Review prescribed drugs and possible adverse effects. Tell the patient to take the drugs exactly as ordered and to complete the prescribed drug regimens.
▶ Instruct the patient to drink at least eight 8-oz glasses of fluid per day (about 2 qt [2 L]).
▶ Review with the patient signs of complications to report to the health care provider as well as prescribed limits on activity.

Psittacosis

Psittacosis (also called ornithosis or parrot fever) is caused by the gram-negative intracellular parasite *Chlamydia psittaci* and is transmitted by infected birds. This disease occurs worldwide and is mainly associated with occupational exposure to birds (such as poultry farming). Most infections result from exposure to psittacine birds (e.g., parrots, parakeets, macaws, cockatiels). With adequate antimicrobial therapy, psittacosis is fatal in less than 1% of patients.

Causes

Psittacine birds, pigeons, and turkeys may harbor *C. psittaci* in their blood, feathers, tissue, nasal secretions, liver, spleen, and feces. Transmission to humans occurs primarily through inhalation of dust from bird droppings that contain *C. psittaci*; less commonly, it results from direct contact with infected secretions or body tissue, as in laboratory personnel who work with birds. Psittacosis is an occupational disease of zoo and pet-shop employees or visitors, poultry farmers, and poultry ranchers. People may acquire the disease by handling sick birds or through mouth-to-beak resuscitation. Person-to-person transmission can happen, but it is rare and can result in severe infection. Infection is thought to develop in the respiratory system after organisms are inhaled from aerosolized dried avian excreta or respiratory secretions from sick birds. *C. psittaci* then attaches to the respiratory epithelial cells. After the initial inoculation, the organism spreads via the bloodstream to the reticuloendothelial system.

Assessment findings

After an incubation period of 4 to 15 days, onset of symptoms may be insidious or sudden. Clinical effects include chills and a low-grade fever that increases to 103° to 105° F (39.4° to 40.6° C) for 7 to 10 days then declines, with treatment, during the second or third week.

Other signs and symptoms include headache, myalgia, sore throat, cough (may be dry, hacking, and nonproductive or may produce blood-tinged sputum), abdominal distention and tenderness, nausea, vomiting, photophobia, decreased pulse rate, slightly increased respiratory rate, secondary purulent lung infection, and a faint macular rash called Horder spots, which resemble the rose spots observed in typhoid fever but appear on the face. Patients may also develop erythema multiforme and erythema nodosum. Epistaxis is common. Renal symptoms include acute glomerulonephritis and tubulointerstitial nephritis. Musculoskeletal symptoms include reactive arthritis that is usually polyarticular and, rarely, rhabdomyolysis. Severe infection also produces delirium, stupor, extensive pulmonary infiltration with cyanosis, acute respiratory failure, sepsis, and septic shock. Psittacosis may recur but is usually milder.

Complications

Complications from psittacosis include pleural effusions, fatal pulmonary embolism, and pulmonary infarction. Bradycardia, pericarditis, culture-negative endocarditis, and myocarditis can occur. Patients may develop anemia secondary to hemolysis.

Disseminated intravascular coagulation may occur in overwhelming infections. Rare complications include meningitis, encephalitis, seizures, and Guillain-Barré syndrome.

Diagnostic tests

▶ According to the Centers for Disease Control and Prevention, confirmed cases require a positive culture result for *C. psittaci* from respiratory secretions, a fourfold increase in antibody titer in two serum samples obtained by complement fixation or microimmunofluorescence 2 weeks apart, or immunoglobulin M antibodies against *C. psittaci*, as detected by microimmunofluorescence to a reciprocal titer of 16. Possible cases show the presence of antibodies against *C. psittaci* with titers of 1:32 by complement fixation or microimmunofluorescence.

SAFETY Culture of *C. psittaci* can be dangerous for laboratory personnel, making serology the preferred method of confirming this diagnosis.

◗ Enzyme-linked immunosorbent assay and direct immunofluorescence can help diagnose *C. psittaci* infection but are still experimental.

◗ Comparison of acute and convalescent serum shows a fourfold rise in *Chlamydia* antibody titers.

◗ A patchy lobar infiltrate appears on chest radiographs during the first week of illness.

TREATMENT

Psittacosis calls for treatment with tetracycline. If the infection is severe, tetracycline may be given via I.V. infusion until the fever subsides. Fever and other symptoms should begin to subside 48 to 72 hours after antibiotic treatment begins, but treatment must continue for 2 weeks after temperature returns to normal. Other antibiotics used to treat psittacosis include doxycycline (Doryx), erythromycin (E-Mycin), and chloramphenicol.

NURSING CONSIDERATIONS

◗ Monitor cough and breath sounds, hoarseness, severity of retractions, inspiratory stridor, cyanosis, respiratory rate and character (especially prolonged and labored respirations), restlessness, fever, and heart rate.

◗ Monitor the patient's fluid and electrolyte balance, laboratory results, and intake and output. Give I.V. fluids as ordered for electrolyte replacement.

◗ Carefully monitor the patient's vital signs. Watch for signs of overwhelming infection or other symptoms of complications.

◗ Reduce fever with tepid alcohol or sponge baths and a hypothermia blanket.

◗ Report all cases of psittacosis to local public health authorities.

Patient teaching

◗ Instruct the patient to use tissues when coughing and to dispose of them in a closed plastic bag. Also instruct the patient to wash his or her hands after using tissues or touching respiratory secretions.

◗ Teach the patient about the infection, including how it is transmitted, causes, and treatment.

◗ Teach the patient about prescribed medications, including drug dosage, schedule of administration, and duration of therapy.

◗ Teach the patient about possible complications, including signs and symptoms of relapse, as well as any symptoms the patient should report to the practitioner immediately.

 PREVENTION Alert persons who raise birds for sale to feed them tetracycline-treated birdseed and follow regulations on bird importation. Imported and exotic birds should be isolated for 30 to 45 days and tested or treated with prophylaxis. Birds that have ocular or nasal discharge, diarrhea, or low body weight should not be purchased or sold; they should be segregated from healthy birds and the housing structures disinfected.

Pyelonephritis

Pyelonephritis, inflammation of the kidney, may be acute or chronic. Acute pyelonephritis (or acute infective tubulointerstitial nephritis) is a sudden inflammation caused by bacteria that primarily affects either the interstitial area and renal pelvis or the renal tubules. It is one of the most common renal diseases; with treatment, the prognosis is good and extensive permanent damage is rare. Chronic pyelonephritis is persistent kidney inflammation that can scar the kidneys and may lead to chronic renal failure. It can result from bacterial, metastatic, or urinogenous origins and is most common in patients who are predisposed to recurrent acute pyelonephritis, such as those with urinary obstructions or vesicoureteral reflux.

CAUSES

Acute pyelonephritis results from bacterial invasion of the renal parenchyma. *Escherichia coli* reigns as the most causative organism, but *Proteus* species, *Pseudomonas* species, *Staphylococcus aureus,* and *Enterococcus faecalis* may also cause this infection. Typically, the infection spreads from the bladder to the ureters then to the kidneys, as in vesicoureteral reflux due to congenital weakness at the junction of the ureter and bladder. Bacteria refluxed to the intrarenal tissue may create colonies of infection within 24 to 48 hours. Infection may also result from instrumentation (catheterization, cystoscopy, or urologic surgery), from hematogenic infection (septicemia or endocarditis), or from lymphatic infection. Pyelonephritis may also result from an inability to empty the bladder (such as in patients with neurogenic bladder), urinary stasis, or urinary obstruction due to tumors, strictures, or benign prostatic hyperplasia. Sexual activity increases the risk of bacterial contamination, particularly the use of diaphragms and other spermicidals, which can result in secondary infection.

Pregnant women and people with diabetes or other renal diseases also seem to be more susceptible.

COMPLICATIONS

Each episode of pyelonephritis can cause significant kidney damage. Acute pyelonephritis can eventually result in chronic pyelonephritis, kidney failure, abscess formation, signs of shock, sepsis, or multiorgan system failure.

ASSESSMENT FINDINGS

Symptoms of pyelonephritis include urinary urgency and frequency, burning during urination, dysuria, nocturia, and hematuria (either microscopic or gross). Urine may appear cloudy and have an ammonia or fishy odor. Other common symptoms include a temperature of 102° F (38.9° C) or higher (although the patient may be afebrile as well), shaking chills, flank pain, anorexia, and general fatigue. These symptoms can develop rapidly over a few hours or within a few days. Although symptoms may disappear within a few days, even without treatment, residual bacterial infection is likely and may cause symptoms to recur later.

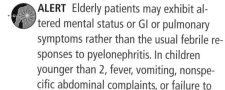 **ALERT** Elderly patients may exhibit altered mental status or GI or pulmonary symptoms rather than the usual febrile responses to pyelonephritis. In children younger than 2, fever, vomiting, nonspecific abdominal complaints, or failure to thrive may be the only signs of acute pyelonephritis.

Patients with chronic pyelonephritis may have symptoms of fever, lethargy, nausea and vomiting, flank pain or dysuria, or failure to thrive (in children). Upon physical exam, hypertension and flank tenderness may be noted.

DIAGNOSTIC TESTS

▶ Urine culture reveals the causative organism with a clean-catch urine specimen, urethral catheterization, or suprapubic sample.
▶ Urinalysis reveals pyuria (pus in the urine) in almost all patients. It may also show hematuria, proteinuria, and bacteriuria.

▶ Excretory urography, computed tomography, or magnetic resonance imaging may also reveal associated kidney abnormalities, such as calculi, tumors, or cysts. It is also helpful in diagnosing chronic pyelonephritis.

TREATMENT

Antibiotic therapy is prescribed appropriate to the specific infecting organism after identification by urine culture and sensitivity studies. When the infecting organism isn't conclusive, a broad-spectrum antibiotic is chosen. Urinary analgesics are also appropriate. Symptoms may disappear after several days of antibiotic therapy, and urine becomes sterile within 48 to 72 hours. However, the patient must continue taking the drug for 14 days in order to eradicate the causative agent. Follow-up treatment may include re-culturing urine 1 week after drug therapy stops and then periodically for the next year to detect residual or recurring infection. In some patients, such as those with vesicoureteral reflux or obstruction, surgery may be necessary. In chronic pyelonephritis, effective treatment requires control of hypertension, elimination of the existing obstruction (when possible), and long-term antimicrobial therapy.

NURSING CONSIDERATIONS

▶ Administer antipyretics for fever.
▶ Encourage fluids to achieve urine output of more than 2,000 ml/day. This helps to empty the bladder of contaminated urine.
▶ Obtain cultures as ordered and monitor results.

Patient teaching

 PREVENTION Instruct women to prevent bacterial contamination by wiping the perineum from front to back after defecation.
▶ Teach proper technique for a clean-catch urine specimen. Be sure to refrigerate or culture the specimen within 30 minutes to prevent overgrowth of bacteria.
▶ Stress the need to complete the prescribed antibiotic therapy, even after symptoms subside. Encourage long-term follow-up care for high-risk patients.

▶ Advise routine checkups for patients with a history of urinary tract infections. Teach them to recognize signs of infection, such as cloudy urine, burning on urination, and urinary urgency and frequency, especially when accompanied by a low-grade fever.
▶ Advise rest, and emphasize activity restrictions. It is usually recommended that the patient not return to work for 2 weeks in order to allow time for the infection to be eliminated and for the patient to regain physical strength. This usually depends on the physical stress and strain of the patient's occupation.
▶ If the patient is using a diaphragm with spermicidal, it is recommended to change to another method of contraception. There is spermicidal-associated colonization of the vagina by uropathogens with diaphragm use.

Q fever

Q fever is a highly infectious rickettsial disease affecting the respiratory system as well as the cardiac and GI systems. It affects people who are exposed to cattle, sheep, or goats. Human-to-human transmission is rare; however, sexual transmission may be possible. The disease has acute and chronic stages. Acute Q fever is often asymptomatic or may be mistaken for influenza or atypical pneumonia. Chronic Q fever is rare, but it carries a 60% mortality rate. It mostly affects patients with pre-existing cardiac valvular disorders.

Q fever occurs worldwide, except in New Zealand; it is most common in France and Australia. Because it is highly infectious, Q fever is considered a potential agent of bioterrorism. Q fever is a reportable illness in the United States.

CAUSES

Q fever is caused by *Coxiella burnetii*, which is excreted in the urine, milk, feces, and amniotic fluid and placenta of infected animals. Excreted fluid or waste contaminates barnyard dust, which may then be inhaled by humans. Once ingested, the microorganism proliferates in macrophages (in the acidic phagolysosome vacuole) and then gains access to the blood, producing a transient bacteremia. It may invade many organs, most commonly the lungs and liver. Inflammation occurs, manifested by granulomas in the liver, spleen, and bone marrow. These classic doughnut-shaped granulomas disappear with convalescence. Risk factors include prolonged or frequent exposure to animals, immune-compromised conditions, or a history of heart valve abnormality.

COMPLICATIONS

Complications of Q fever include heart failure, endocarditis, pneumonia, and hepatitis. Chronic fatigue syndrome may occur 6 months after acquiring the infection.

ASSESSMENT FINDINGS

The patient with Q fever will have a history of exposure to cattle, sheep, or goats; exposure may be indirect via barnyard dust. The incubation period is 2 to 6 weeks after exposure.

For acute Q fever, complaints include headache, myalgia, chills, and fever. Lung auscultation may reveal crackles, which may indicate pneumonia. The patient may have a dry cough. Hepatomegaly and jaundice may be present if the liver is affected. Erythema nodosum may also occur.

With chronic Q fever, patients may complain of the same symptoms as with acute Q fever. Chest auscultation may reveal a heart murmur, or signs of heart failure or endocarditis. These patients usually have a history of an immune-compromising disorder, or illness affecting the heart valves, such as valvular disease or rheumatic heart disease. They may also have a hepatosplenomegaly, a purpuric rash, and clubbing of the fingernails.

DIAGNOSTIC TESTS

▶ Patients during the acute stage may have an elevated white blood cell count, transient thrombocytopenia, and elevated transaminase and alkaline phosphatase levels.
▶ Cerebrospinal fluid evaluation reveals lymphocytosis, an elevated protein level, and a normal glucose level.
▶ Microimmunofluorescence reveals immunoglobulin G (IgG) phase II antibody titers of 200 or more and immunoglobulin M (IgM) phase II antibody titers of 50 or more (acute). The presence of phase II antibodies indicates chronic Q fever; the presence of IgG phase II antibody titers of 800 or more is highly predictive of endocarditis.
▶ Chest radiography may show segmental or lobar opacities, multiple round opacities, and pleural effusions.
▶ Echocardiography may show pericardial effusion with pericarditis.

TREATMENT

Q fever may resolve without any treatment; however, the use of antibiotics has been shown to decrease the duration of the illness. The treatment of choice for the acute stage of Q fever is doxycycline (Doryx) for 14 to 21 days. Ofloxacin and pefloxacin may also be used. The chronic stage is very hard to treat. For Q fever endocarditis, two different drug treatment protocols have been evaluated:

▶ Doxycycline with quinolones, for at least 4 years

▶ Doxycycline with hydroxychloroquine (Plaquenil) for 1½ to 3 years.

The second drug treatment protocol causes fewer relapses but requires routine eye examinations to detect accumulation of chloroquine. Some patients with *C. burnetii* endocarditis or intractable heart failure require surgery to remove damaged valves.

NURSING CONSIDERATIONS

▶ Maintain standard precautions.

▶ After checking for allergies, administer medication and observe for adverse reactions.

▶ Monitor vital signs and pulse oximetry. Perform respiratory assessment every shift and as needed. Note lung sounds, and track chest radiography results.

▶ Assess cardiovascular function every shift and as needed. Observe for murmurs or rubs, and check echocardiogram results, if ordered.

▶ Administer analgesics for pain and evaluate the effect after 30 minutes.

▶ Administer antipyretics for fever and monitor temperature every 4 hours.

Patient teaching

▶ Teach the patient about the disease, including the cause, diagnosis, and treatment.

▶ Review all medication, including dosage and administration, and possible adverse effects. Tell patients who are taking doxycycline to wear sunscreen when outdoors because of the photosensitivity effects of the drug.

▶ Stress the need for follow-up care, which should include blood work at least twice over 6 months for patients with acute Q fever, and monthly (for 6 months) for patients with chronic Q fever. Chronic Q fever patients will then need blood work every 6 months for 2 years, then yearly.

▶ Explain the need for echocardiography and how it is performed. For patients with acute Q fever, a baseline echocardiogram will need to be done; for patients with chronic Q fever, echocardiograms should be done every 3 months when on antibiotics, and then every 6 months for the next 2 years when medication is complete.

▶ Tell patients taking hydroxychloroquine (Plaquenil) that they will need to follow up with an ophthalmologist annually, because this medication may cause serious and potentially permanent eye damage, especially if taken for an extended time.

CONTACT PRECAUTIONS

Rabies

Rabies, also known as hydrophobia, is an acute viral infection of the central nervous system (CNS) that's transmitted by the saliva of an infected animal (especially wild animals). Caregivers may also become infected while treating a rabies-infected patient. If symptoms occur, rabies is almost always fatal. Treatment soon after exposure, however, may prevent fatal CNS invasion.

CAUSES

The rabies virus is usually transmitted to a human through the bite of an infected animal. The virus begins to replicate in the striated muscle cells at the bite site. It then spreads up the nerve to the CNS and replicates in the brain. Finally, it moves through the nerves into other tissue, including the salivary glands.

 PREVENTION In the United States, canine vaccinations have reduced the incidence of rabies transmission to humans. Wild animals, such as skunks, foxes, raccoons, and bats, account for 70% of rabies cases.

COMPLICATIONS

Untreated rabies almost invariably leads to life-threatening complications, including respiratory failure, peripheral vascular collapse, and central brain failure. If intensive support is provided, a number of later complications may occur, including inappropriate secretion of antidiuretic hormone, diabetes insipidus, cardiac arrhythmias, vascular instability, adult respiratory distress syndrome, GI bleeding, thrombocytopenia, and paralytic ileus. Recovery is very rare in patients who show signs of infection; when recovery does occur, it is gradual.

ASSESSMENT FINDINGS

After an incubation period of a few days to several years, but usually 30 to 90 days, ra-

bies typically produces local or radiating pain or burning and a sensation of cold, pruritus, and tingling at the bite site. It also produces prodromal signs and symptoms, such as a slight fever (100° to 102° F [37.8° to 38.9° C]), malaise, headache, anorexia, nausea, sore throat, and persistent loose cough. After this, the patient begins to display nervousness, anxiety, irritability, hyperesthesia, photophobia, sensitivity to loud noises, pupillary dilation, tachycardia, shallow respirations, pain and paresthesia in the bitten area, and excessive salivation, lacrimation, and perspiration.

About 2 to 10 days after the onset of prodromal symptoms, a phase of excitation (neurologic phase) begins. This phase is characterized by agitation, aphasia, incoordination, marked restlessness, anxiety, hoarseness, and apprehension as well as cranial nerve dysfunction that causes ocular palsies, strabismus, asymmetrical pupillary dilation or constriction, absence of corneal reflexes, and weakness of facial muscles. Severe systemic symptoms include tachycardia or bradycardia, cyclic respirations, hypotension, disseminated intravascular coagulation, coma, cardiac arrest, urine retention, and a temperature that exceeds 103° F (39.4° C).

About 50% of affected patients exhibit hydrophobia, in which forceful, painful pharyngeal muscle spasms expel liquids from the mouth and cause dehydration and, possibly, apnea, cyanosis, and death. Difficulty swallowing causes frothy saliva to drool from the patient's mouth. Eventually, even the sight, mention, or thought of water causes uncontrollable pharyngeal muscle spasms and excessive salivation. Between episodes of excitation and hydrophobia, the patient commonly is cooperative and lucid. After about 3 days, excitation and hydrophobia subside, and the progressively paralytic, terminal phase of this illness begins.

 ALERT The patient with rabies experiences progressive, generalized, flaccid paralysis that ultimately leads to peripheral vascular collapse, coma, and death.

Diagnostic tests

▶ Virus isolation from the patient's saliva or throat and examination of the blood for fluorescent rabies antibody (FRA) are diagnostic.
▶ Confinement of the suspected animal for 10 days of observation helps support this diagnosis. If the animal appears rabid, it should be killed and its brain tissue tested for FRA and Negri bodies (oval or round masses that conclusively confirm rabies).

Treatment

Treatment consists of wound care and immunization as soon as possible after exposure. Thoroughly wash all bite wounds and scratches with soap and water to remove any infected saliva. Check the patient's immunization status, and administer tetanus-diphtheria prophylaxis if needed.

After rabies exposure, a patient must receive passive immunization with rabies immune globulin (RIG) and active immunization with human diploid cell vaccine (HDCV). If the patient has already received HDCV and has an adequate rabies antibody titer, he or she needs only an HDCV booster and no RIG immunization. Supportive care is needed for any complications.

Nursing considerations

▶ When injecting rabies vaccine (which consists of a series of three to five injections), rotate injection sites on the deltoid muscle. Watch for and symptomatically treat redness, itching, pain, and tenderness at the injection site. Half of the RIG should be infiltrated into and around the bite wound, with the remainder given I.M.
▶ Cooperate with public health authorities to determine the vaccination status of the animal. If the animal is proven to be rabid, help identify others at risk.

If rabies develops:

▶ Monitor the patient's cardiac and pulmonary function continuously.
◗ Isolate the patient. Wear a gown, gloves, and protection for the eyes and mouth when handling saliva and articles contaminated with saliva. Take precautions to avoid being bitten by the patient during the excitation phase.
▶ Keep the room dark and quiet.

Patient teaching

▶ Reassure the patient who receives prophylactic rabies vaccine that vaccination will prevent rabies infection. Explain how many times and on what dates the patient will need to be vaccinated. Discuss possible adverse effects, such as redness and tenderness at the injection site.
◗ If rabies has developed, explain to the patient and family why contact precautions are needed. Also explain the course of the disease and any treatments.

 PREVENTION Stress the need for vaccination of household pets that may be exposed to rabid wild animals. Warn patients not to try to touch wild animals, especially if the animal appears ill or overly docile (possible signs of rabies).

Recreational water illness

Recreational water illnesses (RWIs) are a group of illnesses that occur secondary to swallowing, breathing, or being exposed to contaminated water from areas where water is enjoyed, such as pools, spas, water parks, lakes, ponds, rivers, oceans, and even decorative water fountains. Depending on the causative organism, illness can affect the GI, respiratory, neurosensory, genitourinary, and integumentary systems, as well as any preexisting wounds. The most common complaint is diarrhea. Although they can affect people of all ages, RWIs are most common in children, pregnant women, and immunocompromised patients, such as those with AIDS, organ transplant recipients, or those receiving chemotherapy.

CAUSES

Different organisms may affect different body systems. Organisms commonly responsible for GI illness include *Cryptosporidium, Giardia, Shigella, Norovirus, Enterococcus,* and *Escherichia coli* O157:H7. Most of these organisms are killed by chlorine in less than an hour; *Cryptosporidium*, however, takes longer to kill and may survive in swimming pools for several days, even with adequate chlorination. Infection may also be caused by organisms that exist naturally in the water or soil.

Pseudomonas may cause skin infections, such as dermatitis, folliculitis, and athlete's foot. It may also be responsible for outer ear and eye infections as well as adenoviruses. Respiratory and central nervous system infections may result from contamination with *Legionella, Mycobacterium,* and echovirus.

Pools and water parks become contaminated when people with existing GI illness submerge in water. They contaminate the water after having an "accident" or from organisms that remain in the anal area after defecation. Diapered babies who experience diarrhea while in the water are also responsible for causing RWI. Spray pools can also cause RWI because that water is simply recycled from underground collection tanks. Transmission via water can result from swallowing or breathing in contaminated water or through breaks in the skin. Illness can result from even a small amount of swallowed water.

Hot tubs more frequently cause "hot tub rash" and respiratory illness. Chlorine evaporates faster in a hot tub, thereby decreasing the disinfectant levels faster. In addition, hot tubs often are not maintained as diligently as swimming pools.

Decorative water fountains are not routinely maintained with chlorine or disinfectant; therefore, they may become contaminated easily if children or diapered babies are permitted to play in them.

Sewage, run-off after rainfall, animal waste, and contamination from individuals (as with swimming pools) causes contamination of lakes, rivers, ponds, and oceans.

 PREVENTION The Centers for Disease Control and Prevention Web site contains design and operation guidelines, disinfection and remediation guidelines, and informational prevention material designed for the general public, aquatic staff, travelers, and health care professionals. There is also a "Healthy Swimming A-Z" index that provides specific information on topics such as safety and specific types of infection (http://www.cdc.gov/healthyswimming/healthy_swimming_a_to_z.htm).

COMPLICATIONS

If infection is not treated in a timely or appropriate manner, it may become widespread depending on the type of microorganism present. Complications from RWI may include septicemia, respiratory failure, and even death.

ASSESSMENT FINDINGS

Signs and symptoms of RWI are based on the type of infection the patient has acquired. Patients with respiratory infections may present with symptoms ranging from flu-like illness to pneumonia 2 to 14 days after exposure.

GI complaints may begin 2 to 10 days after exposure and include watery diarrhea that may last up to 3 weeks, depending on the causative organism. Other symptoms include abdominal cramping and pain, nausea, and vomiting. Fever and weight loss may also occur.

Signs and symptoms of skin infection commonly occur within a few days of swimming. Skin involvement may include a rash consisting of small reddish pimples that develop in areas that have been exposed to the contaminated water. It can cause itching and burning, and small blisters may develop. Open wounds or a break in the skin's integrity, such as a bite or abrasion, may become increasingly reddened, painful, and warm to the touch. Drainage may develop with worsening infection.

Urinary symptoms include frequency and urgency, and possibly painful urination. "Swimmer's ear" may cause progressive ear pain as well as pus and drainage. Eye infections may cause pain, redness, and drainage.

DIAGNOSTIC TESTS

▶ Testing is based on the presenting symptoms. Clinical assessment, such as eye or ear examination, may identify the problem with no need for further tests.
▶ Cultures specific for the type of suspected illness, such as stool, urine, sputum, wound, or blood culture, identify the causative organism.

TREATMENT

Treatment is based on the type of illness contracted. Antimicrobials specific for the type of identified or suspected infection should be prescribed. Supportive care, such

Healthy swimming tips

Give these tips to patients to help prevent RWI:
• When swimming, do not swallow water or even get water in your mouth.
• Do not swim when you have diarrhea.
• Shower before swimming, and assist with washing children before they enter a swimming facility.
• Take children on frequent bathroom breaks.
• Do not change dirty diapers near the pool; use designated changing areas, and dispose of diapers properly. Be sure to clean the child's bottom thoroughly, and wash hands after this activity.
• Always wash hands after using the toilet.
• Monitor for and maintain safe chlorination levels of self-owned pools and spas.

as antipyretics, nonsteroidal anti-inflammatory drugs, analgesics, oxygen therapy, and skin and wound care should be provided as appropriate. For patients with diarrhea, oral fluid replacement is important.

NURSING CONSIDERATIONS

▶ Administer medication as ordered, and evaluate for effectiveness.
▶ Provide supportive measures specific for the illness presented.
▶ Monitor for complications that are specific to the illness.

Patient teaching

▶ Provide information regarding the specific illness present, including the cause, diagnosis, and treatment plan.
▶ Review with the patient all prescribed medication, including dosage, administration, and possible adverse reactions.
▶ Teach patients about healthy swimming practices to prevent further infections. (See *Healthy swimming tips*.)

⬇ CONTACT PRECAUTIONS

Respiratory syncytial virus infection

Respiratory syncytial virus (RSV) infection results from a subgroup of myxoviruses that resemble paramyxovirus. In infants and children, RSV is the leading cause of lower respiratory tract infections and a major cause of pneumonia, tracheobronchitis, and bronchiolitis. Rates of illness are highest among infants ages 1 to 6 months, with the peak incidence between ages 2 and 3 months. Infants in day-care settings are especially susceptible.

CAUSES

The organism that causes RSV is transmitted from person to person through respiratory droplets when an infected person coughs or sneezes. Transmission can also result from direct or indirect contact with the nasal or oral secretions of an infected person. RSV can survive on surfaces, such as tables and cribs, for several hours. The virus is spread when a person touches a contaminated surface and then rubs his or her eye or nose.

Signs and symptoms of RSV usually occur within 4 to 6 days of exposure. Antibody titers seem to indicate that few children younger than age 4 escape contracting some form of RSV, even if it's mild. In fact, RSV is the only viral disease whose maximum impact is during the first few months of life (the incidence of RSV bronchiolitis peaks at age 2 months). School-age children, adolescents, and young adults with mild re-infections are probably the source of infection for infants and young children.

This virus creates annual epidemics during the late winter and early spring in regions with a temperate climate and during the rainy season in the tropics. It can also be seen in immunocompromised adults, especially patients with bone marrow transplants.

COMPLICATIONS

Young children, especially infants, are at increased risk for bronchiolitis, tracheobronchitis, and pneumonia. The child may experience periods of apnea and respiratory failure requiring intubation and mechanical ventilation. Otitis media is a less severe complication of RSV in infants and young children.

ASSESSMENT FINDINGS

The clinical features of RSV infection vary depending on the severity of illness. Initial signs and symptoms may include a runny nose and diminished appetite. Fever, coughing, sneezing, and audible wheezing may develop 1 to 3 days later. Irritability, decreased activity, and breathing difficulties may be the only findings in very young infants. Nasal flaring, retraction, cyanosis, and tachypnea may be present if respiratory involvement is severe. Other findings vary. If otitis media develops, a hyperemic eardrum may be revealed on otoscopic examination.

Although uncommon, signs of central nervous system (CNS) infection, such as weakness, irritability, and nuchal rigidity, may also be observed.

Re-infection is common, producing milder symptoms than the initial infection. RSV has also been identified in patients with a variety of CNS disorders, such as meningitis and myelitis.

DIAGNOSTIC TESTS

Diagnosis is usually based on clinical findings and epidemiologic information.
▶ Rapid antigen testing of a respiratory specimen is positive for RSV.
▶ Real-time reverse transcription–polymerase chain reaction of a respiratory specimen reveals RSV.
▶ Chest radiography helps detect pneumonia.

TREATMENT

Treatment of RSV infection is supportive, aimed at maintaining respiratory function and fluid balance while relieving symptoms.

Ribavirin (Copegus), an antiviral agent in aerosol form, may be administered to severely ill patients or those at high risk for complications.

 PREVENTION Preventive therapy may be indicated for children younger than age 2 who are at high risk for RSV infection (such as children with chronic lung disease and certain infants born prematurely). Prophylactic measures include palivizumab (Synagis) or RSV I.V. immune globulin given once per month for 4 to 5 consecutive months during RSV season (typically November to April). These immunoprophylactic agents are not for use in treating existing RSV infection.

NURSING CONSIDERATIONS

▶ Monitor respiratory status, including rate and pattern. Watch for nasal flaring or retraction, cyanosis, pallor, and dyspnea; listen or auscultate for wheezing, rhonchi, or other signs of respiratory distress. Monitor pulse oximetry and arterial blood gas levels.

▶ Maintain a patent airway, and be especially vigilant when the patient has periods of acute dyspnea. Perform percussion and provide drainage and suction when necessary. Use a croup tent to provide a high-humidity atmosphere. Placing the patient in semi-Fowler's position may help prevent aspiration of secretions.

▶ Monitor intake and output carefully. Observe for signs of dehydration such as decreased skin turgor. Encourage the patient to drink plenty of high-calorie fluids. Administer I.V. fluids as needed.

▶ Promote bed rest. Plan your nursing care to allow uninterrupted rest.

▶ Hold and cuddle infants; talk to and play with toddlers. Offer diversionary activities that are appropriate for the child's age and condition. Encourage parental visits and cuddling. Restrain the child only as necessary.

▶ Institute contact precautions for the duration of the illness. Wear a surgical mask and eye protection when contact with respiratory secretions is likely, according to standard precautions. Encourage hand hygiene before and after contact with the patient or the patient's environment.

 SAFETY To prevent health care–associated infection on pediatric units, don't care for infants with RSV infection if you have a respiratory illness yourself.

Patient teaching

▶ Describe RSV infection transmission methods to parents, and caution them against exposing infants to crowds during RSV season.

▶ Teach the parents about the illness, including diagnostic tests and treatment plan. Review all prescribed medication, including what they are for, how to administer them, and possible adverse reactions.

▶ Teach the parents proper hand hygiene practices. Explain what contact precautions are and why they are necessary.

▶ If the patient is being cared for at home, explain the need for adequate rest, fluids, and nourishment.

▶ Review signs and symptoms of complications and when to seek medical attention.

Rheumatic fever and rheumatic heart disease

A systemic inflammatory disease of childhood, acute rheumatic fever develops after infection of the upper respiratory tract with group A beta-hemolytic streptococci. Rheumatic fever principally involves the heart, joints, central nervous system, skin, and subcutaneous tissue. It commonly recurs.

The term *rheumatic heart disease* refers to cardiac involvement in rheumatic fever—its most destructive effect. Cardiac involvement develops in up to 50% of patients with rheumatic fever and may affect the endocardium, myocardium, or pericardium during the early acute phase. It may later affect the heart valves, causing chronic valvular disease.

The extent of damage to the heart depends on where the disorder strikes. Pericarditis causes a pericardial friction rub and, occasionally, pain and effusion. Myocarditis produces characteristic lesions called Aschoff bodies in the acute stages as well as cellular swelling and fragmentation of interstitial collagen, leading to formation of a progressively fibrotic nodule and interstitial scars. Endocarditis causes valve leaflet swelling, erosion along the lines of leaflet closure, and blood, platelet, and fibrin deposits, which form bead-like vegetation. It usually affects the mitral valve in females and the aortic valve in males; in both, it affects the tricuspid valves occasionally and the pulmonic valve rarely.

Long-term antibiotic therapy can minimize the recurrence of rheumatic fever, reducing the risks of permanent cardiac damage and valvular deformity. Although rheumatic fever tends to be familial, this tendency may reflect contributing environmental factors. For example, in lower socioeconomic groups, the incidence is highest in children between ages 5 and 15, likely due to malnutrition and crowded living conditions.

Rheumatic fever usually strikes during cool, damp weather in winter and early spring. In the United States, it's most common in the northern states.

CAUSES

Rheumatic fever appears to be a hypersensitivity reaction in which antibodies produced to combat streptococci react and produce characteristic lesions at specific tissue sites. How and why group A streptococcal infection initiates the process are unknown. Because few people infected with *Streptococcus* infection ever contract rheumatic fever (about 0.3%), altered host resistance is probably involved in its development or recurrence.

COMPLICATIONS

The long-term effects of rheumatic fever usually destroy the mitral and aortic valves, leading to severe pancarditis and occasionally producing pericardial effusion and fatal heart failure. Of the patients who survive these complications, about 20% die within 10 years.

ASSESSMENT FINDINGS

Nearly all affected patients report having had a streptococcal infection a few days to 6 weeks earlier. They usually have a recent history of fever that spikes to at least 100.4° F (38° C) late in the afternoon, sudden-onset sore throat, pain on swallowing, headache, and abdominal pain; nausea and vomiting may also occur, especially in children. Most patients complain of migratory joint pain in the knees, ankles, elbows, and hips (polyarthritis). Swelling, redness, and signs of effusion typically accompany this pain.

If pericarditis is involved, the patient may complain of sharp, sudden pain that usually starts over the sternum and radiates to the neck, shoulders, back, and arms. The pain is usually pleuritic, increases with deep inspiration, and decreases when the patient sits up and leans forward. (This position pulls the heart away from the diaphragmatic pleurae of the lungs.) The pain may mimic that of a myocardial infarction.

A patient with heart failure caused by severe rheumatic carditis may complain of dyspnea, right upper quadrant pain, and a hacking, nonproductive cough. Inspection may reveal skin lesions, such as erythema marginatum, which is a nonpruritic, macular, and transient rash. The lesions are red with blanched centers and well-demarcated borders and typically appear on the trunk and extremities.

Subcutaneous nodules near tendons or the bony prominences of joints may be noted; these nodules are firm, movable, nontender, and about 1/8″ to 3/4″ (0.3 to 2 cm) in diameter. They occur around the elbows, knuckles, wrists, and knees and, less commonly, on the scalp and backs of the hands. These nodules persist for a few days to several weeks and, like erythema marginatum, commonly accompany carditis.

Edema and tachypnea may be evident if the patient has left-sided heart failure. Up to 6 months after the original streptococcal infection, the patient may experience transient chorea. Mild chorea may produce hyperirritability, deterioration in handwriting, or an inability to concentrate. Severe chorea causes purposeless, nonrepetitive, involuntary muscle spasms and speech disturbances; poor muscle coordination; and weakness. Chorea resolves with rest and causes no residual neurologic damage.

If the patient has pericarditis, palpation may reveal a rapid pulse and auscultation may reveal a pericardial friction rub (a grating sound heard as the heart moves). This can best be heard during forced expiration, with the patient leaning forward or positioned on the hands and knees.

Murmurs and gallops may also occur. With left-sided heart failure, bibasilar crackles and a ventricular or atrial gallop may be heard. The most common murmurs include the following:

▶ Systolic murmur of mitral insufficiency (a high-pitched, blowing, holosystolic murmur, loudest at the apex, possibly radiating to the anterior axillary line)

▶ Midsystolic murmur caused by stiffening and swelling of the mitral leaflet

▶ Occasionally a diastolic murmur of aortic insufficiency (a low-pitched, rumbling, almost inaudible murmur)

Valvular disease may eventually cause chronic valvular stenosis and insufficiency, including mitral stenosis and insufficiency and aortic insufficiency. In children, mitral insufficiency remains the major effect of rheumatic heart disease.

DIAGNOSTIC TESTS

No specific laboratory tests can determine the presence of rheumatic fever, but the following test results support the diagnosis:

▶ Blood studies may reveal an elevated white blood cell count and erythrocyte sedimentation rate (during the acute phase), slight anemia caused by suppressed erythropoiesis during inflammation, and positive C-reactive protein (especially during the acute phase). Cardiac enzyme levels may be increased in patients with severe carditis.

▶ Antistreptolysin-O titer is elevated in 95% of patients within 2 months of onset. (A rising anti-DNase B titer can also determine recurrent streptococcal infection.)

▶ Throat cultures may continue to show the presence of group A streptococci. However, the microorganisms usually occur in small numbers, and isolating them is difficult.

▶ Electrocardiography reveals no diagnostic changes, but 20% of patients show a prolonged PR interval.

▶ Chest radiographs show a normal heart size, except in patients with myocarditis, heart failure, or pericardial effusion.

▶ Echocardiography helps evaluate valvular damage, chamber size, ventricular function, and the presence of a pericardial effusion.

▶ Cardiac catheterization is used to help evaluate valvular damage and left ventricular function in patients with severe cardiac dysfunction.

TREATMENT

Effective management eradicates the streptococcal infection, relieves symptoms, and prevents recurrence, thus reducing the risk of permanent cardiac damage. During the acute phase, treatment includes penicillin or erythromycin (E-Mycin) for patients with penicillin hypersensitivity. Salicylates, such as aspirin, relieve fever and minimize joint swelling and pain; if the patient has carditis or if salicylates fail to relieve pain and inflammation, the physician may prescribe a corticosteroid.

For patients with active carditis, supportive treatment requires strict bed rest for about 5 weeks during the acute phase followed by a progressive increase in physical activity, depending on clinical and laboratory findings as well as the patient's response to treatment. After the acute phase subsides, a monthly I.M. injection of penicillin G benzathine or daily doses of oral sulfadiazine or penicillin G may be used to prevent recurrence. Such preventive treatment usually continues for 5 to 10 years.

Heart failure requires continued bed rest and administration of a diuretic. Severe mitral or aortic valvular dysfunction that causes persistent heart failure requires corrective surgery, such as commissurotomy (separation of the adherent, thickened leaflets of the mitral valve), valvuloplasty (inflation of a balloon within a valve), or valve replacement (with prosthetic valve). Corrective valvular surgery seldom is necessary before late adolescence.

NURSING CONSIDERATIONS

▶ Before giving penicillin, ask the patient or (or, if the patient is a child, his parents) if he or she has ever had a hypersensitivity reaction to it. Warn the patient or parents that such a reaction is possible even in those who have never shown penicillin hypersensitivity.

▶ Administer the prescribed antibiotic at the same time each day to maintain consistent a drug level in the blood.

▶ Stress the importance of bed rest, and assist with bathing as necessary. Provide a bedside commode because using a commode puts less stress on the heart than using a bedpan. Offer the patient diversionary, physically undemanding activities.

▶ Place the patient in an upright position to relieve dyspnea and chest pain, if needed.

▶ Offer an analgesic to relieve pain and provide oxygen to prevent tissue hypoxia, as needed.

▶ To reduce anxiety, allow the patient to express concerns about the effects of activity restrictions on his or her responsibilities and routines. Reassure the patient that the restrictions are temporary.

▶ If the patient is unsteady because of chorea, clear the environment of objects that could make him or her fall.

▶ To minimize boredom after the acute phase, encourage the patient's family and friends to spend as much time as possible with the patient. Advise the parents to secure a tutor to help their child keep up with schoolwork during the long convalescence.

▶ Help the parents overcome any feelings of guilt they may have about their child's illness. Failure to seek treatment for streptococcal infection is common because the illness may seem no worse than a cold.

▶ Encourage the patient and parents to vent their frustrations during the long, tedious recovery. If the child has severe carditis, help the family prepare for permanent changes in the child's lifestyle.

Patient teaching

▶ Explain all tests and treatments to the patient and/or parents.

▶ Tell the patient to resume activities of daily living slowly and to schedule rest periods in his or her routine, as instructed by the physician.

▶ Tell the patient or parents to stop penicillin therapy and call the physician immediately if a rash, fever, chills, or other signs or symptoms of an allergic reaction develop.

▶ Instruct the patient and family to watch for and report early signs and symptoms of left-sided heart failure, such as dyspnea and a hacking, nonproductive cough.

▶ Teach the patient and family about the disease and its treatment. Warn the parents to watch for and immediately report signs and symptoms of recurrent streptococcal infection: sudden sore throat, diffuse throat redness and oropharyngeal exudate, swollen and tender cervical lymph glands, pain on swallowing, temperature of 101° to 104° F (38.3° to 40° C), headache, and nausea. Urge them to keep the child away from people with respiratory tract infections.

▶ Help the patient and family to understand the effects of chorea (such as nervousness, restlessness, poor coordination, weakness, and inattentiveness). Emphasize that these effects are transient.

▶ Make sure the patient and family understand the need to comply with prolonged antibiotic therapy and follow-up care. Arrange for a visiting nurse to oversee home care if necessary.

▶ Explain that an antibiotic must be given prophylactically before any dental work or other invasive procedure is performed.

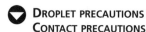

Rhinovirus infection

Rhinovirus, otherwise known as the common cold, is an acute, usually afebrile, viral infection that causes inflammation of the upper respiratory tract. It's the most common type of infection. In temperate climates, colds occur more often in the colder months; in the tropics, colds are more prevalent during the rainy season.

Colds are usually benign and self-limiting, but they cause more lost time from school or work than any other illness. It is estimated that each person in the United States experiences a cold every 1 to 2 years.

Causes

Rhinovirus causes the common cold in 25% to 80% of cases. A cold is communicable for 2 to 3 days after the onset of symptoms. Transmission occurs through airborne respiratory droplets or through contact with contaminated objects, including hands. High rates of infection are found in day-care centers, nurseries, and schools. The virus has been cultured from inanimate objects up to 4 days after exposure. (See *What happens in the common cold.*)

Complications

Secondary bacterial infection may cause sinusitis, otitis media, pharyngitis, or lower respiratory tract infection. Infection may exacerbate underlying pulmonary problems, such as chronic obstructive pulmonary disease. Smokers have longer-lasting, more severe infections than nonsmokers.

Assessment findings

After an incubation period of 1 to 4 days, the patient initially complains of a sore throat, sneezing, coughing, nasal congestion, headache, and mild body aches. Most patients are afebrile, although fever may occur, especially in children.

Clinical features develop more fully as the cold progresses. By the second day (in addition to the initial symptoms), the patient may report copious nasal discharge. About 3 days after onset, major symptoms diminish, but congestion may persist for 7 to 14 days. Re-infection is common, but complications are rare.

Inspection may reveal a reddened nose and eyes and nasal discharge. The nasal and pharyngeal mucous membranes may exhibit increased erythema, and the patient's voice may have a nasal quality.

Diagnostic tests

▶ Diagnosis is typically symptom based.
▶ Blood studies may reveal an elevated white blood cell count.

Treatment

Treatment is symptomatic. Aspirin, acetaminophen (Tylenol), and nonsteroidal anti-inflammatory medications ease myalgia and headache; fluids help loosen accumulated respiratory secretions and maintain hydration; and rest combats fatigue and weakness. Because aspirin has been associated with Reye syndrome in children, acetaminophen or ibuprofen is preferred for a child with a cold and fever.

Decongestants can relieve nasal congestion. Lozenges relieve soreness, and steam encourages expectoration. Nasal douching, sinus drainage, and antibiotics aren't necessary except in patients with complications or chronic illness. Pure antitussives relieve severe coughs but are contraindicated in patients with productive coughs when cough suppression is harmful. In infants, saline drops and mucus aspiration with a bulb syringe may be beneficial in clearing nasal passages.

Nursing considerations

▶ Administer antipyretics and analgesics, as ordered, and evaluate their effects.
◗ Use droplet precautions in all cases. Use additional contact precautions if the patient has copious moist nasal discharge and close contact is likely.

What happens in the common cold

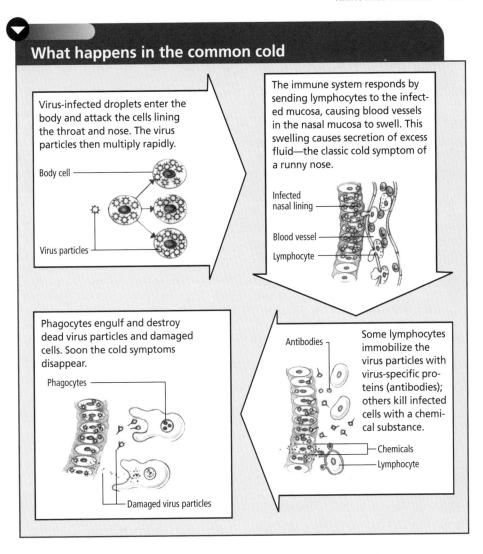

Virus-infected droplets enter the body and attack the cells lining the throat and nose. The virus particles then multiply rapidly.

Body cell

Virus particles

The immune system responds by sending lymphocytes to the infected mucosa, causing blood vessels in the nasal mucosa to swell. This swelling causes secretion of excess fluid—the classic cold symptom of a runny nose.

Infected nasal lining

Blood vessel

Lymphocyte

Phagocytes engulf and destroy dead virus particles and damaged cells. Soon the cold symptoms disappear.

Phagocytes

Damaged virus particles

Some lymphocytes immobilize the virus particles with virus-specific proteins (antibodies); others kill infected cells with a chemical substance.

Antibodies

Chemicals

Lymphocyte

▶ Refer the patient for medical care if he or she has a persistent high fever, changes in level of consciousness, or significant respiratory symptoms.

Patient teaching

▶ Emphasize that antibiotics can't cure the common cold.
▶ Tell the patient to stay in bed for the first few days, to use a lubricant on the nostrils, and to relieve throat irritation with sugarless hard candy, cough drops, or lozenges.
▶ Tell the patient to increase fluid intake.
▶ Recommend a warm bath or heating pad to reduce aches and pains. Suggest a steam

vaporizer to relieve nasal congestion. Commercial expectorants are available, but their effectiveness is questionable.
▶ Advise against overuse of nose drops/sprays, which can cause rebound congestion.

PREVENTION To help prevent rhinovirus, warn patients to minimize contact with people who have colds. To avoid spreading colds, tell patients to perform hand hygiene frequently, to cover the mouth and nose when coughing or sneezing, to avoid sharing towels and drinking glasses, and to dispose of soiled tissues properly.

Rocky Mountain spotted fever

Rocky Mountain spotted fever (RMSF) is a febrile, rash-producing illness caused by the bacterium *Rickettsia rickettsii*. The disease is transmitted to humans by a tick bite. RMSF is fatal in about 5% of patients. Mortality rises in older patients and when treatment is delayed.

CAUSES

R. rickettsii is transmitted to a human or small animal by the prolonged bite (several hours) of an adult tick—the wood tick (*Dermacentor andersoni*) in the western United States and the dog tick (*Dermacentor variabilis*) in the eastern part of the country. Occasionally, *R. rickettsii* is acquired through inhalation (such as in laboratory settings in which aerosolization of blood and specimens may occur) or through the contact of abraded skin with tick excreta or tissue juices. (This explains why people shouldn't crush ticks between their fingers when removing them from other people and animals.) In most tick-infested areas, 1% to 5% of the ticks harbor *R. rickettsii*.

Endemic throughout the continental United States, RMSF is particularly prevalent in the Southeast and Southwest. Because RMSF is associated with outdoor activities, such as camping and backpacking, the incidence of this illness is usually higher in the spring and summer months. Epidemiologic surveillance reports for RMSF indicate that the incidence is also higher in children ages 5 to 9, in men and boys, and in whites.

COMPLICATIONS

Complications of RMSF include lobar pneumonia, pneumonitis, otitis media, parotitis, disseminated intravascular coagulation, shock, renal failure, meningoencephalitis, and hepatic injury.

ASSESSMENT FINDINGS

The incubation period is usually about 7 days but can range from 2 to 14 days. Initial signs and symptoms include fever (102° to 104° F [38.9° to 40° C]), severe headache, nausea, vomiting, neurologic symptoms, and muscle pain. Children may also experience severe abdominal pain, altered mental status, and conjunctival infection. A maculopapular rash commonly develops on the palms of the hands and soles of the feet 4 to 7 days after the onset of symptoms. Blanching, pink maculae develop on the ankles, wrists, or forearms and commonly evolve to maculopapules. In about 50% of cases, the rash becomes petechial over the next several days of illness. The rash may spread to the entire body; however, spread to the face is typically limited. Patients with petechial rash are typically severely ill.

 ALERT A rapid pulse rate and hypotension may lead to death from complete vascular collapse.

Other signs and symptoms include a bronchial cough, a rapid respiratory rate (as high as 60 breaths/minute), anorexia, constipation, abdominal pain, hepatomegaly, splenomegaly, insomnia, restlessness and, in extreme cases, delirium. Urine output decreases to half (or less) of the normal level, is dark in color, and contains albumin.

DIAGNOSTIC TESTS

▶ Diagnosis is based on the patient's history (which usually includes a tick bite or travel to a tick-infested area) and a positive complement fixation test (which shows a fourfold increase in convalescent antibody titer compared with acute titers).
▶ Blood cultures or skin biopsy at the rash site should be performed to isolate the organism and confirm the diagnosis.
▶ Weil-Felix reaction antibody test shows a fourfold increase between the acute and convalescent sera titer levels. Increased titers usually develop after 10 to 14 days and persist for several months.

▶ Laboratory studies reveal decreased platelets (12,000 to 150,000/mm³); the white blood cell count may be elevated (11,000 to 33,000/mm³) during the second week of illness.

TREATMENT

Following careful removal of the tick, treatment involves administration of antibiotics, such as chloramphenicol or doxycycline (Doryx), until 3 days after the fever subsides. Additional treatment is based on the patient's symptoms.

NURSING CONSIDERATIONS

▶ Monitor the patient's intake and output carefully. Watch closely for decreased urine output—a possible indicator of renal failure.
▶ Be alert for signs of dehydration, such as poor skin turgor and dry mouth.
▶ Administer antipyretics as ordered, and provide tepid sponge baths to reduce fever.
▶ Monitor vital signs, and watch for profound hypotension and shock.
▶ Administer oxygen, as prescribed. Endotracheal intubation and mechanical ventilation may be necessary.
▶ Turn the patient frequently to prevent complications of immobility, such as pressure ulcers and pneumonia.
▶ Monitor nutritional status. Administer parenteral nutrition as prescribed or give small frequent meals if needed. Notify the local health department of the patient's condition and treatment regimen.

Patient teaching

▶ Instruct the patient to report any recurrent symptoms to the physician at once so that treatment measures may resume immediately.
▶ Offer printed and illustrated instructions, if available, to teach the patient and family members or other caregivers how to correctly and safely remove a tick. Demonstrate how to use tweezers or forceps and apply steady traction to release the entire tick without leaving its mouth parts in the skin.

▶ Caution the patient not to handle a tick or its fragments after removal.
▶ Instruct the patient to clean his or her skin with alcohol at the point of attachment.

 PREVENTION To prevent RMSF, advise the patient to avoid tick-infested areas (woods, meadows, streams, and canyons) if possible. Teach the patient ways to reduce the risk of becoming infected with RMSF:
- Encourage inspection of the entire body (including the scalp) for ticks every 3 to 4 hours while outdoors.
- Remind the patient to wear protective clothing, such as a long-sleeved shirt, pants securely tucked into laced boots, and a protective head covering such as a cap.
- Advise the patient to apply insect repellant to exposed skin as well as to clothing.

Roseola infantum

Roseola infantum, also known as exanthema subitum or sixth disease, is an acute, benign viral infection that usually affects infants and young children ages 6 months to 2 years, with the peak incidence between 9 and 12 months. Maternal antibodies usually prevent newborns from contracting the illness.

Characteristically, roseola first appears as an upper respiratory illness followed by high fever for 3 to 5 days. The high fever commonly ends abruptly at about the same time a rash develops.

CAUSES

Human herpesvirus 6 (HHV-6) causes roseola. The virus is spread directly through droplets when an infected person coughs or sneezes or indirectly through contact with respiratory secretions. It can also be spread through contact with oral secretions.

COMPLICATIONS

The major complication of roseola is seizures. Rarely, roseola may cause other central nervous system (CNS) complications, such as meningoencephalitis, encephalitis, bulging anterior fontanels, and hemiplegia. HHV-6 has been associated with chronic fatigue syndrome and possibly multiple sclerosis. Exanthem subitum/roseola syndrome may develop with primary infection and cause otitis media, respiratory distress, and gastroenteritis.

However, the virus remains latent and can seriously affect immune-compromised patients. Patients with a history of organ transplantation may develop bone marrow suppression, hepatitis, pneumonitis, or encephalitis. Patients with acquired immunodeficiency syndrome may develop lymphadenopathy, disseminated organ involvement, CNS infection retinitis, and viremia. These complications may be fatal.

The rash of roseola

With roseola, symptoms often take up to 2 weeks to appear following exposure. The first symptom is a high fever, which usually lasts 3 to 7 days. When the fever subsides, the rash usually appears. The rash of roseola consists of multiple small, flat, pink spots or nonpruritic patches. Some of the spots may have a white ring around them. The rash usually starts on the torso and back and then spreads to the neck and arms. It may spread to the face and legs as well, but not always. The rash can take several hours to many days to fade.

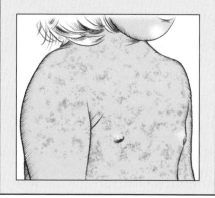

ASSESSMENT FINDINGS

After an incubation period of about 10 days, the patient develops upper respiratory symptoms followed by a high fever (103° to 105° F [39.4° to 40.6° C]), which commonly lasts for 3 to 7 days and then drops suddenly. In the early febrile period, the patient may be anorexic, irritable, and listless but doesn't appear particularly ill. However, because of the high temperature, febrile seizures may occur. Simultaneously with an abrupt drop in temperature, the patient develops a maculopapular, nonpruritic rash that blanches on pressure. The rash is profuse on the trunk, arms, and neck and mild on the face and legs. It fades within 24 hours. (See *The rash of roseola*.)

DIAGNOSTIC TESTS

▶ Diagnosis requires observation of the characteristic rash that appears immediately after fever subsides.

▶ Serologic evidence of primary infection can be determined by checking serum antibody levels in the acute and convalescent phases.

▶ Laboratory studies reveal slight leukocytosis.

TREATMENT

Because roseola is self-limiting, treatment is supportive and symptomatic. Antipyretics, such as acetaminophen (Tylenol), may be given to lower fever. Anticonvulsants are not recommended for febrile seizures.

NURSING CONSIDERATIONS

▶ Monitor temperature; administer antipyretics for fever, and evaluate their effect. Observe for febrile seizures.

▶ Administer tepid baths to help reduce fever and increase comfort.

▶ Encourage oral fluids by offering them frequently.

▶ Monitor for signs of complications.

Patient teaching

▶ Teach parents how to reduce their infant's fever by keeping him or her in lightweight clothes, maintaining normal room temperature, and giving tepid baths.

▶ Stress the need for adequate fluid intake. Strict bed rest and isolation are unnecessary.

▶ Tell parents that a short febrile seizure will not cause brain damage. Explain that seizures will cease after fever subsides; if stupor ensues, tell the parents to call their physician immediately.

▶ Warn parents to avoid giving aspirin to their infant due to risk of Reye syndrome.

▶ Reassure the parents that roseola is not contagious.

CONTACT PRECAUTIONS

Rotavirus infection

Rotavirus is the most common cause of severe diarrhea among children. The infection is characterized by vomiting and watery diarrhea lasting 3 to 8 days, commonly accompanied by fever and abdominal pain.

In the United States and other countries with a temperate climate, the disease has a winter seasonal pattern, with annual epidemics occurring from November to April. The illness occurs most often in infants and young children; most children in the United States are infected by age 2. Rotavirus is responsible for the hospitalization of about 55,000 children each year in the United States.

CAUSES

The primary mode of rotavirus transmission is the fecal-oral route, although low virus titers have been reported in respiratory tract secretions and other body fluids. Because the virus endures in the environment, transmission may also occur through ingestion of contaminated water or food or through contact with contaminated surfaces.

Billions of rotavirus microorganisms are passed in the stool of the infected individual. Small numbers of rotavirus particles may lead to infection if a baby puts fingers or other objects contaminated with the virus into the mouth. Young children can pass it on to siblings and parents.

Rotavirus is the most common diagnosis for young children who have acute diarrhea, but other causes may include bacteria (*Salmonella*, *Shigella*, and *Campylobacter* are the most common), parasites (*Giardia* and *Cryptosporidium* are the most common), localized infection elsewhere in the body, antibiotic-associated adverse effects (such as those related to treatment for *Clostridium difficile*), and food poisoning. Noninfectious causes include overfeeding (particularly of fruit juices), irritable bowel syndrome, celiac disease, milk protein intolerance, lactose intolerance, cystic fibrosis, and inflammatory bowel syndrome.

Immunity after infection is incomplete, but recurrent infections tend to be less severe than the original infection.

 PREVENTION The Rotavirus Vaccine Program—a collaboration between the World Health Organization, the Program for Appropriate Technology in Health, and the U.S. Centers for Disease Control and Prevention—is working to expedite the use of rotavirus vaccines worldwide. A live rotavirus vaccine, oral pentavalent (RotaTeq), may prevent 74% of rotavirus cases, which in turn would decrease hospitalizations due to this infection.

COMPLICATIONS

Complications of rotavirus infection include severe dehydration, shock, and skin breakdown due to severe vomiting and diarrhea. These complications can be detrimental in the immunocompromised patient and can also complicate other conditions, such as cystic fibrosis. About 1 child in 40 infected with rotavirus requires hospitalization for I.V. fluid administration. More than 600,000 children worldwide die each year (80% in poor countries) as a result of rotavirus infection.

ASSESSMENT FINDINGS

The incubation period for rotavirus is about 2 days. Rotavirus gastroenteritis commonly starts with a fever, nausea, and vomiting, followed by watery diarrhea. The illness ranges from mild to severe and can last from 3 to 9 days. Diarrhea and vomiting may cause dehydration. The following guidelines help determine the extent of dehydration as measured by the percentage of body weight lost:
▶ 5% to 6%: Heart rate 10% to 15% above baseline, slightly dry mucous membranes, concentration of the urine, poor tear production
▶ 7% to 8%: Increased severity of the above signs plus decreased skin turgor, oliguria, sunken eyeballs, and sunken anterior fontanel

❱ Greater than 8%: Pronounced severity of above signs plus decreased blood pressure, delayed capillary refill time (>2 seconds), and acidosis (large base deficit)

DIAGNOSTIC TESTS

❱ Rapid antigen stool testing is positive in patients with rotavirus infection.

TREATMENT

For a person with a healthy immune system, rotavirus gastroenteritis is a self-limiting illness, lasting only days. Treatment is nonspecific and consists of oral rehydration therapy to prevent dehydration. If severe dehydration occurs, I.V. therapy may be needed. Oral electrolyte supplements are recommended.

NURSING CONSIDERATIONS

❱ Enforce strict handwashing technique and careful cleaning of all equipment, including the child's toys, to prevent the spread of rotavirus.

⊗ Implement contact precautions.

❱ Help the patient maintain adequate hydration. Remember that dehydration occurs rapidly in infants and young children. Ice pops, gelatin, and ice chips may be included in the diet to maintain hydration. Electrolyte solutions, such as Pedialyte, are also recommended.

❱ Breast-fed infants should continue to nurse without restrictions. Lactose-free soybean formulas may be used for infants who are bottle-fed.

❱ Carefully monitor intake and output (including stools).

❱ Clean the perineum thoroughly to prevent skin breakdown.

Patient teaching

 SAFETY Instruct parents about proper handwashing techniques for themselves and the patient. Provide information about hygienic diaper changing, and instruct parents to clean all affected surfaces after a diaper change.

❱ Teach parents and caregivers how to measure intake and output. Tell them to notify the physician about any increased diarrhea. Explain the signs and symptoms of dehydration and when to notify the physician.

 PREVENTION Suggest the rotavirus vaccine, if appropriate, to parents of infants. It is recommended that the rotavirus doses be completed by age 8 months.

Roundworm infection

Roundworm infection, also known as ascariasis, is caused by *Ascaris lumbricoides*. It's the most common type of intestinal worm infection, occurring worldwide. Most patients recover without treatment, but complications can occur when adult worms move into certain organs and multiply, resulting intestinal obstruction.

Roundworm is most common in tropical areas with poor sanitation and in Asia, where farmers use human feces as fertilizer. In the United States, it's more prevalent in the South, particularly among children ages 4 to 12. However, international travelers and immigrants (especially from Asia and Latin America) are at an increased risk for infection.

CAUSES

A. lumbricoides is a large roundworm that resembles an earthworm. It's transmitted to humans by ingestion of soil contaminated with human feces that harbor *A. lumbricoides* ova. Such ingestion may occur directly (by eating contaminated soil) or indirectly (by eating poorly washed raw vegetables grown in contaminated soil). Hand-to-mouth transmission is also possible—hands that are contaminated by touching soil or other contaminated surfaces transmit the infective eggs to the mouth. The larvae can also enter the human body directly through a break in the skin. Roundworm infection never passes directly from person to person, although whole families may be infected as a result of shared food or living conditions.

After ingestion, *A. lumbricoides* ova hatch and release larvae, which penetrate the intestinal wall and reach the lungs through the bloodstream. After about 10 days in the pulmonary capillaries and alveoli, the larvae migrate to the bronchioles, bronchi, trachea, and epiglottis. There they are swallowed and returned to the intestine to mature into adult worms. This cycle takes approximately 2 to 3 months.

COMPLICATIONS

Complications of roundworm include biliary or intestinal obstruction as well as pulmonary disease. It may also be associated with malnutrition, iron deficiency anemia, and failure to thrive. Death may occur from bowel obstruction or perforation.

ASSESSMENT FINDINGS

The patient's history may reveal ingestion of poorly washed raw vegetables. Most patients with roundworm are asymptomatic. For those who are symptomatic, roundworm produces two phases: early pulmonary and prolonged intestinal.

A patient in the early pulmonary phase (4 to 6 days after ingestion of eggs) may demonstrate a nonproductive cough, fever, wheezing, and dyspnea. During the intestinal phase (6 to 8 weeks after ingestion) the patient may complain of vague stomach discomfort. The first clue may be vomiting a worm or passing a worm in the stool. Patients may complain of a "tingling" in the throat, along with frequent throat clearing. Severe infection, however, causes stomach pain, vomiting, restlessness, disturbed sleep and, in extreme cases, intestinal obstruction. Symptoms may vary when larvae migrate via the lymphatic and circulatory systems; for instance, when they invade the lungs, pneumonitis may result.

Inspection may reveal weight loss and impaired growth. Bowel sounds may be hyperactive above the obstruction and diminished or absent below the obstruction. Auscultation of the chest may detect wheezing. Palpation of the abdomen may identify distention.

DIAGNOSTIC TESTS

▶ Stool culture identifies ova or adult worms.
▶ When migrating larvae invade alveoli, chest radiography will show characteristic bronchovascular markings: infiltrates, patchy areas of pneumonitis, and widening of hilar shadows.

▶ Abdominal radiographs show a whirlpool pattern of intraluminal worms. Intestinal obstruction may be noted.

▶ A complete blood count may show eosinophilia.

TREATMENT

Drug therapy, the primary treatment, consists of albendazole (Albenza) or mebendazole to kill the worms, permitting peristalsis to expel them. No specific treatment exists for migratory infection because anthelmintics affect only mature worms.

Nasogastric suctioning controls vomiting in patients with intestinal obstruction. If the obstruction is caused by a large number of worms, a paralyzing vermifuge can make the worms relax and pass through the intestine to relieve the obstruction. However, surgery may be required if the paralyzed worms continue to block the intestine.

 ALERT Piperazine is contraindicated in patients with seizure disorders and is no longer available in the United States. Albendazole and mebendazole may cause abdominal pain and diarrhea.

NURSING CONSIDERATIONS

▶ Maintain standard precautions. Properly dispose of feces and soiled linen, and carefully wash your hands after patient contact.

▶ If the patient is receiving nasogastric suction, be sure to provide good mouth care.

▶ Administer antipyretics and give tepid sponge baths to reduce fever.

▶ Monitor respiratory status, and administer oxygen or assist ventilation if pulmonary complications develop.

▶ Question family members and other contacts about symptoms.

▶ Weigh the patient daily, and monitor intake and output.

▶ Replace fluids as needed. Provide a nutritionally adequate diet and administer nutritional supplements, as prescribed.

▶ Refer the patient to social services if the cleanliness of living conditions is questionable.

Patient teaching

▶ Teach the patient about prescribed medication, including dosage, administration, and possible adverse effects. Let the patient know that piperazine may cause stomach upset, dizziness, and urticaria.

▶ Tell the patient that the physician will want a follow-up stool specimen to evaluate the effectiveness of treatment.

 PREVENTION Teach the patient to prevent re-infection with proper hand washing, especially before eating and after defecating. Instruct patients to avoid contact with any soil that has been contaminated with human feces or any food that may have been in contact with contaminated soil. Tell them not to defecate outdoors and to dispose of diapers properly. Advise patients to wash, peel, or cook raw vegetables before eating them and to scrub or peel fruit before eating it.

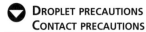

Rubella

Rubella, commonly called German measles, is an acute, mildly contagious viral disease that produces a distinctive 3-day rash accompanied by lymphadenopathy. It usually occurs in children ages 5 to 9, adolescents, and young adults. Rubella flourishes worldwide during the spring, and epidemics occur sporadically.

CAUSES

The rubella virus is transmitted through respiratory droplets when an infected person coughs or sneezes. Transplacental transmission, especially in the first trimester of pregnancy, can cause serious birth defects. The disease is contagious from about 7 days before the rash appears until 5 to 7 days after it has subsided.

COMPLICATIONS

Complications seldom occur in children with rubella; when complications do arise, they commonly appear as hemorrhagic conditions such as thrombocytopenia. Many young women, however, experience transient joint pain or arthritis, usually just as the rash is fading. Fever may then occur, or recur. These complications usually subside spontaneously within 5 to 30 days. In very rare cases, otitis media and encephalitis may develop. When a pregnant woman contracts rubella, complications in the unborn child may be severe. (See *Congenital rubella syndrome*.)

ASSESSMENT FINDINGS

In children, after an incubation period of 12 to 23 days, an exanthematous, maculopapular rash erupts abruptly. In adolescents and adults, prodromal signs and symptoms—headache, malaise, anorexia, low-grade fever, coryza, lymphadenopathy and, sometimes, conjunctivitis—are the first to appear. Suboccipital, postauricular, and postcervical lymph node enlargement is a hallmark of this disease and precedes the rash.

Typically, the rubella rash begins on the face and spreads rapidly, in many cases covering the trunk and extremities within hours. Small, red, petechial macules on the soft palate (Forchheimer sign) may precede or accompany the rash but aren't diagnostic of rubella. By the end of the second day, the facial rash begins to fade, but the rash on the trunk may become confluent and be mistaken for scarlet fever. The rash continues to fade in the downward order, and generally disappears on the third day but may persist for 4 or 5 days—sometimes accompanied by mild coryza and conjunctivitis. In rare cases, rubella can occur without a rash. Low-grade fever may accompany the rash (99° to 101° F [37.2° to 38.3° C]), but it usually doesn't persist after the first day of the rash; rarely, the body temperature may reach 104° F (40° C). A significant number of patients, 20% to 50%, are asymptomatic.

DIAGNOSTIC TESTS

▸ The rubella rash, lymphadenopathy, other characteristic signs, and a history of exposure to infected people usually support a clinical diagnosis without laboratory tests. The rubella rash has been confused with scarlet fever, measles (rubeola), infectious mononucleosis, roseola, and other viral exanthems. Therefore, without exposure history, laboratory confirmation is beneficial.
▸ Cell cultures of the throat, blood, urine, and cerebrospinal fluid can confirm the presence of the virus.
▸ Convalescent serum that shows a fourfold rise in antibody titers corroborates the diagnosis.

TREATMENT

Because the rubella rash is self-limiting and only mildly pruritic, it doesn't require topical or systemic medication. Treatment consists of acetaminophen for fever and joint pain. Bed rest isn't necessary, but the patient should be isolated until the rash disappears.

NURSING CONSIDERATIONS

▸ Make the patient with active rubella as comfortable as possible. If the patient is a

Congenital rubella syndrome

Congenital rubella is by far the most serious form of the disease. Intrauterine rubella infection, especially during the first trimester, can lead to spontaneous abortion or stillbirth or, in fetuses that survive, single or multiple birth defects.

The combination of cataracts, deafness, and heart disease characterizes congenital rubella syndrome. Low birth weight, microcephaly, and mental retardation are other common manifestations. However, researchers now believe that congenital rubella can cause more disorders, many of which don't appear until later in life. These include dental abnormalities, thrombocytopenic purpura, hemolytic and hypoplastic anemia, encephalitis, giant-cell hepatitis, seborrheic dermatitis, and diabetes mellitus. Indeed, it now appears that congenital rubella may be a lifelong disease.

Neonates born with congenital rubella should be isolated immediately because they excrete the virus for several months to a year after birth. Cataracts and cardiac defects may require surgery. The prognosis depends on the particular malformations that occur. The overall mortality for neonates with rubella is 6%, although it's higher for neonates born with thrombocytopenic purpura, congenital heart disease, or encephalitis.

child, provide books or games to keep him or her occupied.

◗ Explain to the patient or, if the patient is a child, the parents why droplet precautions are necessary. Maintain contact precautions for the patient with congenital rubella syndrome until age 1. Make sure female patients understand how important it is to avoid exposure to this disease when pregnant.

▶ Report confirmed cases of rubella to local public health officials.

▶ Before giving the rubella vaccine:
- Obtain a history of allergies, especially to neomycin. If the patient has this allergy or has had a reaction to immunization in the past, check with the physician before giving the vaccine.
- Ask women of childbearing age if they're pregnant. If they are pregnant or think they may be, perform a pregnancy test before giving the vaccine or don't give the vaccine at all. Warn women who receive rubella vaccine to use an effective means of birth control for at least 3 months after immunization.
- Give the vaccine at least 3 months after administration of any immune globulin or blood, which could have antibodies that neutralize the vaccine.
- Don't vaccinate patients who are immunocompromised, patients with immunodeficiency diseases, or those receiving immunosuppressive, radiation, or corticosteroid therapy. Instead, administer immune serum globulin, as ordered, to prevent or reduce infection.
- After giving the rubella vaccine, observe the patient for at least 30 minutes for signs of anaphylaxis.

Patient teaching

▶ Warn the patient about possible mild fever, slight rash, transient arthralgia (in adolescents), and arthritis (in elderly patients). Suggest acetaminophen for fever.

▶ If lymphadenopathy persists after the initial 24 hours, suggest a cold compress to promote vasoconstriction and prevent antigenic cyst formation.

 PREVENTION Immunization with the live virus vaccine RA 27/3 (Meruvax II)—the only rubella vaccine available in the United States—is necessary for prevention, and this vaccine appears to be more immunogenic than previous vaccines. To decrease the cost and number of injections, the rubella vaccine should be given with measles and mumps vaccines at age 15 months.

AIRBORNE PRECAUTIONS

Rubeola

Rubeola, also known as measles or morbilli, is an acute, highly contagious paramyxovirus infection that may be one of the most common and most serious of all communicable childhood diseases. Vaccine use has reduced its occurrence during childhood. In the United States, the prognosis is usually excellent; however, rubeola is a major cause of death in children in underdeveloped countries.

Generally, one bout of rubeola provides immunity (a second infection is extremely rare and may indicate a misdiagnosis); infants younger than age 4 months may be immune because of circulating maternal antibodies. Under normal conditions, rubeola vaccine isn't administered to children younger than age 15 months. However, during an epidemic, infants as young as 6 months may receive the vaccine and then be re-immunized at age 15 months. An alternative preventive approach calls for administering gamma globulin to infants between ages 6 and 15 months who are likely to be exposed to rubeola.

CAUSES

Rubeola is spread by direct contact or by contaminated airborne respiratory droplets. The portal of entry is the upper respiratory tract.

COMPLICATIONS

Complications of rubeola include otitis media, cervical adenitis, laryngitis, pneumonia, and encephalitis.

ASSESSMENT FINDINGS

Incubation is from 10 to 12 days. Initial symptoms begin and greatest communicability occurs during the prodromal phase, about 11 days after exposure to the virus. This phase lasts from 4 to 5 days; signs and symptoms include fever, photophobia, malaise, anorexia, conjunctivitis, coryza, hoarseness, and a hacking cough.

At the end of the prodrome, Koplik spots—the hallmark of the disease—appear. These spots, which resemble tiny, bluish white specks surrounded by a red halo, are found on the oral mucosa opposite the molars and occasionally bleed. About 5 days after Koplik spots appear, temperature rises sharply, spots slough off, and a slightly pruritic rash appears. This characteristic rash starts as faint maculae behind the ears and on the neck and cheeks. The maculae become papular and erythematous, rapidly spreading over the entire face, neck, eyelids, arms, chest, back, abdomen, and thighs. When the rash reaches the feet 2 to 3 days later, it begins to fade in the same sequence in which it appeared, leaving a brownish discoloration that disappears in 7 to 10 days.

The disease climax occurs 3 to 4 days after the rash appears and is marked by a fever of 103° to 105° F (39.4° to 40.6° C), severe cough, puffy red eyes, and rhinorrhea. About 5 days after the rash appears, other symptoms disappear and communicability ends. More severe symptoms and complications are more likely to develop in young infants, adolescents, adults, and patients who are immunocompromised than in young children.

Atypical rubeola may appear in patients who received the killed rubeola vaccine. These patients become acutely ill, either with a fever and maculopapular rash that's most obvious in the arms and legs or with pulmonary involvement and no skin lesions.

Severe infection may lead to secondary bacterial infection and to autoimmune reaction or organ invasion by the virus, resulting in otitis media, pneumonia, and encephalitis. Subacute sclerosing panencephalitis, a rare and invariably fatal complication, may develop several years after rubeola but is less common in patients who have received the rubeola vaccine.

DIAGNOSIS

▶ Diagnosis rests on recognizing distinctive clinical features, especially the pathognomonic Koplik spots.

Administering rubeola vaccine

- Ask the patient about known allergies, especially to neomycin (each dose contains a small amount). However, a patient who's allergic to eggs may receive the vaccine because it contains only minimal amounts of albumin and yolk components.
- Avoid giving the vaccine to pregnant women (ask for the date of last menstrual period). Warn female patients to avoid pregnancy for at least 3 months following vaccination.
- Don't vaccinate children who have untreated tuberculosis, immunodeficiencies, leukemia, or lymphoma or those receiving immunosuppressants. If such children are exposed to the virus, recommend that they receive gamma globulin (which won't prevent measles but will lessen its severity). Older unimmunized children who have been exposed to measles for more than 5 days may also require gamma globulin. Be sure to immunize these children again 3 months later.
- Delay vaccination for 8 to 12 weeks after administration of whole blood, plasma, or gamma globulin because measles antibodies in these components may neutralize the vaccine.
- Watch for signs of anaphylaxis for 30 minutes after vaccination. Keep epinephrine 1:1,000 handy.
- Warn the patient or parents that mild adverse effects of vaccination may occur, usually within 7 to 10 days, and include anorexia, malaise, rash, mild thrombocytopenia or leukopenia, and fever. If swelling occurs within 24 hours after vaccination, advise the application of cold compresses to the injection site to promote vasoconstriction and prevent antigenic cyst formation.

▶ If necessary, rubeola virus may be isolated from the blood, nasopharyngeal secretions, and urine during the febrile period. Serum antibodies appear within 3 days after onset of the rash and reach peak titers 2 to 4 weeks later.

TREATMENT

Treatment for rubeola requires bed rest, relief of symptoms, and airborne precautions throughout the communicable period. Vaporizers and a warm environment help reduce respiratory irritation, and antipyretics can reduce fever. I.V. ribavirin has reduced the severity of illness in adults.

 PREVENTION Administration of the rubeola vaccine prevents contraction of the infection. The vaccine is given in two doses—the first dose at age 12 to 15 months and the second before the start of kindergarten, at age 4 to 6. (See *Administering rubeola vaccine*.)

NURSING CONSIDERATIONS

▶ Administer medications as ordered, and evaluate the patient's response.

◯ Maintain standard and airborne precautions. Place the patient in a negative pressure room. Utilize appropriately sized respirator masks when entering the room.

▶ Provide tepid baths to decrease temperature and increase comfort.

Patient teaching

▶ Teach the patient or the patient's parents supportive measures, and stress the need for isolation, plenty of rest, and increased fluid intake. Advise them to cope with photophobia by darkening the room or providing the patient with sunglasses and to reduce fever with antipyretics and tepid sponge baths.

 SAFETY Discuss airborne and standard precautions with the family and visitors. Demonstrate how to use respirator masks correctly. Stress the need for proper hand washing technique.

▶ Warn the patient or the patient's parents to watch for and report the early signs of complications, such as encephalitis, otitis media, and pneumonia.

CONTACT PRECAUTIONS

Salmonellosis

A common infection in the United States, salmonellosis is caused by gram-negative bacilli of the genus *Salmonella*, a member of the Enterobacteriaceae family. About 40,000 cases of salmonellosis are reported yearly in the form of enterocolitis, bacteremia, localized infection, typhoid fever, or paratyphoid fever. Nontyphoidal forms can produce mild to moderate illness that lasts 4 to 7 days and carries a low mortality.

Typhoid fever, caused by *Salmonella typhi*, is the most severe form of salmonellosis and can last up to 4 weeks. Mortality is about 3% in those who receive treatment. Ten percent of untreated cases result in fatality. An attack of typhoid fever confers lifelong immunity, although the patient may become a carrier. Salmonellosis is 20 times more common in patients with acquired immunodeficiency syndrome.

CAUSES

Of an estimated 1,700 serotypes of *Salmonella*, serotypes *typhimurium* and *enteritidis* are the most common in the United States. Nontyphoidal salmonellosis generally follows the ingestion of contaminated or inadequately processed foods, especially eggs, chicken, turkey, and duck. Cooking foods to an appropriate temperature reduces the risk of contracting salmonellosis. Other causes include contact with infected people or animals or ingestion of contaminated dry milk or drugs of animal origin. Salmonellosis may occur in children younger than age 5 via the fecal-oral route. Enterocolitis and bacteremia are common (and more virulent) among infants, elderly persons, and people already weakened by other infections; paratyphoid fever is rare in the United States.

Typhoid fever usually results from drinking water contaminated by the excretions of a carrier or from ingesting contaminated shellfish. (Contamination of shellfish occurs by leakage of sewage from offshore disposal depots.) Most typhoid patients are younger than age 30; most carriers are women older than age 50. The incidence of typhoid fever in the United States is on the rise as a result of increased travel to endemic areas.

COMPLICATIONS

Salmonellosis may result in such complications as intestinal perforation or hemorrhage, cerebral thrombosis, pneumonia, endocarditis, myocarditis, meningitis, pyelonephritis, osteomyelitis, cholecystitis, hepatitis, septicemia, and acute circulatory failure.

ASSESSMENT FINDINGS

Clinical manifestations of salmonellosis vary but usually include fever, abdominal pain, and severe diarrhea with enterocolitis. Headache, increasing fever, and constipation are more common in typhoidal infection.

DIAGNOSTIC TESTS

▶ Blood or stool culture identifies the organism. Other appropriate culture specimens include urine, bone marrow, pus, and emesis. In endemic areas, clinical symptoms of enterocolitis allow a working diagnosis before the cultures are positive. The presence of *S. typhi* in stool 1 or more years after treatment indicates that the patient is a carrier, which is true of 3% of patients.

▶ Widal reaction, an agglutination reaction against somatic and flagellar antigens, may suggest typhoid with a fourfold rise in titer. However, drug use or hepatic disease can also increase these titers and invalidate test results.

▶ Other supportive laboratory values may include transient leukocytosis during the first week of typhoidal salmonellosis, leukopenia during the third week, and leukocytosis in patients with local infection.

TREATMENT

Nontyphoidal *Salmonella* infections usually resolve in 4 to 7 days and commonly don't require treatment other than maintaining hydration with oral fluids. Patients with

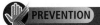

PREVENTION

Preventing recurrence of salmonellosis

Take the following actions to help your patients prevent a recurrence of salmonellosis:
- Explain the causes of *Salmonella* infection.
- Show the patient how to wash the hands by wetting them under running water, lathering with soap and scrubbing, rinsing under running water with the fingers pointing down, and drying with a clean towel or paper towel.
- Tell the patient to wash the hands after using the bathroom and before eating.
- Tell the patient to cook foods thoroughly—especially eggs and chicken—and to refrigerate them at once after eating.

- Teach the patient how to avoid cross-contaminating foods by cleaning preparation surfaces after use with hot, soapy water and drying them thoroughly; cleaning surfaces between tasks when preparing more than one food; and washing the hands before and after handling each food.
- Tell the patient with a positive stool culture to avoid handling food and to use a separate bathroom or clean the bathroom after each use.
- Tell the patient to report dehydration, bleeding, or recurrence of signs of *Salmonella* infection.

---

severe diarrhea may require I.V. fluids. Antibiotics, such as ampicillin, trimethoprim-sulfamethoxazole (Bactrim), or ciprofloxacin (Cipro), aren't typically necessary unless the infection spreads from the intestines. *Salmonella* has become resistant to many antibiotics as a result of antibiotic use in the food supply. Antibiotic therapy for typhoid fever, paratyphoid fever, and bacteremia depends on organism sensitivity and may include amoxicillin, chloramphenicol and, in severely toxemic patients, trimethoprim-sulfamethoxazole, ciprofloxacin, or ceftriaxone (Rocephin). Localized abscesses may also need surgical drainage. Enterocolitis requires a short course of antibiotics only if it causes septicemia or prolonged fever. Other treatments include bed rest and fluid and electrolyte replacement. The administration of camphorated tincture of opium, kaolin with pectin, diphenoxylate, codeine, or small doses of morphine may be necessary to relieve diarrhea and control cramps in patients who must remain active.

NURSING CONSIDERATIONS

▶ Report all infections caused by *Salmonella* to the state health department.
◕ Follow contact precautions with diapered or incontinent patients; otherwise, standard precautions are appropriate.

▶ Observe the patient closely for signs and symptoms of bowel perforation resulting from erosion of intestinal ulcers.
▶ Record intake and output accurately, and maintain adequate I.V. hydration. When the patient can tolerate oral feedings, encourage high-calorie fluids such as milkshakes. Watch for constipation.
▶ Provide good skin and mouth care. Turn the patient frequently, and perform mild passive exercises as indicated. Apply mild heat to the abdomen to relieve cramps.

Patient teaching

▶ If the patient has positive stool cultures on discharge, tell him or her to be sure to wash the hands after using the bathroom and to avoid preparing uncooked foods, such as salads, for family members. These patients shouldn't work as food handlers until culture results are negative. (See *Preventing recurrence of salmonellosis*.)

CONTACT PRECAUTIONS

Scabies

Scabies is a highly transmissible skin infection that is characterized by burrows, pruritus, and excoriations with secondary bacterial infection. It occurs worldwide, is associated with overcrowding and poor hygiene, and can be endemic. The mites that cause this disorder can live their entire life cycle in human skin, causing chronic infection. The female mite burrows into the skin to lay eggs, from which larvae emerge to copulate and then re-burrow under the skin.

CAUSES

Infestation with *Sarcoptes scabiei* var. *hominis* (itch mite) causes scabies. (See *Scabies: cause and effect*.) Transmission is via direct, prolonged skin contact. It is most often seen in nursing home residents, school-age children and their families, and the intimate contacts of those with scabies. The adult mite can live for 2 to 3 days without a human host; therefore, inanimate objects can't be ruled out as a means of transmission.

COMPLICATIONS

Persistent pruritus caused by secondary mite sensitization is a complication of scabies. Intense scratching can lead to excoriation, tissue trauma, and secondary bacterial infection.

ASSESSMENT FINDINGS

The patient history may uncover predisposing factors. The patient may first present with asymptomatic lesions. The patient who has been infected for several weeks will complain of intense itching that becomes more severe at night.

Inspection may reveal characteristic gray-brown burrows, which may appear as erythematous nodules when excoriated. These threadlike lesions, about 1 cm long, occur between the fingers, on the flexor surfaces of the wrists, on the elbows, in axillary folds, at the waistline, on the nipples in females, and on the genitalia in males. In infants, the burrows (lesions) may appear on the head and neck. Secondary infection may develop, resulting in the formation of papules and vesicles as well as crusting.

DIAGNOSTIC TESTS

▶ Superficial scraping and examination under a low-power microscope of material that has been expressed from a burrow may reveal the mite, ova, or mite feces. However, excoriation or inflammation of the burrow can make such identification difficult.

▶ If scabies is strongly suspected but diagnostic tests offer no positive identification of the mite, skin clearing following a therapeutic trial of a pediculicide helps confirm the diagnosis.

TREATMENT

Treatment of scabies generally involves applying a pediculicide—permethrin (Nix) or crotamiton (Eurax)—in a thin layer over the affected area. Permethrin is left on for 8 to 12 hours. Crotamiton is applied nightly for 2 consecutive nights and washed off 24 hours after the second application. In severe cases, Crotamiton should be applied 1 additional time, 1 week later. Other topical treatments for scabies include benzyl benzoate, malathion, and sulfur in petrolatum. Oral administration of ivermectin, an anthelminthic drug, is also effective, especially in resistant cases.

Lindane is an effective scabicide but is recommended only as an alternative therapy in patients who cannot tolerate other therapies or when other therapies have failed.

Persistent pruritus (from mite sensitization or contact dermatitis) may develop from repeated use of a pediculicide rather than from continued infection. An antipruritic emollient or topical steroid can reduce itching; an intralesional steroid may resolve erythematous nodules.

Scabies: cause and effect

Infestation with *Sarcoptes scabiei*—the itch mite—causes scabies. This mite (shown enlarged below) has a hard shell and measures a microscopic 0.1 mm. The bottom illustration shows the erythematous nodules with excoriation that appear in patients with scabies. These lesions are usually highly pruritic.

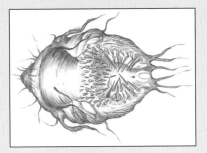

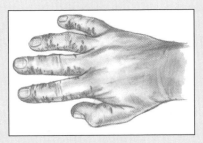

NURSING CONSIDERATIONS

▶ Have the patient's fingernails cut short to minimize skin breaks from scratching, which may lead to secondary bacterial infection.

◐ To prevent transmission, isolate the patient until treatment is completed; use meticulous handwashing technique; observe contact precautions for 24 hours after treatment with a pediculicide; sterilize blood pressure cuffs in a gas autoclave before using them on other patients; isolate linens, towels, clothing, and personal articles until the patient is noninfectious; thoroughly disinfect the patient's room after discharge; and have all contaminated clothing and personal articles washed and disinfected.

▶ Be alert for complications associated with treatment, including contact dermatitis and hypersensitivity reactions from repeated use of pediculicides. Remember that prolonged use of pediculicides may lead to excessive central nervous system stimulation and seizures.

▶ Encourage the patient to verbalize his or her feelings about the infestation, including embarrassment, fear of rejection by others, and disturbed body image.

Patient teaching

▶ Teach the patient and family to identify characteristic lesions and the modes of transmission. Assure the patient and family that the infestation can be treated successfully with good hygiene and the use of pediculicides. Stress the importance of meticulous handwashing to prevent the spread and recurrence of infection.

▶ Instruct the patient to apply cream or lotion from the neck down, covering the entire body. (Assistance may be needed to reach all body areas.) Tell the patient to wait 15 minutes after applying a pediculicide before dressing and to avoid bathing for 12 hours.

▶ Tell the patient not to apply lotion to raw or inflamed skin. Explain the signs of skin irritation and hypersensitivity reaction. Advise the patient to notify the physician immediately, discontinue using the drug, and wash the drug from the skin.

▶ Suggest that the patient's family and other close personal contacts be checked for symptoms. Have the patient notify sexual contacts about the infection. If the patient is a school-age child, notify the school of his or her condition.

DROPLET PRECAUTIONS

Scarlet fever

Scarlet fever, also known as scarlatina, is an illness that results from group A beta-hemolytic streptococcal infection. It occurs most frequently as a complication of streptococcal pharyngitis but may also result from wound infections, urosepsis, sinusitis, bronchopneumonia, meningitis, and puerperal sepsis. A more lethal illness prior to the 19th century, scarlet fever currently follows a more benign course with decreased mortality resulting from the use of antibiotics. It's most common in children ages 4 to 8. The incubation period usually lasts 2 to 4 days but may be as short as 1 day or as long as 7 days. Scarlet fever occurs mainly in the summer and fall and in areas where the temperature is warmer.

CAUSES

Group A beta-hemolytic streptococci cause scarlet fever. The infecting strain produces one of three erythrogenic toxins that trigger a sensitivity reaction in the patient. Transmission occurs by inhalation of respiratory droplets from infected patients. Risk factors include crowded conditions, such as in schools and institutions. Immunity is type specific and occurs after infection, and 80% of people have developed protective antibodies by age 10. The presence of maternal antiexotoxin antibodies protects children younger than age 2; therefore, scarlet fever is very rare in this age group.

COMPLICATIONS

Scarlet fever can lead to severe disseminated toxic illness, septicemia, rheumatic heart disease, and liver damage. Glomerulonephritis may develop if the patient contracts a nephritogenic strain of group A beta-hemolytic *Streptococcus*. Other complications include otitis media, bronchopneumonia, brain abscess, intracranial venous sinus thrombosis, vasculitis, and uveitis.

ASSESSMENT FINDINGS

After a 1- to 4-day incubation period, signs and symptoms appear suddenly, with the patient reporting a sore throat, headache, chills, anorexia, abdominal pain, nausea, vomiting, and malaise. The patient is likely to have a sudden temperature of 100° to 103° F (37.8° to 39.4° C) and commonly has had contact with a person with a sore throat.

Initial inspection of the patient's mouth shows an inflamed and heavily coated tongue. As the infection progresses, a strawberry-like tongue is noted, with reddened papillae covered with a white coating. As it progresses further, the coating begins to peel and the tongue becomes raspberry red. It returns to normal by the end of the second week. The uvula, tonsils, and posterior oropharynx appear red and edematous, with mucopurulent exudate.

Inspection of the skin may reveal a fine, erythematous rash that appears first on the upper chest and back. It later spreads to the neck, abdomen, legs, and arms but doesn't appear on the soles of the feet or palms of the hands. The rash is more noticeable in the skin folds; it resembles sunburn with goose bumps and blanches when pressure is applied. The patient's face appears flushed, except around the mouth, which remains pale. During convalescence, desquamation of the skin occurs at the tips of the fingers and toes, axilla, and groin and, occasionally, over wide areas of the trunk and limbs. Desquamation is more pronounced where the erythematous rash was most severe.

The cervical lymph nodes feel enlarged and tender on palpation. The liver may also feel slightly enlarged and tender, and tachycardia may be noted.

DIAGNOSTIC TESTS

▶ Pharyngeal culture is positive for group A beta-hemolytic streptococci.
▶ Streptolysin O antibody testing confirms previous group A streptococcal infection (this test is not indicated during acute infection).

A complete blood count reveals an increased white blood cell count, granulocytosis and, possibly, a reduced red blood cell count.

TREATMENT

Penicillin is the drug of choice for patients with group A streptococcal infections. Erythromycin (E-mycin) may be given as an alternative, with therapy lasting for 10 days. Antipyretics, such as acetaminophen (Tylenol), are given to reduce fever but may also be used to ease throat soreness and decrease myalgia. The patient should be isolated until 24 hours of antibiotic treatment has been administered.

NURSING CONSIDERATIONS

⬇ Maintain droplet precautions until 24 hours after starting antibiotic therapy; then follow standard precautions.

▶ Keep the patient on complete bed rest while he or she is febrile to prevent complications, promote recovery, and help conserve energy.

▶ Offer frequent oral fluids and oral hygiene, and give antipyretics as ordered.

▶ Apply topical anesthetics on the patient's tongue and throat to relieve pain.

▶ Provide skin care to relieve discomfort from the rash.

▶ Provide emotional support to the patient and family.

Patient teaching

▶ Review all medication, including dosage, administration, and possible side effects. Instruct the patient or parents to ensure that oral antibiotics are taken for the prescribed length of time, even if the patient is feeling better.

▶ Teach the patient or parents about the signs and symptoms of possible complications and when to notify the physician.

▶ Tell the patient to follow up with the physician as recommended.

 SAFETY If the patient remains at home for treatment, stress the need to isolate eating utensils, drinking glasses, napkins, tissues, and towels from the rest of the family in order to prevent spread of the infection.

Septicemia

Septicemia, also known as bacteremia or blood poisoning, is an overwhelming bacterial infection that invades the bloodstream. The infection quickly progresses to sepsis, a serious condition characterized by an inflammatory state called systemic inflammatory response syndrome (SIRS). Sepsis can lead to adult respiratory distress syndrome, septic shock, multiorgan dysfunction syndrome, and death. It is the second leading cause of noncardiac deaths in intensive care units.

CAUSES

Septicemia can be caused by infection that originates from anywhere in the body, primarily in the lungs, urinary tract, bones, abdomen, and central nervous system. Up to 70% of cases of septic shock are caused by gram-negative bacteria, such as *Escherichia coli*, *Klebsiella pneumoniae*, *Serratia*, *Enterobacter*, and *Pseudomonas*.

COMPLICATIONS

Complications of septicemia include septic shock, respiratory failure requiring ventilator support, circulatory system collapse, renal failure, and death (mortality exceeds 50% if septic shock develops). Other complications include disseminated intravascular coagulation, heart failure, GI ulcers, and abnormal liver function.

ASSESSMENT FINDINGS

The patient with septicemia typically presents with malaise, spiking fevers and chills, and an extremely ill appearance. Vital signs may reveal tachycardia and tachypnea along with decreased blood pressure. The source of infection may be evident (such as an infected wound or cellulitis) or elusive (such as pneumonia, urinary tract infection, meningitis, or peritonitis). The patient's condition can quickly deteriorate to sepsis, which is categorized into several levels according to the

Society of Critical Care Medicine and the American College of Chest Physicians:

▶ SIRS (two or more of the following symptoms): Temperature less than 97° F (36° C) or greater than 100° F (38° C); heart rate greater than 90 bpm; respiratory rate greater than 20 breaths/min; white blood cell count less than 4,000 or greater than 12,000/mm^3; and partial pressure of arterial carbon dioxide less than 32 mm Hg

▶ Sepsis: SIRS with a confirmed infection

▶ Severe sepsis: Sepsis with organ dysfunction

▶ Septic shock: Sepsis with hypotension despite aggressive fluid resuscitation; composed of two phases:

- Hyperdynamic phase: Skin possibly pink and flushed; altered level of consciousness (LOC; reflected in agitation, anxiety, irritability, and a shortened attention span); rapid, shallow respirations; decreased urine output; and normal or slightly elevated blood pressure

- Hypodynamic phase: Pale skin resulting from inadequate tissue perfusion; cyanosis; decreased LOC (possibly obtundation and coma); urine output less than 25 ml/hr; cold, clammy skin; hypotension; and an irregular pulse (if arrhythmias are present)

DIAGNOSTIC TESTS

▶ Blood cultures identify the specific organism causing infection. Cultures of sputum, urine, wounds, and cerebrospinal fluid may also show the causative organism and source of infection. The clinical signs of sepsis—fever, chills, and hypotension—are a response to endotoxins or exotoxins being released from the organism; these signs occur up to 1 hour after organisms have been cleared from the bloodstream. Thus, the worst time to collect blood samples for culture is when the patient develops a fever. Two or three blood samples should be collected at random times over a 24-hour period; additional samples are not necessary, even in patients receiving antibiotics.

‣ A complete blood count shows the presence or absence of anemia and leukopenia, severe or absent neutropenia and, usually, the presence of thrombocytopenia. Lactate levels are elevated.

‣ In the early stages of septicemia, arterial blood gas (ABG) analysis demonstrates metabolic alkalosis, which may proceed to metabolic acidosis.

TREATMENT

Locating and treating the underlying infection are essential. Aggressive antimicrobial therapy appropriate for the causative organism must be initiated immediately. Culture and sensitivity test results help determine the most effective antimicrobial drug.

Oxygen therapy should be initiated to maintain arterial oxygen saturation greater than 95%. Mechanical ventilation may be required if respiratory failure occurs. Colloid or crystalloid infusions are given to increase intravascular volume and maintain blood pressure. If fluid resuscitation fails, a vasopressor may be needed. Drotrecogin alfa (Xigris) may also be given if the patient meets the criteria for use. Hemodynamic monitoring may be used to assess treatment outcomes and for diagnostic purposes.

 PREVENTION Sepsis and septic shock may be prevented with early recognition and appropriate treatment of existing infections.

NURSING CONSIDERATIONS

‣ Remove and send for culture any I.V., intra-arterial, or urinary drainage catheters. Insert new catheters.

‣ Monitor vital signs, including pulse oximetry. Monitor hemodynamic parameters, if indicated. Monitor cardiac rhythm for arrhythmias.

‣ Administer I.V. fluids as ordered. Monitor blood pressure and urine output following fluid administration. If the patient continues to be hypotensive, administer vasopressors and titrate according to blood pressure parameters provided by the physician.

‣ Provide oxygen therapy as needed. Assist with endotracheal intubation and ventilation support, if necessary.

‣ Monitor laboratory values, including ABGs, and report abnormal values to the physician.

‣ Administer antibiotics as ordered, and observe for any allergic response.

‣ Measure output hourly. If output is less than 30 ml/hr in adults, increase the fluid infusion rate; however, watch for signs of fluid overload. Administer diuretics as ordered. If acute renal failure develops, continuous renal replacement therapy may be required.

‣ Follow guidelines for administration of drotrecogin alfa; obtain blood for appropriate laboratory testing, as ordered. Monitor for signs of bleeding.

‣ Monitor for complications, such as abnormal bleeding, renal failure, respiratory failure, heart failure, and signs of GI disturbances.

‣ Provide emotional support to the patient and family.

Patient teaching

‣ Explain the illness to the patient and family, including the cause, diagnosis, and treatment plan.

‣ Review all prescribed medication with the patient, including dosage and administration as well as possible adverse effects.

Shellfish poisoning

Shellfish poisoning, recognized for several hundred years, is infection resulting from the ingestion of shellfish contaminated with a virus or bacteria. Shellfish poisoning includes four primary syndromes that are commonly caused by ingestion of bivalve mollusks (oysters, clams, mussels, and scallops) but may also result from ingestion of shrimp, crabs, and salted raw fish. These syndromes include paralytic shellfish poisoning (PSP), neurologic shellfish poisoning (NSP), diarrheal shellfish poisoning (DSP), and amnesic shellfish poisoning (ASP). PSP affects children more often than adults and is considered the most severe of the four syndromes, with a mortality rate of 1% to 12% in isolated outbreaks. All reported deaths from ASP have been in elderly patients. NSP and DSP have not been known to cause any deaths.

CAUSES

Bivalve mollusks accumulate toxins produced by microscopic algae. Offending toxins include saxitoxin (PSP), brevetoxin (NSP), okadaic acid (DSP), and domoic acid (ASP). These toxins are not inactivated by regular cooking and are also water soluble. Poisoning generally occurs after ingestion, although brevetoxin may become aerosolized by the surf. Outbreaks occur more often in warm weather but have decreased in the United States as a result of education and regulation by public health officials. Hepatitis A virus, Norwalk virus, *Vibrio parahaemolyticus* infection, and *Vibrio vulnificus* infection have also been implicated in shellfish toxicity.

 PREVENTION Shellfish poisoning may be prevented by routine surveillance of shellfish beds, including preventing the consumption of shellfish harvested outside of regulated areas.

COMPLICATIONS

Complications from PSP include respiratory failure and death. Complications from ASP include seizures, coma, hemiparesis, severe cognition dysfunction, and death. Dehydration may occur with all syndromes.

ASSESSMENT FINDINGS

Some symptoms are common among all syndromes, while others are distinct according to the type of toxicity. Signs and symptoms may appear quickly and last a few minutes to several hours after ingestion of contaminated shellfish.

With PSP, symptoms usually present within 30 minutes of ingestion and include paresthesia of the lips, tongue, and gums. Other central nervous system signs may include headache, ataxia, central nerve dysfunction, and a sensation of floating. Muscle weakness and paralysis may occur with signs of respiratory failure. GI symptoms are less common and may include nausea, vomiting, diarrhea, and abdominal pain. Muscle weakness may last for weeks, but symptoms generally subside after 3 days.

Patients with NSP present with symptoms anywhere from 15 minutes to 18 hours after ingesting contaminated shellfish; symptoms generally resolve within 3 days. Similar to PSP, paresthesia of the face, limbs, and trunk can occur, without progression to paralysis. Rectal burning, gastroenteritis, myalgia, vertigo, and hot/cold sensation reversal may also occur. Signs of an upper respiratory tract infection, such as cough, bronchospasm, and rhinorrhea, may occur from aerosolized toxins. Less common signs include bradycardia, tremor, and decreased reflexes.

DSP may last up to 2 days and include GI symptoms of diarrhea, nausea, vomiting, and abdominal pain. ASP is rare and includes GI symptoms along with headache and short-term memory loss.

Patients shellfish poisoning that is caused by a bacterium, such as *V. parahaemolyticus*, may present with watery diarrhea, blood in the stool, nausea, vomiting, and a fever with chills.

Diagnostic tests

▶ Enzyme-linked immunosorbent assay screening identifies saxitoxin, brevetoxin, and domoic acid.
▶ Liquid chromatography identifies saxitoxin and domoic acid.
▶ Antibody radioimmunoassay identifies brevetoxin.
▶ Mass spectrometry can identify domoic acid.
▶ Cultures of stool or blood may identify a bacterial cause of shellfish poisoning.

Treatment

Treatment for shellfish poisoning is supportive according to the presenting signs and symptoms. Respiratory support is crucial in patients with PSP. Although not routinely done, gastric lavage may be performed in patients with shellfish poisoning who present with symptoms within 1 hour of ingestion. Activated charcoal may be given within 4 hours of ingestion. Fluid and electrolyte replacement should be provided as needed. Antibiotics are not usually prescribed unless a specific bacterium is identified. Medications that control diarrhea and vomiting should be avoided as they may decrease intestinal motility and prolong the illness. Bismuth may be given for abdominal pain.

Nursing considerations

▶ Monitor the patient's respiratory status, including pulse oximetry. Initiate emergency measures to maintain an adequate airway and ventilation, if necessary.
▶ Monitor intake and output. To prevent dehydration, encourage oral fluids or, if the patient is unable to drink, administer I.V. fluids.
▶ Monitor laboratory results, and provide electrolyte replacements if indicated.
▶ Provide comfort measures to help decrease abdominal pain. Provide assistance with toileting if needed.

Patient teaching

▶ Teach the patient about the infection, including its cause, diagnosis, and treatment.
▶ Explain all procedures and why they are done. Answer all questions.
▶ Review the signs and symptoms of complications, such as lethargy, thirst, and decreased urine output. Tell the patient to seek medical attention immediately if signs and symptoms of respiratory distress occur.

 PREVENTION Instruct patients to avoid eating raw or undercooked shellfish. If illness occurs after eating shellfish, report it to the state health department. Refer patients to the Food and Drug Administration for more information about illness resulting from shellfish ingestion.

CONTACT PRECAUTIONS

Shigellosis

Shigellosis, also known as bacillary dysentery, is an acute intestinal infection characterized by severe diarrhea and caused by the bacterium *Shigella*, a short, nonmotile, gram-negative rod. *Shigella* can be classified into four groups, all of which may cause shigellosis: group A (*S. dysenteriae*), which is most common in Central America and causes particularly severe infection and septicemia; group B (*S. flexneri*); group C (*S. boydii*); and group D (*S. sonnei*). Typically, shigellosis causes a high fever (especially in children) along with acute, self-limiting diarrhea with tenesmus and, possibly, electrolyte imbalance and dehydration. Shigellosis is most common in children ages 1 to 4; however, many adults acquire the illness from children.

The prognosis is good. Mild infections usually subside within 10 days; severe infections may persist for 2 to 6 weeks. With prompt treatment, shigellosis is fatal in only 1% of cases, although mortality may reach 8% in a severe *S. dysenteriae* epidemic.

CAUSES

Transmission occurs through the fecal-oral route, by direct contact with contaminated objects, or through ingestion of contaminated food or water. Occasionally, the housefly is a vector.

Shigellosis is endemic in North America, Europe, and the tropics. In the United States, about 20,000 to 30,000 cases are reported annually, usually in children or in elderly, debilitated, or malnourished adults. Worldwide, 150 million cases are reported each year. Shigellosis commonly occurs among confined populations, such as in mental institutions and day-care centers.

COMPLICATIONS

Although not common, complications may be fatal in children and in those who are debilitated. Such complications include electrolyte imbalances (especially hypokalemia), metabolic acidosis, and shock. Less common complications include conjunctivitis, iritis, arthritis, rectal prolapse, secondary bacterial infection, acute blood loss from mucosal ulcers, and toxic neuritis.

ASSESSMENT FINDINGS

The patient's history commonly reveals crowded living conditions and family members or close contacts with acute diarrhea. After an incubation period of 12 hours to 2 weeks (3 days is the average), *Shigella* organisms invade the intestinal mucosa and cause inflammation. In children, shigellosis usually produces a high fever, diarrhea with tenesmus, nausea, vomiting, irritability, drowsiness, and abdominal pain and distention. Within a few days, the child's stool may contain pus, mucus, and—from the superficial intestinal ulceration typical of this infection—blood. Without treatment, dehydration and weight loss are rapid and overwhelming.

In adults, shigellosis produces sporadic, intense abdominal pain, which may be relieved at first by passing formed stools. Eventually, however, it causes rectal irritability, tenesmus and, in severe infection, headache and prostration. Stools may contain pus, mucus, and blood. Fever may be present.

Inspection will reveal a patient in considerable discomfort, with signs of dehydration—dry mucous membranes, poor skin turgor, and decreased urine output. Central venous pressure and blood pressure may be below normal, and the pulse may be rapid and thready. Auscultation may detect hyperactive bowel sounds. Palpation may elicit abdominal tenderness, especially over the abdominal quadrants, with accompanying distention.

DIAGNOSTIC TESTS

▌ Microscopic examination of a fresh stool specimen may reveal mucus, red blood cells, and polymorphonuclear leukocytes.
▌ Direct immunofluorescence with specific antisera will demonstrate *Shigella*. Severe infection increases hemagglutinating antibodies.

▶ Sigmoidoscopy or proctoscopy may reveal typical superficial ulcerations.

▶ Stool cultures must rule out other causes of diarrhea, such as enteropathogenic *Escherichia coli* infection, malabsorption diseases, and amebic or viral diseases.

TREATMENT

Treatment of shigellosis includes enteric precautions, a low-residue diet and, most important, replacement of fluids and electrolytes with I.V. infusions of normal saline solution in sufficient quantities to maintain a urine output of 40 to 50 ml/hour. Antibiotics are of questionable value but may be used in an attempt to eliminate the pathogen and thereby prevent further spread. Ampicillin or ceftriaxone (Rocephin) may be useful in severe cases, especially in children with overwhelming fluid and electrolyte loss. Trimethoprim-sulfamethoxazole (Bactrim) and ciprofloxacin (Cipro) are also used.

Antidiarrheals that slow intestinal motility are contraindicated in shigellosis because they delay fecal excretion of *Shigella* and prolong fever and diarrhea. An investigational vaccine containing attenuated strains of *Shigella* appears promising in preventing shigellosis.

NURSING CONSIDERATIONS

▶ To prevent dehydration, administer I.V. fluids as ordered. Measure intake and output (including stools) carefully.

▶ Correct identification of *Shigella* requires examination and culture of fresh stool specimens. Therefore, hand-carry specimens directly to the laboratory. If shigellosis is suspected, include this information on the laboratory slip.

▶ Use a disposable warming pad to relieve abdominal discomfort, and schedule care to conserve patient strength.

 SAFETY To help prevent the spread of this disease, maintain contact precautions until microscopic bacteriologic studies confirm that the stool specimen is negative. Contact precautions are also necessary for diapered or incontinent patients for the duration of illness and to control institutional outbreaks. Keep the patient's (and your own) nails short to avoid harboring organisms. Change soiled linens promptly, and store them in an isolation container.

▶ During shigellosis outbreaks, obtain stool specimens from all potentially infected staff, and instruct infected employees to remain away from work until two stool specimens are negative for *Shigella*.

▶ Report cases of shigellosis to the local health department.

Patient teaching

▶ Teach the patient and family about the illness, including its cause, diagnostic testing, and treatment.

 SAFETY Explain preventive measures, including proper handwashing technique and basic hygiene practices. Stress the need to isolate the linens and any soiled clothing of an infected person.

Sinusitis

Infection and inflammation of the paranasal sinuses may be acute, subacute, chronic, allergic, or hyperplastic. Acute sinusitis usually results from the common cold and can occur in patients of all ages; in about 10% of patients, it lingers in subacute form. Chronic sinusitis follows persistent bacterial infection, usually occurring when a cold spreads to the sinuses.

Allergic sinusitis accompanies allergic rhinitis. Hyperplastic sinusitis is a combination of purulent acute sinusitis and allergic sinusitis or rhinitis. For all types, the prognosis is good.

CAUSES

Sinusitis usually results from a bacterial infection (*Streptococcus pneumoniae*, *Haemophilus influenzae*, anaerobes) or, less frequently, from a viral infection. Viral sinusitis usually follows an upper respiratory infection in which the virus penetrates the normal mucous membrane, decreasing ciliary transport.

Fungal sinusitis is uncommon and found more often in immunocompromised patients. The most common types are aspergillosis, mucormycosis, candidiasis, histoplasmosis, and coccidioidomycosis. The spores causing these infections are usually found in soil and enter through the respiratory tract.

Acute sinusitis is caused most commonly by *H. influenzae*, *Staphylococcus aureus*, *S. pneumoniae*, and *Streptococcus pyogenes*. Predisposing factors include any condition that interferes with sinus drainage and ventilation, such as chronic nasal edema, a deviated septum, and viscous mucus. Bacterial invasion also may result from swimming in contaminated water. Generalized debilitating conditions, including chemotherapy, malnutrition, diabetes, blood dyscrasias, long-term steroids, and immunodeficiency, may also predispose an individual to sinusitis.

COMPLICATIONS

Complications—typically resulting from inadequate therapy during the acute phase or from a delay in treatment—may include meningitis, cavernous sinus thrombosis syndrome, bacteremia or septicemia, brain abscess, frontal lobe abscess, osteomyelitis, mucocele, and orbital cellulitis or abscess.

ASSESSMENT FINDINGS

A patient with acute sinusitis typically complains of nasal congestion that preceded a gradual buildup of pressure in the affected sinus. There may also be nasal discharge for 24 to 48 hours after onset that later becomes purulent. A sore throat, localized headache, and general feeling of malaise may also occur.

The patient may point to pain specific to the affected sinus: in the cheeks and upper teeth (maxillary sinusitis); over the eyes (ethmoid sinusitis); over the eyebrows (frontal sinusitis); or behind the eyes, over the occiput, or at the top of the head (sphenoid sinusitis, a rare condition).

The patient also may report purulent nasal drainage that continues more than 3 weeks after an acute infection subsides; this usually suggests subacute sinusitis. The patient with chronic sinusitis may report continuous mucopurulent discharge. In the acute form, the patient may complain of a stuffy nose, vague facial discomfort, edematous nasal mucosa, fatigue, and a nonproductive cough. Assessment of vital signs may reveal a low-grade fever of 99° to 99.5° F (37.2° to 37.5° C).

The areas over the sinuses may appear swollen (as a result of bacterial growth on diseased tissue in hyperplastic sinusitis). Inspection also may reveal enlarged turbinates and thickening of the mucosal lining and mucosal polyps (hyperplastic sinusitis). Palpation may cause pain and pressure over the affected sinus areas. Transillumination may expose diminished areas of light, which indicate areas of purulent drainage that prevent the passage of light.

DIAGNOSTIC TESTS

▶ Sinus radiographs reveal cloudiness in the affected sinus, air-fluid levels, or a thickened mucosal lining.

▶ Ultrasonography and computed tomography may uncover suspected complications or recurrent, chronic, or unresolved sinusitis.

▶ Antral puncture, in addition to promoting drainage of purulent material, may be used to collect a specimen for culture and sensitivity identification of the infecting organism, but this test is rarely performed.

▶ Sinus endoscopy reveals purulent nasal drainage, nasal edema, and ostial obstruction.

TREATMENT

Antibiotics are the primary treatment for acute and subacute sinusitis. An analgesic may be prescribed to relieve pain. Other appropriate measures include a vasoconstrictor, such as epinephrine or phenylephrine, to decrease nasal secretions. Steam inhalation also promotes vasoconstriction and encourages drainage.

Antibiotic therapy—usually with amoxicillin (Amoxil) or ampicillin—combats persistent infection. Local heat application may help to relieve pain and congestion.

Treatment of allergic sinusitis must include treatment of allergic rhinitis: administration of an antihistamine, identification of allergens by skin testing, and desensitization by immunotherapy. Severe allergic symptoms may require treatment with a corticosteroid and epinephrine.

In both patients with chronic sinusitis and in those with hyperplastic sinusitis, an antibiotic and a steroid nasal spray may relieve pain and congestion.

If a subacute infection persists, the maxillary sinus may be irrigated. If irrigating techniques fail to relieve symptoms, one or more sinuses may require surgery.

NURSING CONSIDERATIONS

▶ To relieve pain and promote drainage, apply warm compresses continuously or four times daily at 2-hour intervals. Encourage oral fluids.

▶ After surgery, monitor the patient for excessive drainage or bleeding. Frequently change the drip pad, recording the consistency, amount, and color of drainage (expect scant, bright red drainage with some clots).

Patient teaching

▶ Inform the patient about prescribed medications, including their intended effects, dosage, and potential adverse reactions. Tell the patient to complete the full course of therapy for the prescribed antibiotic, even if symptoms subside.

▶ Reinforce the patient's understanding of sinusitis, review signs and symptoms of complications, and emphasize the importance of medical follow-up.

▶ Discuss proper disposal of tissues and review handwashing technique to prevent the spread of infection.

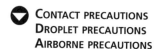

CONTACT PRECAUTIONS
DROPLET PRECAUTIONS
AIRBORNE PRECAUTIONS

Smallpox

Smallpox, also known as variola, is an acute, highly contagious infectious disease caused by the poxvirus variola. After a global eradication program, the World Health Organization pronounced smallpox eradicated on October 26, 1979, 2 years after the last naturally occurring case was reported in Somalia. Vaccination is no longer recommended, except for certain laboratory workers. The last known case in the United States was reported in 1949. Although naturally occurring smallpox has been eradicated, variola virus preserved in laboratories remains an unlikely source of infection. In response to bioterrorism concerns, smallpox vaccination was offered to members of the military, health department officials, first responders, and key health care providers. If a bioterrorism event involving smallpox is suspected or occurs, vaccination programs can be initiated.

Naturally occurring smallpox exists in two major forms: variola major (classic smallpox) and variola minor. Variola major is classified into four types—ordinary (accounts for 90% of cases), modified (a mild variant of smallpox that occurs in previously vaccinated people who have only partial immunity), flat, and hemorrhagic; the flat and hemorrhagic forms of variola are both rare and usually fatal. Variola minor is a mild form of smallpox that occurs in nonvaccinated people and results from a less virulent strain.

Smallpox can affect people of all ages. In the past, the incidence was highest during the winter months in temperate zones; in the tropics, it occurred primarily during the hot, dry months.

CAUSES

Smallpox is transmitted either directly, by respiratory droplets or dried scales of virus-containing lesions, or indirectly, through contact with contaminated linens or other objects. Variola major is contagious from onset until after the last scab is shed.

COMPLICATIONS

Complications of smallpox may include arthritis, encephalitis, blindness, and respiratory problems, such as pneumonia, bronchitis, and pneumonitis. Death may occur. Healed smallpox lesions may cause permanent scarring.

ASSESSMENT FINDINGS

After an incubation period of 7 to 14 days, smallpox characteristically causes an abrupt onset of chills (and possible seizures in children), high fever (above 104° F [40° C]), headache, backache, severe malaise, vomiting (especially in children), marked prostration and, occasionally, violent delirium, stupor, or coma. Symptoms become more severe 2 days after onset, but by the third day the patient begins to feel better.

A few days after onset of the initial signs and symptoms, a sore throat and cough develop as well as lesions on the mucous membranes of the mouth, throat, and respiratory tract. These lesions break open and spread the virus further. Smallpox is most contagious during this phase, which lasts about 4 days. A few days later, lesions also appear on the skin, first on the face, hands, and forearms and later on the torso. Usually most noticeable on the palms of the hands and soles of the feet, the lesions progress from macular to papular, vesicular, and pustular (pustules can be as large as 8.5 mm in diameter). During the pustular stage, the patient's temperature rises, and early symptoms return. By day 10, the pustules begin to rupture and eventually dry and form scabs. Symptoms finally subside about 14 days after onset. Desquamation of the scabs takes another 1 to 2 weeks; desquamation may cause intense pruritus and commonly leaves permanently disfiguring scars. The patient is considered contagious until all the scabs have fallen off.

Smallpox is fatal in about 30% of cases. In these patients, a diffuse dusky appearance comes over the face and upper chest. Death results from encephalitic manifestations, from extensive bleeding from any or all body orifices, or from secondary bacterial infections.

DIAGNOSTIC TESTS

▶ Culture of vesicles and pustules isolates variola virus.

▶ Other laboratory tests include microscopic examination of smears from lesion scrapings and complement fixation to detect virus or antibodies to the virus in the patient's blood.

TREATMENT

Treatment for smallpox requires hospitalization with airborne, droplet, and contact precautions; antimicrobial therapy to treat bacterial complications; vigorous supportive measures; and symptomatic treatment of lesions with antipruritics, starting during the pustular stage. If the smallpox vaccination is given within 1 to 4 days of exposure to the disease, it may lessen symptoms or prevent illness altogether. Once the disease has started, treatment is limited. The drug cidofovir is being studied for use in smallpox infection.

 PREVENTION In the case of a bioterrorism attack with smallpox, the Centers for Disease Control and Prevention currently has a stockpile of smallpox vaccine— enough to vaccinate every person in the United States.

NURSING CONSIDERATIONS

▶ Nonvaccinated health care workers should not provide care when immune health care workers are available; vaccination administered within 4 days of exposure may be protective.

◗ Initiate strict contact, droplet, and airborne precautions. N95 or higher respiratory protection should be worn by both susceptible and successfully vaccinated individuals. Place the patient in a negative airflow room, and limit visitors as much as possible.

▶ Give aspirin, codeine, or (as needed) morphine to relieve pain.

▶ Because pharyngeal lesions make swallowing difficult, administer I.V. infusions and gastric tube feedings to provide fluids, electrolytes, and calories.

▶ Monitor vital signs, intake and output, and pulse oximetry. Assess for signs and symptoms of complications.

▶ If smallpox is suspected, the state health department should be notified immediately.

▶ Encourage the patient to verbalize fears and concerns about the disease, and provide emotional support.

Patient teaching

▶ Provide information about the disease, including its cause, means of transmission, diagnostic tests, and treatment.

▶ Review all prescribed medication, including dosage, administration, and possible adverse effects.

 PREVENTION Refer those who are in direct contact with an infected person for pre-exposure and post-exposure vaccination if more than 3 years have passed since their last vaccination or if they have never been vaccinated.

Southern tick-associated rash illness

Southern tick-associated rash illness (STARI), also known as Masters disease, is a newly recognized tickborne disease that produces a rash similar to that caused by Lyme disease. STARI is associated with the bite of the lone star tick, *Amblyomma americanum*, which is found in the south-central and southeast United States, including Texas and Oklahoma, and along the Atlantic coastline, all the way to Maine.

CAUSES

Deoxyribonucleic acid analysis of the spirochetes found in the *A. americanum* tick has indicated that these ticks differ from *Borrelia burgdorferi*—the agent of Lyme disease. *A. americanum* ticks have three life stages, all of which have been found to aggressively bite people. (See *The lone star tick*.)

COMPLICATIONS

There are no known complications of STARI.

ASSESSMENT FINDINGS

Patients may present with some symptoms similar to those of Lyme disease, such as an expanding red rash with central clearing, similar to a "bull's-eye," that usually appears within 7 days of the tick bite. It may have a diameter of 3″ (8 cm) or larger. Mild illness, characterized by such signs and symptoms as fatigue, headache, joint and muscle pain, stiff neck and, occasionally, fever, may accompany the rash.

DIAGNOSTIC TESTS

▸ Although there are no current specific diagnostic tests for STARI, the illness is strongly suspected if diagnostic tests rule out Lyme disease, if the patient lives in or has travelled

The lone star tick

The lone star tick gets its name from the star or dot on its back. The rash of STARI, similar to the rash that accompanies Lyme disease, is a red "bulls-eye" lesion that develops within 7 days around the site of a lone star tick bite and can cover an area 3″ (8 cm) in diameter or larger. The rash may be confused with much smaller areas of redness and discomfort that can occur commonly at tick bite sites. Unlike Lyme disease, STARI has not been linked to any arthritic, neurologic, or chronic symptoms. The rash and accompanying symptoms respond well to oral antibiotics.

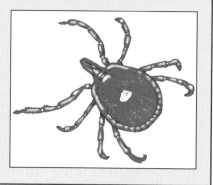

to an area where the tick is commonly found, or if a known lone star tick bite has been reported or the patient has participated in activities that may have resulted in exposure to ticks.

TREATMENT

No recommendations currently exist for treating STARI, but the rash and other accompanying signs and symptoms usually resolve with doxycycline therapy. The Centers for Disease Control and Prevention (CDC) does not recommend treatment of a patient who presents after a tick bite without accompanying symptoms. In order to learn more about the illness, the CDC wishes to study STARI patients more closely under an Institutional Review Board–approved investigational protocol. Other treatment would be symptomatic, such as wound care and administration of analgesics (ibuprofen or acetaminophen) for muscle aches or fever.

Nursing considerations

▶ If the tick is still present, remove it appropriately. Place the tick in a container in order to identify it, if able.
▶ Administer analgesics or antipyretics, as ordered, for muscle pain or fever, and evaluate the response.

Patient teaching

▶ Teach the patient about the illness, including its cause, diagnosis, and treatment.
▶ Review any prescribed medication, including dosage, administration, and possible adverse effects. Stress the importance of completing the prescribed antibiotics, as ordered, even if symptoms subside.
▶ Instruct the patient to report any recurring symptoms to the physician at once so that treatment measures may resume immediately.
▶ Offer printed and illustrated instructions, if available, to teach the patient and family or other caregivers how to correctly and safely remove a tick. Demonstrate how to use fine-pointed tweezers or forceps and apply steady traction to release the entire tick, including the mouth parts, from the skin. The tick should be removed as close as possible to where its mouth parts are attached to the skin.
  - Tell the patient not to place petroleum jelly, a hot match, nail polish, or alcohol on the tick to aid removal.
  - Caution the patient not to handle the tick or its fragments after removal but rather to kill the tick by placing it in a vial filled with alcohol.
  - Instruct the patient to clean the skin with alcohol at the point of attachment.

 PREVENTION To prevent STARI, advise the patient to avoid tick-infested areas (woods, meadows, streams, and canyons) if possible. Teach the patient ways to reduce the risk of becoming infected with a tick bite:
- Encourage inspection of the entire body (including the scalp) every 3 to 4 hours while outdoors.
- Remind the patient to wear protective clothing, such as a long-sleeved shirt, pants securely tucked into laced boots, and a protective head covering such as a cap.
- Advise the patient to apply insect repellant to exposed skin as well as to clothing.
- Advise the patient to avoid sitting on stone walls or directly on the ground because ticks may hide on or around ground cover, lawns, gardens, and stone walls.
- Advise the patient to travel on cleared paths as much as possible when hiking.

CONTACT PRECAUTIONS

Staphylococcal scalded skin syndrome

Staphylococcal scalded skin syndrome (SSSS) is a severe skin disorder marked by epidermal erythema, peeling, and necrosis that give the skin a scalded appearance. This disorder is most prevalent in infants ages 1 to 3 months but may develop in children younger than age 5 years; it is uncommon in adults. It follows a consistent pattern of progression, and most children recover fully; however, the mortality rate for adults with SSSS secondary to toxigenic *Staphylococcus aureus* in the blood is more than 60%. SSSS affects males more than females.

CAUSES

S. aureus phage group 2 (types 3A, 3B, 3C, 55, or 71) is the causative organism of SSSS. This penicillinase-producing organism releases exotoxins (epidermolytic toxins A and B) that are widely disseminated from a systemic site into the lower layers of the skin. Transmission usually occurs from an asymptomatic carrier.

Predisposing factors may include impaired immunity and renal insufficiency, which are present to some extent in the normal neonate because of immature development of these systems. Rarely, this disorder may affect adults undergoing immunosuppressant therapy.

COMPLICATIONS

SSSS causes death in 2% to 3% of affected children as a result of complications of fluid and electrolyte loss, sepsis, and involvement of other body systems. Septicemia and secondary infections from *Candida* species and gram-negative bacteria may also occur. Cellulitis, sepsis, and pneumonia may result from SSSS.

ASSESSMENT FINDINGS

The patient history includes a prodromal upper respiratory tract infection, possibly with concomitant purulent conjunctivitis, or otitis media. Usually, the patient appears profoundly ill. Inspection reveals characteristic lesions. Exfoliation may appear within 24 to 48 hours of onset. Assessment of vital signs typically reveals a fever. Palpation may reveal tenderness over the lesions.

Visible cutaneous changes progress through the following three stages:
▶ Erythema: Erythema becomes visible usually around the mouth and other orifices; it may spread in widening circles over the entire body surface.
▶ Exfoliation (24 to 48 hours later): With the more common, localized form of the disease, superficial erosions and minimal crusting occur, usually around body orifices, and may spread to exposed skin areas. With the more severe form of SSSS, large, flaccid bullae erupt and may spread to cover extensive body areas. When they rupture, these bullae expose sections of tender, oozing, denuded skin. Intact lesions may not be found because the bullae are fragile; only the erosions may be visible. At first, the patient with this disorder may appear to be sunburned or to have scarlet fever, but inspection of the mouth shows the lack the oral lesions characteristic of scarlet fever.
▶ Desquamation: In this final stage, affected areas dry up and powdery scales form. Sheets of epidermis shed, and the skin appears reddish in 5 to 7 days. Residual scarring is rare.

During the initial disease stages, palpation of the affected areas results in Nikolsky sign (sloughing of the skin when friction is applied). Bullae are so fragile that minimal palpation produces tender, red, moist areas.

DIAGNOSTIC TESTS

▶ Diagnosis requires careful observation of the three-stage progression of this disease as well as exfoliative cytology and biopsy, which aid in the differential diagnosis by ruling out erythema multiforme and drug-induced toxic epidermal necrolysis, both of which are similar in appearance to SSSS.

❱ Isolation of group 2 *S. aureus* on cultures of skin lesions confirms the diagnosis; however, skin lesions sometimes appear sterile.

❱ Blood cultures may be used to recover some causative organisms in patients who are very ill. If this disorder occurs in a nursery setting, cultures from the nose, throat, and skin breaks of nursing personnel can be used to identify potential carriers of the organism.

TREATMENT

Treatment of SSSS includes a systemic antibiotic to treat the originating infection. Cloxacillin (a penicillinase-resistant anti-staphylococcal antibiotic) is the drug of choice and is used to prevent secondary infection. In severe cases, fluid and electrolyte replacement measures are also instituted to maintain fluid and electrolyte balance.

 PREVENTION In neonatal intensive care units, identification and treatment of infected nursing personnel is important. Strict handwashing using chlorhexidine, use of barrier protection, and application of mupirocin ointment to nasal passages (with persistent infection) will help prevent SSSS in the neonates they are caring for.

NURSING CONSIDERATIONS

◔ Observe contact precautions with any patient in whom SSSS is suspected.

❱ Consider health care workers as a potential source of nursery or neonatal intensive care unit outbreaks.

❱ Provide special care for the neonate with SSSS, including placement in an isolette to maintain body temperature and provide isolation.

❱ Monitor intake and output carefully, and assess for fluid and electrolyte balance. In severe cases, provide I.V. fluid and electrolyte replacement as ordered.

❱ Check vital signs per your facility's policy. Be especially alert for a sudden rise in temperature, indicating sepsis, which requires prompt, aggressive treatment.

❱ Maintain skin integrity. Use strict aseptic technique to preclude secondary infection, especially during the exfoliation stage (because of open lesions). To prevent friction and sloughing of the skin, leave affected areas uncovered or loosely covered. Place cotton between severely affected fingers and toes to prevent webbing.

❱ Administer warm baths and soaks during the recovery period. Gently debride exfoliated areas.

Patient teaching

❱ Reassure parents that complications are rare and residual scars are unlikely.

❱ Instruct parents to use meticulous handwashing and aseptic techniques when changing the patient's dressings and providing comfort measures, such as warm soaks and baths.

❱ Stress the importance of avoiding friction on the skin surface during the exfoliation stage and picking or rubbing scales during the desquamation stage.

❱ Instruct the parents to contact the physician if adverse reactions to antibiotic therapy occur. Explain the importance of completing the prescribed course of antibiotic therapy, even after the lesions appear to have healed.

Strongyloidiasis

Strongyloidiasis, also called threadworm infection, is a parasitic intestinal infection caused by the helminth *Strongyloides stercoralis*. This worldwide infection is endemic in the tropics and subtropics as well as in areas associated with poor hygiene. Susceptibility to strongyloidiasis is universal. Infection doesn't confer immunity, and people who are immunocompromised may suffer overwhelming disseminated infection. Because the threadworm's reproductive cycle may continue in the untreated host for up to 45 years, autoinfection is highly probable. Most patients with strongyloidiasis recover, but debilitation from protein loss may result in death.

CAUSES

Transmission to humans usually occurs through contact with soil that contains infective *S. stercoralis* filariform larvae; such larvae develop from noninfective rhabdoid (rod-shaped) larvae in human feces. The filariform larvae penetrate the human skin, usually at the feet. They migrate by way of the lymphatic system to the bloodstream and lungs. Once they enter the pulmonary circulation, the filariform larvae break through the alveoli and migrate upward to the pharynx, where they are swallowed. They then lodge in the small intestine, where they deposit eggs that mature into noninfectious rhabdoid larvae. Next, the rhabdoid larvae migrate into the large intestine and are excreted in feces, starting the cycle again. The threadworm life cycle, from penetration of the skin by filariform larvae to the excretion of rhabdoid larvae, takes 17 days.

In autoinfection, rhabdoid larvae mature within the intestine to become infective filariform larvae.

COMPLICATIONS

If autoinfection is severe (disseminated strongyloidiasis), malnutrition from substantial fat and protein loss, anemia, and lesions resembling ulcerative colitis may result in secondary bacterial infection. Ulcerated intestinal mucosa may lead to perforation. Potentially fatal septicemia and massive invasion of organs can occur. These effects of autoinfection are most likely to develop in immunocompromised patients. (See *Signs of disseminated strongyloidiasis*.)

ASSESSMENT FINDINGS

The patient's resistance and the extent of infection determine the severity of symptoms. Some patients have no symptoms, but many develop an erythematous maculopapular rash at the site of penetration that produces swelling and pruritus that may be confused with an insect bite. As the larvae migrate to the lungs, pulmonary signs develop, including minor hemorrhage, pneumonitis, and pneumonia; later, intestinal infection produces frequent, watery, bloody diarrhea accompanied by intermittent abdominal pain.

DIAGNOSTIC TESTS

▶ Diagnosis requires observation of *S. stercoralis* larvae in a fresh stool specimen (2 hours after excretion); rhabdoid larvae resemble hookworm larvae.
▶ Duodenal aspiration shows larvae in duodenal fluid, and antigen testing is positive for *S. stercoralis*.
▶ During the pulmonary phase, sputum shows *S. stercoralis*; marked eosinophilia also occurs in disseminated strongyloidiasis.

TREATMENT

The goal of treatment is to eliminate the larvae with an anthelmintic, such as ivermectin (Stromectol) or thiabendazole. Patients may need protein replacement, blood transfusions, and I.V. fluid replacement. Re-treatment is necessary if *S. stercoralis* remains in the stool after therapy.

NURSING CONSIDERATIONS

▶ Strict infection prevention measures must be enforced when caring for patients with hyperinfection syndrome due to the

Signs of disseminated strongyloidiasis

Disseminated strongyloidiasis is a potentially fatal disease that occurs in immunocompromised patients—such as those with lymphoma, leukemia, lepromatous leprosy, or human immunodeficiency virus infection—and in those taking corticosteroids.

If your patient is at risk for this disorder, be alert for severe generalized abdominal pain, diffuse pulmonary infiltrates, pericarditis, myocarditis, herpetic granulomas, cholecystitis, ileus, shock, and signs of meningitis or sepsis from gram-negative bacilli. (Note that diagnostic tests may not show eosinophilia.)

▶ Review the need for a nutritious diet that contains adequate amounts of protein.
▶ Emphasize the need for follow-up stool examination, continuing for several weeks after treatment.

PREVENTION To prevent re-infection, teach the patient proper handwashing technique. Stress the importance of proper hand hygiene before eating and after defecating, and instruct the patient to wear shoes when in endemic areas.

presence of infectious filariform larvae in the stool, saliva, emesis, and body fluids. Use standard precautions when handling bedpans or giving perineal care, and dispose of feces promptly.
▶ Keep accurate intake and output records. Ask the dietary department to provide a high-protein diet. The patient may need tube feedings to increase caloric intake.
▶ Because direct person-to-person transmission doesn't occur, contact precautions are not required.
▶ In pulmonary infection, reposition the patient frequently, encourage coughing and deep breathing, and administer oxygen as ordered.
▶ Check the patient's family and close contacts for signs of infection.

Patient teaching
▶ Teach the patient about the infection, including its cause, diagnosis, and treatment.
▶ Review all prescribed medication, including dosage, administration, and possible adverse effects.
▶ Discuss signs and symptoms of possible complications and when to contact the physician.

Subacute sclerosing panencephalitis

Classified as a persistent immune-resistant form of rubeola (measles), subacute sclerosing panencephalitis (SSPE) is a rare infection that results from a defective variant of rubeola that was generated during the acute phase of disease. The SSPE virus is slow-growing and causes cytopathologic effects in neurons; symptoms occur many years after acute disease. SSPE is a chronic illness that causes progressive encephalitis, mainly in children and young adults. Approximately 1 in every 100,000 people infected with rubeola develops SSPE. The illness consists of two stages; if SSPE reaches stage 2, it is fatal. SSPE is also known as Dawson disease, Dawson encephalitis, and measles encephalitis.

CAUSES

SSPE is caused by the rubeola virus, a member of the genus *Morbillivirus* in the Paramyxoviridae family. The highly contagious rubeola virus is transmitted by respiratory droplets. Although the incidence of rubeola declined vastly following the introduction of the rubeola vaccine, the vaccine is not available in all areas of the world. Therefore, the disease still affects approximately 30 million people annually, with the highest percentage of cases occurring in Africa. Fewer than 10 cases of SSPE are reported each year in the United States. SSPE seems to affect males more than females with a ratio of 3:1.

 PREVENTION Administration of the rubeola (measles) vaccine to prevent the development not only of rubeola but also of SSPE.

COMPLICATIONS

SSPE causes psychoneurological problems, with death resulting from heart failure or autonomic nervous system failure within 3 months to 3 years if treatment is not provided.

ASSESSMENT FINDINGS

The patient's history will reveal infection with rubeola early in life, usually before age 2. After the initial infection, the patient may appear to have recovered and be without symptoms for possibly 6 to 8 years. During stage 1, the patient will begin to display erratic, abnormal behavior, such as ataxia and myoclonic jerks of the head, trunk, or extremities. Personality changes, such as irritability, memory loss, and intellectual problems then ensue. If left untreated, more severe neurologic problems develop. Muscle spasms become so severe that normal daily activities and walking become difficult. Seizures may be noted, along with ocular abnormalities and photosensitivity. As the patient advances into stage 2, speech becomes impaired and comprehension declines. Blindness may occur, along with muteness. Finally, the patient may slip into a coma before death occurs.

DIAGNOSTIC TESTS

▶ Cerebrospinal fluid is normal, showing only an elevation in immunoglobulin.
▶ Rubeola immunoglobulin G antibody titers are elevated.
▶ Electroencephalography shows characteristic periodic activity (Radermecker complex) with cortical dysfunction.

TREATMENT

There is no cure for SSPE; with lifelong medication, however, the patient may remain in remission with no symptom recurrence. For treatment to be effective it needs to be initiated during stage 1; therefore, early diagnosis is crucial. Medication includes combination therapy with interferon alpha (given intrathecally or intraventricularly) and antiviral medication, such as ribavirin (Copegus) or isoprinosine. For patients who progress to stage 2, anticonvulsants and antispasmodics may be given along with palliative, supportive care, such as tube feedings and safety measures.

The rate of progression of the illness is different for each patient, although the signs and symptoms that develop are predictable. During either stage, treatment with interferon and an antiviral medication can cause a 50% improvement rate. The National Institute of Neurological Disorders and Stroke is currently conducting and supporting research related to the treatment and cure of SSPE.

Nursing considerations

▶ SSPE is not transmitted from person to person; therefore, standard precautions are adequate.
▶ Administer medication as ordered. Provide anticonvulsants and antispasmodics for patients with progressive disease.
▶ Institute seizure precautions and provide safety measures to prevent patient injury caused by spastic movements.
▶ Assist the patient with activities of daily living as needed, based on the severity of myoclonus and spasticity.
▶ Provide passive range-of-motion exercise as indicated by the level of decline.
▶ Reposition the patient every 2 hours to prevent skin breakdown.
▶ Administer tube feedings as ordered, and assess nutritional status regularly. Record daily weight.
▶ Assess neurologic status, and note any deterioration in mental function. If the patient has visual disturbances or blindness, be sure to place items close to the patient and let him or her know where the items are located.
▶ Provide emotional support to the patient and family, especially if the patient deteriorates into a coma or vegetative state.
▶ Provide information regarding long-term, home health, or hospice care, as appropriate for the patient's condition or stage of illness. Refer the patient and family to social services for assistance as needed.

Patient teaching

▶ Teach the patient and family about the disease, including its cause, diagnosis, and treatment. Be sure to answer all questions. If SSPE is diagnosed late in stage 1 or has progressed to stage 2, be sure to explain the prognosis as well as the supportive care that will be provided.
▶ Discuss end of life care, if appropriate and if the family is open to the discussion.
▶ Review all prescribed medication, including dosage, administration, and possible adverse effects. Tell the patient and family that lifelong medication will be required.
▶ Describe safety measures to prevent injury, especially for the patient with pronounced muscle spasticity.

Syphilis

Syphilis is a chronic, infectious, sexually transmitted infection (STI) that begins in the mucous membranes and quickly becomes systemic, spreading to nearby lymph nodes and the bloodstream. Untreated syphilis progresses in four stages: primary, secondary, latent, and late (formerly called tertiary).

The incidence of syphilis in the United States is highest in people between ages 15 and 39, in drug users, and in those infected with human immunodeficiency virus (HIV). Untreated syphilis can lead to crippling or death. With early treatment, however, the prognosis is excellent. The incubation period varies but typically lasts about 3 weeks.

CAUSES

The spirochete *Treponema pallidum* causes syphilis. Transmission occurs primarily through sexual contact during the primary, secondary, and early latent stages of infection. Prenatal transmission is also possible.

COMPLICATIONS

Aortic regurgitation or aneurysm, meningitis, and widespread central nervous system damage can result from advanced syphilis.

ASSESSMENT FINDINGS

The typical patient history points to unprotected sexual contact with an infected person or with multiple or anonymous sexual partners. A patient with primary syphilis may present with one or more chancres (small, fluid-filled lesions) on the genitalia, anus, fingers, lips, tongue, nipples, tonsils, or eyelids. In female patients, chancres may develop on the cervix or vaginal wall. These usually painless lesions start as papules and then erode. They have indurated, raised edges and clear bases and typically heal after 3 to 6 weeks, even when untreated. In the primary stage, palpation may reveal enlarged unilateral or bilateral regional lymph nodes (adenopathy).

In secondary syphilis (beginning within a few days or up to 8 weeks after the initial chancres appear), the patient may complain of headache, nausea, vomiting, malaise, anorexia, weight loss, sore throat, and a slight fever.

Inspection may reveal symmetrical mucocutaneous lesions. The rash of secondary syphilis may appear macular, papular, pustular, or nodular. Lesions are uniform, well defined, and generalized. Macules typically erupt between rolls of fat on the trunk and proximally on the arms, palms, soles, face, and scalp. In warm, moist body areas the lesions enlarge and erode, producing highly contagious, pink or grayish white lesions (condylomata lata).

Alopecia, which is usually temporary, may occur with or without treatment. The patient may also complain of brittle, pitted nails. Palpation may disclose generalized lymphadenopathy.

In latent syphilis, physical signs and symptoms are absent except for the possible recurrence of mucocutaneous lesions that resemble those of secondary syphilis. In late syphilis, the patient's complaints vary with the involved organ. Late syphilis has three subtypes: neurosyphilis, late benign syphilis, and cardiovascular syphilis.

If neurosyphilis affects meningovascular tissue, the patient may report headache, vertigo, insomnia, hemiplegia, seizures, and psychological difficulties. If it affects parenchymal tissue, the patient may report paresis, alteration in intellect, paranoia, illusions, and hallucinations. Inspection may reveal Argyll Robertson pupil (a small, irregular pupil that's nonreactive to light but accommodates for vision), ataxia, slurred speech, trophic joint changes, positive Romberg sign, and facial tremor. A patient with late benign syphilis may complain of gummas—lesions that develop between 1 and 10 years after infection. A single gumma may be a chronic, superficial nodule or a deep, granulomatous lesion that's solitary, asymmetrical, painless, indurated, and large or small. Visible on the skin and mucocutaneous tissue, gummas commonly affect bones and can develop in any organ. In cardiovascular syphilis, decreased cardiac output may cause decreased urine output and decreased sensorium related to hypoxia. Auscultation may reveal pulmonary congestion.

DIAGNOSTIC TESTS

▶ Dark-field microscopy identifies *T. pallidum* from lesion exudate and provides an immediate diagnosis.

▶ Nontreponemal serologic tests include the Venereal Disease Research Laboratory (VDRL) slide test, the rapid plasma reagin test, and the automated reagin test. These tests can detect nonspecific antibodies that become reactive within 1 to 2 weeks after the primary syphilis lesion appears or 4 to 5 weeks after the infection begins.

▶ Treponemal serologic studies include the fluorescent treponemal antibody absorption test, the *T. pallidum* hemagglutination assay, and the microhemagglutination assay. These tests detect the specific antitreponemal antibody and can confirm positive screening results.

▶ Cerebrospinal fluid examination identifies neurosyphilis when the total protein level is higher than 40 mg/dl, the VDRL slide test is reactive, and the white blood cell count exceeds 5 mononuclear cells/μl.

TREATMENT

In early syphilis, treatment may consist of a single injection of I.M. penicillin G benzathine. Syphilis lasting longer than 1 year may respond to additional doses of penicillin G benzathine I.M.

Patients who are allergic to penicillin may be treated successfully with tetracycline or erythromycin. Tetracycline is contraindicated during pregnancy.

NURSING CONSIDERATIONS

▶ Follow standard precautions when assessing the patient, collecting specimens, and treating lesions.

▶ Check for a history of drug sensitivity before administering the first dose of medication.

▶ Assess for complications of late syphilis if the patient's infection is older than 1 year. In late syphilis, provide symptomatic care during prolonged treatment.

 SAFETY Report all cases of syphilis to the appropriate health authorities.

Patient teaching

▶ Teach the patient about the prescribed medication, including dosage, administration, and possible adverse effects.

 SAFETY Urge the patient to inform his or her sexual partners about the infection and to encourage them to seek testing and treatment.

▶ Counsel the patient and his or her sexual partners about HIV infection, and recommend HIV testing.

 PREVENTION Inform the patient that using condoms may provide protection against STIs.

Tapeworm infection

Tapeworm infection, also called taeniasis or cestodiasis, is a parasitic infestation by *Taenia saginata* (beef tapeworm), *Taenia solium* (pork tapeworm), *Diphyllobothrium latum* (fish tapeworm), or *Hymenolepis nana* (dwarf tapeworm). Tapeworm is usually a chronic, benign intestinal infection; however, infection with *T. solium*, also called cysticercosis, may cause dangerous systemic and central nervous system symptoms if larvae invade the brain, eyes, or striated muscle of vital organs. A single tapeworm can produce 50,000 eggs in a single day and may live for 25 years. The incidence of tapeworm infection is higher in countries with poor public hygiene.

CAUSES

T. saginata, *T. solium*, and *D. latum* are transmitted to humans through ingestion of beef, pork, or fish, respectively, that contains tapeworm cysts. Gastric acids break down these cysts in the stomach, allowing them to mature. Mature tapeworms attach to the intestinal wall and produce ova that are passed in the feces. *H. nana*, naturally found in beetles and mice, can be transmitted directly from person to person and thus requires no intermediate host. *H. nana* completes its life cycle in the intestine. (See *Common tapeworm infections*.)

COMPLICATIONS

Severe tapeworm infection can lead to dehydration and malnutrition. Intestinal obstruction, obstructed bile or pancreatic ducts, and appendicitis may also occur. Central nervous system complications, such as hydrocephalus, seizures, and stroke, may result from infection with *T. solium*. Some cases may be fatal.

ASSESSMENT FINDINGS

Signs and symptoms vary with the type of infection. Symptoms may be absent or mild, such as nausea, flatulence, hunger, weight loss, diarrhea, and increased appetite. Occasionally, worm segments may exit through the anus and appear on bed clothes. A patient with beef tapeworm may complain of a crawling sensation in the perianal area; and pork tapeworms may cause seizures, headaches, and personality changes. Neurologic symptoms may include hemiparesis and sensory disturbances. If cysticercosis affects the eyes, intraocular larvae may be seen.

DIAGNOSTIC TESTS

▶ Tapeworm ova or body segments can be identified in feces. (Because ova aren't excreted continuously, confirmation may require multiple specimens.)
▶ A supporting dietary or travel history aids confirmation of the diagnosis.

TREATMENT

The drug of choice for tapeworm infection is niclosamide, but praziquantel (Biltricide) and albendazole (Albenza) can also be used. Laxative use and induced vomiting are contraindicated because of the danger of autoinfection and systemic disease. In patients with cysticercosis, a glucocorticosteroid may also be prescribed for its anti-inflammatory effects. Surgery may be required for intestinal obstruction. If ocular cysticercosis occurs, surgery is the treatment of choice.

A follow-up laboratory examination of stool specimens is required following treatment (3 to 5 weeks for *T. solium* and 3 months for *T. saginata*) to check for any remaining ova or worm segments. Persistent infection typically requires a second course of medication.

NURSING CONSIDERATIONS

▶ Obtain a complete history, including recent travel to endemic areas, dietary habits, and physical symptoms.
▶ Follow strict standard precautions: Always wear gloves when giving personal care and when handling fecal excretions, bedpans, and bed linens; wash your hands thoroughly, and tell the patient to do the same. Dispose of the patient's excretions carefully.

Common tapeworm infections

Source of infection	Incidence	Clinical features
D. latum (fish tapeworm): Uncooked or undercooked freshwater fish, such as pike, trout, salmon, and turbot	Highest in cool lake regions where raw and pickled fish consumption is common: Finland, parts o˙ the former Soviet Union, Japan, Alaska, Australia, U.S. Great Lakes region, Switzerland, Chile, and Argentina	Anemia (hemoglobin level as low as 6–8 g/100 dl)
H. nana (dwarf tapeworm): Mice and beetles are intermediate hosts; parasite may pass directly from person to person via ova passed in stool; inadequate handwashing facilitates spread; autoinfection can occur without passing through the intermediate host	Most common tapeworm infection in humans; particularly prevalent among institutionalized mentally retarded children and in underdeveloped countries	Depend on nutritional status of patient and parasite load; commonly no symptoms with mild infection; with severe infection, anorexia, diarrhea, restlessness, dizziness, and apathy
T. saginata (beef tapeworm): Uncooked or undercooked beef	Found worldwide, but most prevalent in Europe and East Africa; most common cestode infection in United States	Crawling sensation in the perianal area caused by worm segments that have been passed rectally; intestinal obstruction and appendicitis due to long worm segments that have twisted in the intestinal lumen
T. solium (pork tapeworm): Uncooked or undercooked pork; in areas where prevalent, directly related to human fecal contamination	Highest in Mexico and Latin America; lowest among Muslims and Jews	Cysticercosis: seizures, headaches, personality changes; commonly overlooked in adults

▶ In order to prevent infecting other patients, pediatric patients require a private room, as do patients who are incontinent.
▶ Administer medication as ordered.

Patient teaching
▶ Teach the patient about the infection, including the cause, diagnosis, and treatment.
▶ Review all prescribed medication with the patient, including dosage, administration, and possible adverse effects.

▶ Stress the need for follow-up evaluations to monitor the success of therapy and to detect possible re-infection.

 PREVENTION To prevent re-infection, teach the patient proper hand hygiene technique. Stress the importance of washing the hands before eating and after defecating and of wearing shoes in endemic areas. Review the need to cook meat and fish thoroughly before eating it.

Tetanus

Tetanus, also known as lockjaw, is an acute exotoxin-mediated infection caused by the anaerobic, spore-forming, gram-positive bacillus *Clostridium tetani*. This infection is usually systemic; less commonly, it is localized. Tetanus is fatal in up to 60% of nonvaccinated people, usually within 10 days of onset. When symptoms develop within 3 days after exposure, the prognosis is poor.

CAUSES

Normally, transmission occurs through a puncture wound that's contaminated by soil, dust, or animal excreta containing *C. tetani* or by way of burns and minor wounds. After *C. tetani* enters the body, it causes local infection and tissue necrosis. It also produces toxins that then enter the bloodstream and lymphatics and eventually spread to central nervous system tissue.

Tetanus occurs worldwide but is more prevalent in agricultural regions and in developing countries that lack mass immunization programs. It's one of the most common causes of neonatal death in developing countries, where infants of nonvaccinated mothers are delivered under nonsterile conditions. In these infants, the unhealed umbilical cord is the portal of entry.

In the United States, about 75% of all tetanus cases occur between April and September.

COMPLICATIONS

Atelectasis, pneumonia, pulmonary emboli, acute gastric ulcers, seizures, flexion contractures, and cardiac arrhythmias can result from tetanus.

ASSESSMENT FINDINGS

The incubation period ranges from 3 to 4 weeks in mild tetanus to less than 2 days in severe tetanus. Death is more likely when symptoms occur within 3 days following injury. If tetanus remains localized, signs of onset are spasm and increased muscle tone near the wound. Indications of generalized (systemic) tetanus include marked muscle hypertonicity, hyperactive deep tendon reflexes, tachycardia, profuse sweating, low-grade fever, and painful, involuntary muscle contractions:

▶ Neck and facial muscles, especially cheek muscles: Lockjaw (trismus), painful spasms of masticatory muscles, difficulty opening the mouth, and risus sardonicus, a grotesque, grinning expression produced by spasm of facial muscles
▶ Somatic muscles: Arched-back rigidity (opisthotonos) and boardlike abdominal rigidity
▶ Intermittent tonic seizures lasting several minutes, which may result in cyanosis and sudden death by asphyxiation
Despite such pronounced neuromuscular signs, cerebral and sensory functions remain normal.

Neonatal tetanus is always generalized. The first clinical sign is difficulty sucking, which is usually noted 3 to 10 days after birth. This progresses to a total inability to suck with excessive crying, irritability, and nuchal rigidity.

DIAGNOSTIC TESTS

▶ In many cases, diagnosis must rely on clinical features, a history of trauma, and no previous tetanus immunization.
▶ Blood cultures and tetanus antibody tests are often negative; only a third of patients have a positive wound culture.
▶ Cerebrospinal fluid pressure may rise above normal.
▶ Diagnosis must also rule out meningitis, rabies, phenothiazine or strychnine toxicity, and other conditions that mimic tetanus.

TREATMENT

Within 72 hours after receiving a puncture wound, a patient with no previous history of tetanus immunization first requires tetanus immune globulin (TIG) or tetanus antitoxin to neutralize the toxins and confer temporary protection. This is followed by active immunization with tetanus toxoid. If the patient hasn't had a tetanus immunization within the past 10 years, a booster injection of tetanus toxoid is necessary. If tetanus develops despite immediate postinjury treatment, the patient will require airway maintenance and a muscle relaxant, such as diazepam (Valium), to decrease muscle rigidity and spasm. If muscle contractions aren't relieved by muscle relaxants, a neuromuscular blocker, such as metocurine iodide, may be prescribed. The patient with tetanus needs high-dose antibiotics (penicillin administered I.V. if he or she isn't allergic to it or such alternatives as clindamycin, erythromycin, and metronidazole.) The source of the toxin needs to be removed and destroyed through surgical exploration and wound debridement.

 PREVENTION The tetanus vaccine is usually given to children as part of the diphtheria-tetanus-pertussis (DTP) vaccine. It's recommended that adolescents receive a booster shot between the ages of 11 and 18 and that adults receive a routine tetanus booster shot every 10 years. In the event of a deep or dirty wound in a patient who has not had a tetanus booster in more than 5 years, another booster should be given as part of treatment.

Nursing considerations

▶ Thoroughly debride and clean the injury site, and check the patient's immunization history. Record the cause of injury. If it's an animal bite, report the case to local public health authorities.

▶ Before giving penicillin, TIG, tetanus antitoxin, or tetanus toxoid, obtain an accurate history of allergies to immunizations or penicillin.

▶ If tetanus develops:
- Maintain an adequate airway and ventilation to prevent pneumonia and atelectasis. Suction often, and watch for signs of respiratory distress.
- Maintain an I.V. line for medications and emergency care, if necessary.
- Monitor for arrhythmias. Record intake and output accurately, and check vital signs often.
- Because even minimal external stimulation provokes muscle spasms, keep the patient's room quiet and dimly lit. Warn visitors not to upset or overly stimulate the patient.
- Give muscle relaxants and sedatives, as ordered, and schedule patient care, such as passive range-of-motion exercises, to coincide with periods of heaviest sedation.
- Provide adequate nutrition to meet the patient's increased metabolic needs. The patient may require nasogastric feedings or total parenteral nutrition.

Patient teaching

▶ Stress the importance of maintaining active immunization with a booster dose of tetanus toxoid every 10 years.

▶ Teach the patient or family about proper wound care. Review signs and symptoms of complications and when to notify the physician.

Tonsillitis

Tonsillitis, sometimes referred to as pharyngitis, is inflammation of the pharyngeal tonsils that may also extend to the adenoids. The condition can be acute, recurrent, or chronic. The uncomplicated acute form, which often follows an upper respiratory infection, usually lasts 4 to 6 days and affects children between ages 5 and 10. Tonsillitis is considered recurrent if the patient experiences seven episodes in 1 year, five episodes in 2 consecutive years, or three episodes yearly for 3 consecutive years. Chronic tonsillitis is persistent infection of the tonsils.

CAUSES

Tonsillitis generally results from infection with beta-hemolytic streptococci but can also result from other bacteria or viruses, such as herpesvirus, cytomegalovirus, or adenovirus.

COMPLICATIONS

Chronic tonsillitis may result in chronic upper airway obstruction, causing sleep apnea or sleep disturbances, cor pulmonale, failure to thrive, eating or swallowing disorders, and speech abnormalities. Febrile seizures, otitis media, cardiac valvular disease, abscesses, glomerulonephritis, subacute bacterial endocarditis, and abscessed cervical lymph nodes may also be noted. Scarlet fever, rheumatic fever, and heart disease may also occur, but these conditions are not as common as they were before the widespread use of antibiotics.

ASSESSMENT FINDINGS

The patient with acute tonsillitis may complain of mild to severe sore throat. In a child who is too young to complain about throat pain, the parents may report that the child has stopped eating. The patient or parents also may report muscle and joint pain, chills, malaise, headache, and pain that is frequently referred to the ears. Because of excess secretions, the patient may complain of a constant urge to swallow and a constricted feeling in the back of the throat. Such discomfort usually subsides after 72 hours. Fever of 100° F (37.8° C) or higher may be present, and palpation may reveal swollen, tender lymph nodes in the submandibular area.

Inspection of the throat may reveal generalized inflammation of the pharyngeal wall, with swollen tonsils that project from between the pillars of the fauces and exude white or yellow follicles. Purulent drainage becomes apparent when pressure is applied to the tonsillar pillars. The uvula may also be edematous and inflamed.

Patients with chronic tonsillitis may report recurrent sore throats and attacks of acute tonsillitis. They may present with purulent drainage in the tonsillar crypts, foul breath, and persistently tender cervical nodes.

DIAGNOSTIC TESTS

▶ Throat culture may reveal the infecting organism and indicate appropriate antibiotic therapy.
▶ A complete blood count usually reveals leukocytosis.
▶ Needle biopsy helps differentiate cellulitis from abscess.

TREATMENT

Management of acute tonsillitis stresses symptom relief and requires rest, adequate fluid intake, aspirin or acetaminophen and, for bacterial infection, an antibiotic. For infection with group A beta-hemolytic *Streptococcus*, penicillin is the drug of choice. (Erythromycin or another broad-spectrum antibiotic may be given if the patient is allergic to penicillin.) To prevent complications, antibiotic therapy should continue for 10 days.

Patients with chronic tonsillitis or complications may require tonsillectomy—but only after they are free of tonsillar or respiratory tract infections for 3 to 4 weeks.

Nursing considerations

▶ Despite dysphasia, urge the patient to drink plenty of fluids, especially if fever is present. Offer young patients ice cream and flavored drinks and ices. Assess hydration status, and increased humidification to provide comfort.

▶ Monitor the effect of pain medication.

▶ Suggest gargling to soothe the throat.

▶ Before surgery, assess the patient for bleeding abnormalities.

▶ After surgery:
- Maintain a patent airway. To prevent aspiration, place the patient on his or her side. Keep suction equipment nearby.
- Monitor vital signs frequently, and check for bleeding. Immediately report excessive bleeding, increased pulse rate, or decreased blood pressure.
- When the patient is fully alert and the gag reflex has returned, offer water. Later, encourage the patient to drink nonirritating fluids. Avoid milk products, which coat the throat, leading to throat clearing and an increased risk for bleeding.
- Provide an analgesic for pain relief. Because crying irritates the operative site, keep the child comfortable.
- Encourage deep-breathing exercises to prevent pulmonary complications.

Patient teaching

▶ Tell the patient to complete the entire course of the prescribed antibiotic, even if symptoms subside.

▶ Instruct the adult patient to avoid smoking and drinking alcohol because they irritate the throat.

▶ Review the patient's medications, including dosage, administration, and adverse effects. (See *Promoting recovery from tonsillitis.*)

▶ For patients undergoing surgery:
- Before tonsillectomy, explain the procedure to the pediatric patient in a simple, nonthreatening way. Show the patient the operating and recovery rooms and briefly explain the facility routine. Note whether a

Promoting recovery from tonsillitis

For a patient recovering from tonsillitis, provide these guidelines:
• Make sure the patient (or parents) understand the importance of completing the prescribed course of antibiotic.
• Explain possible adverse effects of the prescribed medications, especially those that demand medical attention.
• Instruct the patient (or parents) to avoid spicy, irritating foods; eat primarily soft, nutritious foods; and avoid using straws or forks.
• Advise the patient (or parents) to restrict activities and avoid aspirin and products that contain aspirin for 7 to 10 days postoperatively.

parent may stay with the child during the procedure.
- Explain to the adult patient that a local anesthetic prevents pain but allows a sensation of pressure during surgery.
- Warn the patient to expect considerable throat discomfort and some bleeding after surgery.
- Before discharge, provide written home care instructions. Explain that a white scab will form in the throat 5 to 10 days postoperatively, and instruct the patient or parents to report bleeding, ear discomfort, or a fever lasting for 3 days or longer.

Toxic shock syndrome

Toxic shock syndrome (TSS) is an acute bacterial infection caused by toxin-producing, penicillin-resistant strains of *Staphylococcus aureus*, such as TSS toxin-1 and staphylococcal enterotoxins B and C. Initially, TSS was thought to affect primarily menstruating women younger than age 30 as a result of continuous use of tampons during the menstrual period; however, only about 55% of cases are associated with menstruation. TSS is fatal in 50% of cases.

Causes

Theoretically, tampons may contribute to the development of TSS by introducing *S. aureus* into the vagina during insertion (insertion with fingers instead of the supplied applicator increases the risk) or by traumatizing the vaginal mucosa during insertion, thus leading to infection.

When TSS isn't related to menstruation, it appears to be linked to *S. aureus* infections, such as abscesses, osteomyelitis, and postsurgical infections. It's also associated with prior antibiotic use.

Risk factors include recent use of barrier contraceptives (diaphragms or vaginal sponges), childbirth, and surgery.

Complications

TSS can complicate the patient's use of contraceptives, the puerperium, septic abortion, and gynecologic surgery. Postoperative infections can develop hours to weeks after a surgical procedure. TSS has also been associated with musculoskeletal and respiratory infections caused by *S. aureus* and with staphylococcal bacteremia.

Complications of organ hypoperfusion related to TSS include renal and myocardial dysfunction, massive edema, acute respiratory distress syndrome, and desquamation of the skin. Late signs include peripheral gangrene, reversible hair and nail loss, muscle weakness, and neuropsychiatric dysfunction. Death may also occur.

Assessment findings

TSS symptoms typically are abrupt in onset and produce intense myalgia, fever higher than 104° F (40° C), vomiting, diarrhea, headache, bruising, decreased level of consciousness, rigors, conjunctival hyperemia, and vaginal hyperemia and discharge. Severe hypotension occurs with hypovolemic shock. Within a few hours of onset, a deep red rash develops—especially on the palms of the hands and soles of the feet—that later desquamates.

Diagnostic tests

▶ Isolation of *S. aureus* from vaginal discharge or the infection site helps support the diagnosis, but a confirmed diagnosis must follow the criteria set by the Centers for Disease Control and Prevention. (See *Guidelines for diagnosing TSS.*)

Treatment

Treatment involves examination and removal of foreign material, such as tampons, vaginal sponges, or nasal packing, and drainage of any identified infection site, such as surgical wounds. One or more antistaphylococcal antibiotics, such as clindamycin (Cleocin), oxacillin (Bactocill), or nafcillin, are given I.V. Penicillin may also be given until the causative organism is identified. To reverse shock, fluids are replaced with large amounts of saline solution and colloids, as ordered. Blood pressure support and dialysis may be necessary. Respiratory support may be needed with the use of a ventilator, and nutritional needs should be addressed. In some cases, I.V. immune globulin may be required. Surgical exploration and debridement may be necessary.

Nursing considerations

▶ Monitor the patient's vital signs frequently.
▶ Administer antibiotics slowly and strictly on time. Be sure to watch for signs of penicillin allergy.

Guidelines for diagnosing TSS

TSS is typically diagnosed based on the following criteria set by the Centers for Disease Control and Prevention:
- Fever of 102° F (38.9° C) or higher
- Widespread red, flat rash
- Hypotension (including fainting or dizziness on standing)
- Shedding of skin, especially on the palms and soles, 1 to 2 weeks after the onset of illness
- Involvement of at least three organ or body systems:
  - GI (vomiting, profuse diarrhea)
  - Muscular (severe muscle pain, fivefold or greater increase in creatine kinase level)
  - Mucous membranes (conjunctiva, vagina, or oropharyngeal hyperemia)
  - Renal (blood urea nitrogen or creatinine elevated to at least twice normal levels)
  - Hepatic (bilirubin, aspartate aminotransferase, or alanine aminotransferase elevated to at least twice normal levels)
  - Hematologic (bruising due to a platelet count <100,000/μl)
  - Central nervous system (disorientation, confusion)
- Other conditions ruled out

medication, dosage, and possible adverse effects with them.

▶ Discuss any necessary follow-up care.

 PREVENTION Instruct women to change tampons frequently and to always wash their hands before and after doing so. To prevent recurrence, antistaphylococcal antibiotics may be required for several months before and during each menstrual cycle.

▶ Check the patient's fluid and electrolyte balance. Administer replacement fluids as ordered.

▶ Obtain specimens of vaginal and cervical secretions (or from other sites of infection) for culture of *S. aureus*.

▶ Implement standard precautions.

Patient teaching

▶ Teach the patient about the infection, including the cause, diagnosis, and treatment.

▶ Review all prescribed medication, including dosage, administration, and possible adverse effects. If household members are required to take medication as prophylaxis against re-infecting the patient, review the

Toxoplasmosis

Toxoplasmosis, one of the most common infectious diseases, is caused by the protozoan *Toxoplasma gondii*. Depending on their environment and eating habits, up to 70% of people in the United States are infected with *T. gondii* at any given time. Distributed worldwide, the infection is less common in arid climates (cold or hot) and at high elevations. It usually causes localized infection but may produce significant generalized infection, especially in neonates and in patients who are immunocompromised. Congenital toxoplasmosis, characterized by central nervous system lesions, may result in stillbirth or serious birth defects. For this reason, pregnant women are advised to avoid cleaning cat litter boxes because fecal-oral contamination from infected cats transmits toxoplasmosis.

CAUSES

T. gondii exists in trophozoite forms in the acute stages of infection and in cystic forms (tissue cysts and oocysts) in the latent stages. In addition to possible fecal-oral transmission from infected cats, ingestion of tissue cysts in raw or uncooked meat (heating, drying, or freezing destroys these cysts) can also transmit toxoplasmosis. However, toxoplasmosis also occurs in vegetarians who aren't exposed to cats, so other means of transmission may exist. Congenital toxoplasmosis follows transplacental transmission from a chronically infected mother or one who acquired toxoplasmosis shortly before or during pregnancy.

Once infected, the patient may carry the organism for life. Reactivation of the acute infection can occur.

COMPLICATIONS

Toxoplasmosis may cause encephalitis, myocarditis, pneumonitis, hepatitis, or polymycosis. If the disease is acquired in the first trimester of pregnancy, it commonly results

Ocular toxoplasmosis

Ocular toxoplasmosis (active chorioretinitis), which is characterized by focal necrotizing retinitis, accounts for about 25% of all cases of granulomatous uveitis. It's usually the result of congenital infection but may not appear until adolescence or young adulthood, when infection is reactivated. Symptoms include blurred vision, scotoma, pain, photophobia, and impairment or loss of central vision. Vision improves as inflammation subsides, but lost visual acuity is usually not recovered. Ocular toxoplasmosis may subside after treatment with prednisone.

in stillbirth. About one-third of infants who survive have congenital toxoplasmosis. The later in pregnancy that maternal infection occurs, the greater the risk will be of congenital infection in the infant. Other defects, which may become apparent months or years later, include strabismus, blindness, epilepsy, and mental retardation. (See *Ocular toxoplasmosis*.)

ASSESSMENT FINDINGS

The patient history may reveal an immunocompromised state, exposure to cat feces, or frequent ingestion of poorly cooked meat. Acquired toxoplasmosis may cause localized (mild lymphatic) or generalized (fulminating, disseminated) infection. Localized infection produces fever and a mononucleosis-like syndrome (malaise, myalgia, headache, fatigue, and sore throat) and lymphadenopathy. Generalized infection produces encephalitis, fever, headache, vomiting, delirium, seizures, and a diffuse maculopapular rash (except on the palms, soles, and scalp). Auscultation of a patient with toxoplasmosis may reveal coarse crackles.

Obvious signs of congenital toxoplasmosis include chorioretinitis, hydrocephalus or microcephalus, cerebral calcification, seizures, lymphadenopathy, fever, hepatosplenomegaly, jaundice, and rash.

ALERT Don't palpate an infected patient's abdomen vigorously, as this could lead to a ruptured spleen. For the same reason, discourage vigorous activity.

DIAGNOSTIC TESTS

▶ Identification of *T. gondii* in an appropriate tissue specimen confirms the diagnosis of toxoplasmosis.

▶ Serologic tests may be useful in patients with toxoplasmosis encephalitis and are required for diagnosis in patients with acute active infection.

▶ Computed tomography and magnetic resonance imaging disclose central nervous system lesions.

TREATMENT

Treatment of acute toxoplasmosis consists of drug therapy with sulfonamides, pyrimethamine (Daraprim), folinic acid, clindamycin (Cleocin), or co-trimoxazole. In patients who also have acquired immunodeficiency syndrome, treatment continues indefinitely. No safe, effective treatment exists for chronic toxoplasmosis or toxoplasmosis occurring in the first trimester of pregnancy.

NURSING CONSIDERATIONS

▶ Because sulfonamides cause blood dyscrasias and pyrimethamine depresses bone marrow, closely monitor the patient's hematologic values. Also emphasize the importance of regularly scheduled follow-up care.

▶ Patients who are receiving immunosuppressants are very susceptible to toxoplasmosis. Warn them of the risks, and suggest having all cats that go outdoors tested for toxoplasmosis.

▶ Report all cases of toxoplasmosis to the local public health department.

Patient teaching

▶ Teach the patient about the infection, including the cause, diagnosis, and treatment.

▶ Review all medications, including dosage, administration, and possible adverse effects. Discuss the need for blood tests.

 PREVENTION Teach all patients to wash their hands after working with soil (because it may be contaminated with oocysts shed in cat feces); to cook meat thoroughly and freeze it promptly if it isn't for immediate use; to change cat litter daily (oocysts don't become infective until 1 to 4 days after excretion); to cover children's sandboxes when not in use; and to keep flies away from food (flies transport oocysts).

▶ Advise all pregnant women to avoid cleaning or handling cat litter boxes. If this can't be avoided, advise them to wear gloves.

Trichinosis

Trichinosis (also known as trichiniasis or trichinellosis) is an infection caused by larvae of the intestinal roundworm *Trichinella spiralis*. It occurs worldwide, especially in populations that eat pork or bear meat. Trichinosis may produce multiple symptoms; respiratory, central nervous system (CNS), and cardiovascular complications; and, rarely, death. In the United States, trichinosis is rare and usually mild with few symptoms.

CAUSES

Transmission is through ingestion of uncooked or undercooked meat that contains *T. spiralis* cysts. Such cysts are found primarily in swine and less commonly in dogs, cats, bears, foxes, wolves, and marine animals. These cysts result from the animals' ingestion of similarly contaminated flesh. In swine, infection results from eating table scraps or garbage consisting of raw food.

After gastric juices free the worm from the cyst capsule, the worm reaches sexual maturity within a few days. The female roundworm burrows into the intestinal mucosa and reproduces. Larvae are then transported through the lymphatic system and bloodstream and become embedded as cysts in striated muscle. The muscles most commonly invaded are the extraocular muscles of the eye; the tongue; the deltoid, pectoral, and intercostal muscles; the diaphragm; and the gastrocnemius muscle. Human-to-human transmission doesn't take place.

Although common worldwide, trichinosis is seldom seen in the United States because of regulations regarding animal feed and meat processing.

COMPLICATIONS

Trichinosis can cause such complications as encephalitis, myocarditis, pneumonia, and respiratory failure. Death is rare but may occur 2 to 8 weeks after infection.

ASSESSMENT FINDINGS

The patient's history may reveal ingestion of uncooked or undercooked meat, especially pork. When symptoms do occur, they vary with the stage and degree of infection:

▶ Stage 1 (intestinal trichinosis) occurs 1 week after ingestion. Release of larvae and reproduction of adult *T. spiralis* may cause anorexia, nausea, vomiting, diarrhea, abdominal pain, and cramps. The patient may develop a petechial rash or splinter hemorrhages beneath the nails.

▶ Stage 2 (disseminated or invasive trichinosis) occurs 7 to 10 days after ingestion. *T. spiralis* penetrates the intestinal mucosa and begins to migrate to striated muscle. Signs and symptoms include edema, especially of the eyelids or face; muscle pain, particularly in the extremities; and, occasionally, itching and burning skin, sweating, skin lesions or rash, a temperature of 102° to 104° F (38.9° to 40° C), and delirium. In severe respiratory, cardiovascular, or CNS infections, palpitations and lethargy can occur, as well as paresis and focal paralysis.

▶ Stage 3 (encystment or convalescent trichinosis) occurs during convalescence, generally 1 week after stage 2. *T. spiralis* larvae invade muscle fibers and become encysted. Dehydration may occur, along with cachexia. The patient may complain of weakness and chronic headache. Recovery after heavy infection may take 2 to 3 months.

DIAGNOSTIC TESTS

▶ A history of ingesting raw or improperly cooked pork or pork products, with typical clinical features, suggests trichinosis, but infection may be difficult to prove.

▶ Stools may contain mature worms and larvae during the invasive stage.

▶ Skeletal muscle biopsies can show encysted larvae 10 days after ingestion; if available, analyses of contaminated meat also show larvae.

▶ Skin testing may show a positive histamine-like reactivity 15 minutes after intradermal injection of the antigen (within 17 to

20 days after ingestion). However, such a result may remain positive for up to 5 years after exposure.

▶ Elevated acute and convalescent antibody titers (determined by flocculation tests 3 to 4 weeks after infection) confirm the diagnosis.

▶ Other abnormal results include elevated aspartate aminotransferase, alanine aminotransferase, creatine kinase, and lactate dehydrogenase levels during the acute stages and an elevated eosinophil count (up to 15,000/μl) during stage 2 (though occasionally seen during stage 1 as well). A normal or increased cerebrospinal fluid lymphocyte level (up to 300/μl) and increased protein levels indicate CNS involvement.

TREATMENT

Mebendazole or albendazole (Albenza) effectively combats this *T. spiralis* during the intestinal stage; severe infection (especially CNS invasion) may warrant glucocorticoids to combat possible inflammation. There's no treatment for trichinosis once the parasite is in the muscles, but analgesics may be used to relieve muscle pain.

NURSING CONSIDERATIONS

▶ Question the patient about recent ingestion of pork products and the methods used to store and cook them.

▶ Reduce fever with tepid baths, cooling blankets, or antipyretics; relieve muscle pain with analgesics, enforced bed rest, and proper body alignment.

▶ To prevent pressure ulcers, reposition the patient frequently and gently massage bony prominences.

▶ Report all cases of trichinosis to local public health authorities.

Patient teaching

▶ Teach the patient about the infection, including its cause, diagnosis, and treatment.

▶ Review all prescribed medication, including dosage, administration, and possible adverse effects.

▶ Discuss the signs and symptoms of complications and when to notify the physician.

▶ Explain the importance of bed rest. Sudden death from cardiac involvement may occur in a patient with moderate to severe infection who has resumed activity too soon. Warn the patient to continue bed rest into the convalescent stage to avoid a serious relapse and possible death.

 PREVENTION Take these actions to help prevent trichinosis:

- Educate the public about proper cooking and storing methods not only for pork and pork products but also for meat from other carnivores. To kill trichinae, internal meat temperatures should reach 150° F (65.9° C) and meat color should change from pink to gray unless the meat has been cured or frozen for at least 10 days at low temperatures.

- Warn travelers to foreign countries or to poor areas in the United States to avoid eating pork; swine in these areas are commonly fed raw garbage.

Trichomoniasis

Trichomoniasis, also referred to as "trich," is one of the most common sexually transmitted infections (STIs) in the United States, with approximately 8 million cases reported annually. It also has a high incidence worldwide, especially in Africa, with 180 million cases reported to date. It is more common in women, ages 16 to 35, than in men.

CAUSES

Trichomoniasis is caused by the protozoan *Trichomonas vaginalis*. It damages the epithelium of vaginal and urethral tissue and more than doubles the risk of acquiring human immunodeficiency virus (HIV). This infection has an incubation period of 4 to 28 days and is associated with other STIs, such as gonorrhea, chlamydia, and HIV.

It was once thought that trichomoniasis resulted from common water in hot tubs, wet bathing suits, and wet towels because trichomonads can survive for 45 minutes outside the body; however, this is now thought to be unlikely. It is transmitted by penis-to-vagina intercourse or vulva-to-vulva contact with an infected person. Trichomoniasis is not transmitted by oral or anal sex.

Risk factors for contracting trichomoniasis include the following:
▶ Past or present infection with other STIs
▶ Multiple sexual partners
▶ Unsafe sex practices
▶ Bacterial vaginosis
▶ High vaginal pH
▶ Being of African descent

COMPLICATIONS

Complications of trichomoniasis include prostatitis, urethral stricture disease, and epididymitis in men. In women, pelvic inflammatory disease may occur. Trichomoniasis may also play a role in cervical neoplasia and postoperative infection as well as in acquiring herpes simplex type 2. Infertility can be a complication for both men and women. For pregnant women, preterm birth or adverse fetal outcomes may result from untreated trichomoniasis.

ASSESSMENT FINDINGS

Symptoms are different in men and women. Some patients, especially men, are asymptomatic. When symptoms do occur, women may have a history of dyspareunia and dysuria, along with a frothy, foul-smelling, yellow-green vaginal discharge. A patient may complain of vaginal soreness and itching, and there may be vulvar or vaginal redness. If cervicitis is present, purulent discharge and bleeding may occur. The patient may also complain of abdominal pain or tenderness. On gynecologic inspection, the cervix may show a patchy macular erythematous lesion. Men may complain of urethral discharge and itching as well as dysuria. (See *Symptoms in trichomoniasis.*)

DIAGNOSTIC TESTS

▶ On microscopy, vaginal secretions reveal trichomonads, the number of which corresponds to the severity of infection.
▶ Culture of urethral tissue, urine, or semen (in men) identifies *T. vaginalis.*
▶ Polymerase chain reaction identifies the infection.
▶ The OSOM Trichomonas Rapid Test identifies infection within 10 to 45 minutes, but it is less sensitive and specific than culture.

TREATMENT

An antiprotozoal agent is the treatment for trichomoniasis. Metronidazole (Flagyl), taken orally, is the treatment of choice, with tinidazole (Tindamax) as an alternative drug. The preferred administration is a single 2-g dose of metronidazole; however, it may also be given twice per day over 7 days. Topical medication may be used, such as clotrimazole (Mycelex), povidone-iodine, or metronidazole; however, this type of treatment is not as effective as oral dosing. With

Symptoms in trichomoniasis

Trichomoniasis is a common STI that affects both men and women, although usually only women exhibit symptoms. While most men who have trichomoniasis don't have any symptoms, some may experience irritation inside the penis, sometimes accompanied by a mild discharge, and burning following urination or ejaculation.

Women may exhibit signs and symptoms of infection, such as a foul-smelling, yellow-green discharge. The infection may cause pain during intercourse and with urination, and it may be accompanied by genital itching and irritation.

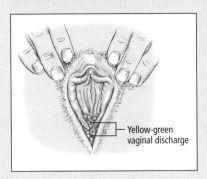

Yellow-green vaginal discharge

Patient teaching

▶ Teach the patient about the infection, including its cause, diagnosis, and treatment. Encourage the patient to inform any sexual partners about the infection so that they may also be tested and treated appropriately.

▶ Review all prescribed medication, including dosage, administration, and possible adverse effects. Tell the patient to avoid ingesting alcohol while taking metronidazole (and for 48 hours after completing the prescription), as the combination may cause severe nausea and vomiting, abdominal pain, headaches, and flushing.

▶ Tell the patient to avoid sexual intercourse until the course of medication is completed, and advise the patient to insist that his or her sexual partner be treated in order to avoid re-infection.

▶ Review with the patient the signs and symptoms of recurrence, and tell the patient to seek medical attention if they occur.

 PREVENTION Provide information regarding safe sex practices. Educate the patient about the proper use of condoms to help avoid STIs. Teach patients, especially adolescents, that abstinence from sexual intercourse is the ultimate preventive measure.

treatment, trichomoniasis has an 86% to 100% cure rate, according to the Centers for Disease Control and Prevention.

If other STIs are identified with testing, appropriate treatment should be initiated.

NURSING CONSIDERATIONS

▶ Follow standard precautions. Trichomoniasis is a reportable disease. Follow facility policy to report this infection if identified.

▶ Assist with obtaining appropriate specimens for culture or testing.

▶ Provide emotional support, as needed.

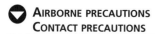

Tuberculosis

Tuberculosis (TB) is an acute or chronic infection characterized by pulmonary infiltrates and by the formation of granulomas with caseation, fibrosis, and cavitation. The incidence of TB has been declining in the United States, but its prevalence is increasing worldwide. According to the World Health Organization, approximately 2 billion people—one-third of the world's population—have latent TB. Globally, TB is the leading infectious cause of morbidity and mortality, generating 8 to 10 million new cases each year and causing 3 million deaths.

The disease is twice as common in males as in females and four times as common in nonwhites as in whites. The incidence is highest in people who live in crowded, poorly ventilated, unsanitary conditions, such as prisons, tenement housing, and homeless shelters. The typical newly diagnosed patient with TB is a single, homeless, nonwhite man. With proper treatment, the prognosis is usually excellent. However, mortality is 50% in those with strains of TB that are resistant to two or more of the major antitubercular agents.

CAUSES

TB results from exposure to *Mycobacterium tuberculosis* and, sometimes, other strains of mycobacteria. Transmission occurs when an infected person coughs or sneezes, spreading infected droplets. After exposure to *M. tuberculosis*, roughly 5% of infected people develop active TB within 2 years. In the remainder, the microorganisms cause a latent infection. The host's immunologic defense system usually destroys the bacillus or walls it up in a tubercle. However, the live, encapsulated bacilli may lay dormant within the tubercle for years, reactivating later to cause active infection. In this respect, the disease is an opportunistic infection.

The following at-risk populations incur a high incidence of TB with presenting symptoms:

▶ Black and Hispanic males ages 25 to 44
▶ People in close contact with a newly diagnosed patient with TB
▶ Those who have already had TB
▶ People with multiple sexual partners
▶ Recent immigrants from Africa, Asia, Mexico, and South America
▶ Gastrectomy patients
▶ People with silicosis, diabetes, malnutrition, cancer, Hodgkin's disease, or leukemia
▶ Drug and alcohol abusers
▶ Smokers
▶ Patients in mental health facilities
▶ Nursing home residents (they are 10 times more likely to contract TB than anyone in the general population)
▶ Those receiving treatment with immunosuppressants or corticosteroids
▶ People with weak immune systems or diseases that affect the immune system, especially acquired immunodeficiency syndrome (AIDS)
▶ Prisoners
▶ Homeless people

COMPLICATIONS

TB can cause massive pulmonary tissue damage, with inflammation and tissue necrosis eventually leading to respiratory failure. Bronchopleural fistulas can develop from lung tissue damage, resulting in pneumothorax. The disease can also lead to hemorrhage, pleural effusion, and pneumonia. Small mycobacterial foci can infect other body organs and systems, including the kidneys and the central nervous and skeletal systems. The patient also might develop complications such as liver involvement from drug therapy.

ASSESSMENT FINDINGS

The patient with a primary TB infection after an incubation period of 4 to 8 weeks is usually asymptomatic but may complain of weakness and fatigue, anorexia and weight loss, low-grade fever, and night sweats. The patient with reactivated TB may report chest pain and a cough that produces blood or mucopurulent or blood-tinged sputum. He or she may also have a low-grade fever.

Percussion may reveal dullness over the affected area (a sign of consolidation or the presence of pleural fluid). On auscultation, crepitant crackles, bronchial breath sounds, wheezes, and whispered pectoriloquy may be heard.

DIAGNOSTIC TESTS

Several of the following tests may be necessary to distinguish TB from other diseases that may mimic it, such as lung carcinoma, lung abscess, pneumoconiosis, and bronchiectasis.

▶ Chest radiography shows nodular lesions, patchy infiltrates (mainly in the upper lobes), cavity formation, scar tissue, and calcium deposits. Radiography may not help distinguish between active and inactive TB.

▶ A tuberculin skin test reveals that the patient has been infected with TB at some point, but it doesn't indicate active disease. A positive reaction (an induration 10 mm or larger) develops within 2 to 10 weeks after infection with the tubercle bacillus in both active and inactive TB. However, patients who are severely immunosuppressed may not develop a positive reaction.

▶ Stains and cultures of sputum, cerebrospinal fluid, urine, drainage from an abscess, or pleural fluid show heat-sensitive, nonmotile, aerobic, acid-fast bacilli.

▶ Computed tomography and magnetic resonance imaging allow the evaluation of lung damage and can confirm a difficult diagnosis.

▶ Bronchoscopy may be performed if the patient can't produce an adequate sputum specimen.

TREATMENT

Antitubercular therapy consists of four drug prescriptions, with daily oral doses of isoniazid, rifampin (Rimactane), pyrazinamide, and either ethambutol (Myambutol) or streptomycin added for drug-resistant strains. After 2 to 4 weeks, the disease is no longer infectious and the patient can resume normal activities while continuing to take medication. Treatment may be intermittent if the TB isolate is fully susceptible to the medication. If the isolate is found to be a multidrug-resistant strain, daily treatment may be required for up to 2 years. A longer course of treatment may also be necessary if the patient is slow to respond to treatment or has AIDS.

The patient with atypical mycobacterial disease or drug-resistant TB may require second-line drugs, such as capreomycin (Capastat), streptomycin, para-aminosalicylic acid, cycloserine (Seromycin), amikacin, or quinolone drugs.

NURSING CONSIDERATIONS

▶ Administer antibiotics and antitubercular agents, as ordered.

◐ Isolate the infectious patient in a negative airflow room, as per Centers for Disease Control and Prevention guidelines, and maintain airborne precautions with use of a properly fitting respirator mask. Make sure that visitors and other health care workers also maintain proper contact precautions.

 SAFETY Place a covered trash can near the patient or tape a waxed bag to the bedside for used tissues. Tell the patient to wear a mask when outside the room. Visitors and health care personnel should also take proper precautions while in the patient's room.

▶ Discontinue precautions only when patient is on effective therapy, is improving clinically, and three consecutive sputum smears collected on separate days test negative for acid-fast bacilli.

▶ Make sure the patient gets plenty of rest. Provide for periods of rest and activity to promote health as well as to conserve energy and reduce oxygen demands.

▶ Provide the patient with a well-balanced, high-calorie diet, preferably in small, frequent meals to conserve energy. (Small, frequent meals may also encourage the anorexic patient to eat more.) Record the patient's

Preventing TB

The best way to prevent TB is to detect it early. Hospitalized patients with TB should be isolated from other patients in a negative airflow room and placed on airborne precautions. Staff members should also use disposable HEPA filter masks (N95), which serve as adequate respiratory protection when caring for patients who are under airborne precautions.

Other ways to prevent the spread of TB include the following:

• Patients who have a weakened immune system or human immunodeficiency virus should receive annual TB testing. Annual testing is also recommended for health care workers, for people who work in prisons or long-term care facilities, and for those with a substantially increased risk of exposure to the disease.

• Patients who test positive for latent TB infection but have no evidence of active TB may be able to reduce their risk of developing active TB by taking a course of isoniazid therapy.

• To prevent the spread of disease from those with active TB or from those who are receiving treatment, give the patient the following recommendations:

- Stress the need to maintain the medication regimen without stopping or skipping doses. When the medication is discontinued prematurely, the TB bacteria can mutate and become drug resistant.

- Explain that patients who are receiving treatment are still contagious until they have been taking all their medications for 2 to 3 weeks. Encourage the patient to stay indoors and home from school or work during this period. If a patient must leave the home, a mask is recommended during the initial treatment time to lessen the risk of transmission.

- The patient should tell all health care providers he or she sees, including the dentist and optometrist, that he or she has TB so they can institute appropriate infection-control precautions.

- Teach the patient other specific precautions to avoid spreading the infection, including coughing and sneezing into tissues and disposing of the tissues properly. Stress the importance of thorough handwashing with hot, soapy water after handling secretions. Also instruct the patient to wash his or her eating utensils separately in hot, soapy water.

---

weight weekly. If oral supplements are needed, consult with the dietitian.

❱ Watch for adverse reactions to the medications.

❱ Administer isoniazid with food. This drug can cause hepatitis or peripheral neuritis, so monitor levels of aspartate aminotransferase and alanine aminotransferase. To prevent or treat peripheral neuritis, give pyridoxine (vitamin B₆) as ordered.

❱ If the patient receives ethambutol, give the medication with food and report signs of optic neuritis to the physician, who likely will discontinue the drug. Check the patient's vision monthly.

❱ If the patient receives rifampin, watch for signs of hepatitis, purpura, and a flu-like syndrome as well as other complications

such as hemoptysis. Monitor liver and kidney function throughout therapy.

❱ Perform chest physiotherapy, including postural drainage and chest percussion, several times per day.

❱ Give the patient supportive care, and help him or her adjust to lifestyle changes that may be necessary during the illness. Include the patient in care decisions, and let the family take part in the patient's care whenever possible.

Patient teaching

❱ Teach the patient and family about the infection, including its cause, diagnosis, treatment, and manner of transmission.

❱ Explain to the patient the prescribed medication regimen, which can be complicated.

Review drug dosage and administration as well as potential adverse effects, and tell the patient to report adverse effects immediately. Emphasize the importance of regular follow-up examinations, and instruct the patient and family members concerning the signs and symptoms of recurring TB. Stress the importance of faithfully following the long-term treatment plan.

▶ Show the patient and family how to perform postural drainage and chest percussion, and teach the patient coughing and deep-breathing exercises. Instruct the patient to maintain each position for 10 minutes and then to perform percussion and cough.

▶ Advise anyone who is exposed to an infected patient to receive tuberculin tests. If a positive reaction occurs, obtain chest radiographs and administer prophylactic isoniazid. (See *Preventing TB*.)

▶ Warn the patient taking rifampin that the drug temporarily makes body secretions such as urine appear orange; reassure the patient that this effect is harmless. Caution the female patient who is taking an oral contraceptive that the contraceptive may be less effective while she's taking rifampin.

▶ Teach the patient the signs and symptoms that require medical assessment, including increased cough, hemoptysis, unexplained weight loss, fever, and night sweats.

▶ Stress the importance of eating high-calorie, high-protein, balanced meals.

▶ Emphasize the importance of scheduling and keeping follow-up appointments.

▶ Refer the patient to support groups and organizations, such as the American Lung Association.

Tularemia

Tularemia (also called glandular fever, rabbit fever, tick fever, and deer fly fever) is a highly infectious disease that can be caused by as few as 10 organisms of *Francisella tularensis*, a gram-negative coccobacillus. There are seven forms of tularemia: ulceroglandular, glandular, oculoglandular, oropharyngeal, pneumonic, GI, and typhoidal (septicemic) tularemia. The disease is fatal in about 5% of patients who don't receive treatment and in less than 1% of patients who do receive treatment.

F. tularensis is considered a potential bioterrorism agent. If dispersed in aerosol form (the most likely method of dispersion), infected persons would generally develop signs and symptoms of severe respiratory illness, including pneumonia and systemic infection.

CAUSES

Tularemia is transmitted by the bites of infected ticks and deer flies, via consumption of contaminated food or water, and through contact with the blood of an infected animal (such as by skinning or handling infected carcasses), especially rabbits. The organism gains access to the host by skin or mucous membrane inoculation, inhalation, or ingestion. After inoculation, a papule and high fever develop. (The papule eventually develops into an ulcer.) The incubation period is 3 to 4 days.

In the United States, about 200 human cases of tularemia are reported annually, with most occurring in the south-central and western parts of the country.

COMPLICATIONS

Complications of tularemia include pneumonia, lung abscess, respiratory failure, rhabdomyolysis, meningitis, pericarditis, and osteomyelitis. Death may also occur.

ASSESSMENT FINDINGS

Common signs and symptoms present 3 to 4 days after infection but may not present until 14 days. Ulcer at the inoculation site and fever are common, as are weakness and muscle and joint pain. Signs and symptoms also vary according to the form of tularemia the patient is infected with:

▶ Ulceroglandular: This is the most common form of tularemia, with ulcers occurring at the site of inoculation and accompanied by swollen regional lymph nodes, commonly the armpit or groin.

▶ Glandular: This form is similar to ulceroglandular tularemia but without ulcer formation. Swollen regional lymph nodes are present.

▶ Oculoglandular: Infection occurs in the eye; the patient exhibits a painful, red eye with purulent exudates and swollen submandibular, preauricular, or cervical lymph nodes.

▶ Oropharyngeal and GI: These types of infection follow eating or drinking contaminated water or food. The patient complains of a sore throat, abdominal pain, nausea, vomiting, diarrhea and, occasionally, GI bleeding. The lymph nodes in the neck may be swollen.

▶ Pneumonic: Infection occurs from inhalation of infected dust or aerosols but can also result when other forms of tularemia are left untreated and the infection advances into the blood and lungs. The patient presents with a dry cough, dyspnea, and pleuritic chest pain. With septicemia, the patient has fever, chills, myalgia, malaise, and weight loss.

▶ Typhoidal: This rare form of the disease can affect a number of body organs. It usually causes fever, exhaustion, and weight loss.

DIAGNOSTIC TESTS

▶ Diagnosis is based on presenting signs and symptoms as well as the patient's history, which may include a tick bite and exposure to contaminated food, water, or blood.

▶ The white blood cell count is normal or elevated.

▶ Blood cultures may be negative, but cultures of lymph nodes, skin scrapings, sputum, gastric aspirate, or pharyngeal washings may be positive for *F. tularensis*.

▶ Chest radiography may show pneumonia.

TREATMENT

General treatment involves proper skin care and increased fluid intake or supportive therapy with I.V. fluids. Medications include I.V., I.M., or oral antibiotic therapy with streptomycin, gentamicin, doxycycline (Doryx), or ciprofloxacin (Cipro). Treatment may be required for up to 2 weeks, with most patients recovering. Antipyretics may be administered for fever.

NURSING CONSIDERATIONS

▶ Maintain standard precautions. Tularemia is not transmitted from person to person, so stricter precautions are not necessary.

▶ Laboratory personnel are at significant risk for infection through direct contact or inhalation of the organism. Specimens must be labeled accordingly to alert the lab.

▶ Administer medications as ordered, and monitor for adverse reactions. Administer fluids to prevent dehydration.

▶ Monitor the patient's intake and output as well as vital signs.

▶ Assess the patient for signs of dehydration, such as tachycardia, tachypnea, and decreased urine output.

▶ Monitor for complications, such as meningitis, pneumonia, pericarditis, and osteomyelitis.

Patient teaching

▶ Teach the patient about the infection, including its cause, diagnosis, treatment, and transmission.

▶ Review all prescribed medication, including dosage, administration, and possible adverse effects. Urge the patient to take the full course of antibiotics exactly as prescribed.

▶ Teach the patient signs and symptoms of complications, such as dehydration, and when to report them to the physician.

 PREVENTION To prevent tularemia, advise the patient to avoid tick-infested areas (woods, meadows, streams, and canyons) if possible. Teach the patient ways to reduce the risk of becoming infected with tularemia:

- Remind the patient to wear protective clothing, such as a long-sleeved shirt, pants securely tucked into laced boots, and a protective head covering such as a cap.

- Advise the patient to apply insect repellant to exposed skin as well as to clothing.

- Tell the patient to wear gloves if handling a dead or sick animal and to avoid running over dead animals with a lawn mower.

- Warn the patient not to drink untreated water.

- Tell the patient to use fine-tipped tweezers to remove any ticks found on the body.

- Advise the patient to cook all game thoroughly before eating it.

CONTACT PRECAUTIONS

Typhoid fever

Also known as enteric fever, typhoid fever is a multisystem infection that causes the classic symptoms of fever, malaise, diffuse abdominal pain, and constipation. It occurs in areas where there is poor sanitation and unsafe water conditions. Most infections diagnosed in the United States were acquired during international travel. Approximately 200 to 400 cases are reported annually in the United States, but worldwide it affects over 21 million people. Mortality is about 3% in patients who receive treatment. Ten percent of untreated cases may result in fatality, usually as a result of complications. An attack of typhoid fever confers lifelong immunity, although the patient may become a carrier. Most typhoid fever patients are younger than age 30; most carriers are women older than age 50.

CAUSES

Typhoid fever is caused by *Salmonella typhi*, which can only live in humans. *S. typhi* enters the GI tract and invades the bloodstream via the lymphatics, setting up intracellular sites. During this phase, infection of the biliary tract leads to intestinal seeding with millions of bacilli. Involved lymphoid tissue (especially Peyer patches in the ileum) becomes enlarged, ulcerated, and necrotic, resulting in hemorrhage. The incubation period usually lasts 1 to 2 weeks.

S. typhi is transmitted through stool. A person who eats or drinks food or beverages handled by someone infected with *S. typhi* who does not practice good hygiene can become infected. Infection may also occur through contaminated water.

COMPLICATIONS

Complications of typhoid fever include intestinal perforation or hemorrhage, abscesses, thrombophlebitis, cerebral thrombosis, pneumonia, osteomyelitis, myocarditis, and acute circulatory failure. Studies have shown

that close to 6% of treated patients become chronic carriers. Pancreatitis, acute renal failure, subclinical disseminated intravascular coagulation, and neuropsychiatric manifestations, such as seizures, spastic paraplegia, mania, and depression, may also occur.

ASSESSMENT FINDINGS

Abdominal pain and tenderness may develop within hours of ingestion of *S. typhi* and usually subside before onset of typhoid fever symptoms, which begin 7 to 14 days after ingestion:

▶ First week: Patients present with a gradually increasing fever, anorexia, myalgia, malaise, headache, and slow pulse.

▶ Second week: There is a remittent fever up to 104° F (40° C) usually in the evening, chills, diaphoresis, weakness, delirium, increasing abdominal pain and distention, diarrhea or constipation, cough, moist crackles, tender abdomen with an enlarged spleen, and a rose rash (especially on abdomen) that is salmon-colored in appearance with maculopapules that generally resolve in 2 to 5 days.

▶ Third week: Persistent fever, increasing fatigue and weakness, and weight loss usually subside by end of third week, although relapses may occur. The patient may also demonstrate infected conjunctivae, a thready pulse, tachypnea with audible basilar crackles, or severe abdominal distention with green-yellow, foul smelling, and liquid diarrhea. A typhoid state—apathy, confusion, and psychosis—may ensue.

▶ Fourth week: Slow improvement is noted in the fever and GI state, with mental status also improving. Weakness and weight loss may persist for months. In some cases, symptoms resolve but the patient becomes a chronic carrier.

DIAGNOSTIC TESTS

▶ Diagnosis of typhoid fever is based largely on clinical presentation and history.

▶ Cultures of blood, intestinal secretions, and stool are positive for *S. typhi*.

▶ Polymerase chain reaction identifies typhoid fever.

▶ Bone marrow aspiration identifies *S. typhi.*

TREATMENT

Antimicrobial therapy for typhoid fever depends on organism sensitivity. The drug of choice is cefixime (Suprax) or azithromycin (Zithromax), although treatment may include ampicillin, trimethoprim-sulfamethoxazole (Bactrim), or chloramphenicol. Ceftriaxone (Rocephin) is recommended for complicated cases. Increasing resistance to antimicrobials may prove challenging to treatment. Antipyretics and analgesics may be given for symptomatic treatment. Supportive treatment is provided based on complications that develop. A localized abscess may need surgical drainage. Other treatments include bed rest and fluid and electrolyte replacement. The administration of camphorated tincture of opium, kaolin with pectin, diphenoxylate, codeine, or small doses of morphine may be necessary to relieve diarrhea and control cramps in patients who must remain active.

NURSING CONSIDERATIONS

◯ Maintain standard precautions unless the patient is incontinent or in diapers or if an outbreak develops in an institution; initiate contact precautions for these patients.

▶ Report cases of typhoid fever to the state health department.

▶ Observe the patient for signs and symptoms of bowel perforation, including sudden pain in the lower right side of the abdomen and abdominal rigidity.

▶ Administer medication as ordered, and observe for adverse effects.

▶ Provide good skin and mouth care. Turn the patient frequently, and perform mild passive exercises, as indicated. Apply mild heat to the abdomen to relieve cramps.

Patient teaching

▶ Teach the patient about the infection, including its cause, diagnosis, and treatment.

▶ Review all prescribed medication, including dosage, administration, and possible adverse effects.

 SAFETY Teach the patient to use proper handwashing technique, especially after defecating and before eating or handling food.

▶ Encourage participation in follow-up care, as ordered by the physician. Monitoring for relapse may be required for 3 months after treatment is finished. Repeat stool cultures may be required.

 PREVENTION Review with the patient measures to prevent contracting typhoid fever when traveling:

- Avoid ingesting water that has not been bottled or boiled. Ask for drinks without ice, unless the ice is made with bottled water.

- Only eat vegetables that can be peeled, or peel them yourself. Be sure to wash your hands after handling the peel, as it may be contaminated.

- Avoid eating food and vegetables purchased from street vendors.

- Consider being vaccinated before traveling.

Typhus

Typhus is a group of febrile illnesses caused by rickettsial organisms. Epidemic (or louse-borne), murine, and scrub typhus are the more common types. Murine typhus, also called endemic typhus, is a mild form, and epidemic typhus is the most severe. The rare cases of epidemic typhus that have been reported in the United States have been related to exposure to flying squirrels. Epidemic typhus, also known as jail or prison fever, camp fever, famine fever, and hospital fever, has been found in areas of natural disaster, war, or poverty, where sanitation is difficult to maintain. Epidemic typhus occurs more often in colder months, when clothes are not laundered as frequently.

Worldwide, murine typhus is the most common type of typhus. In the United States, it occurs mostly in southern California during the summer and fall and in southern Texas during the spring and summer. Scrub typhus has not been reported in the United States but is endemic in northern Japan, Southeast Asia, and eastern Australia.

CAUSES

Murine typhus is caused by *Rickettsia typhi* and is transmitted by fleas, usually on rats or cats. *Rickettsia prowazekii* causes epidemic typhus and is transmitted by human body lice and the ectoparasites of flying squirrels. Epidemic typhus has a milder form, called Brill-Zinsser disease or Brill disease, which is actually a relapse of epidemic typhus that can occur years after the primary attack. Scrub typhus, also known as tsutsugamushi disease, is caused by *Orientia tsutsugamushi* (formerly *Rickettsia tsutsugamushi*) and transmitted by mites.

COMPLICATIONS

Complications of epidemic typhus include vasculitis (which may result in gangrene), central nervous system dysfunction, multi-system organ failure, and death, with a mortality rate of 3% to 4%. Mortality rates from murine and scrub typhus are 1% to 4% and less than 1%, respectively.

ASSESSMENT FINDINGS

Patients found to have typhus may have a history of exposure to an endemic area, overcrowded living conditions, or inadequate personal hygiene. The patient may be knowledgeable of having a flea bite. Signs and symptoms may be similar to those of Rocky Mountain spotted fever, also a rickettsial infection, and appear 1 to 2 weeks after exposure.

The patient experiences an abrupt high fever, up to 105.8° F (41° C), along with a severe headache. A macular or petechial rash appears initially on the trunk and axilla and then spreads to the rest of the body, avoiding the palms of the hands, soles of the feet, and face. Lymphadenopathy occurs. With scrub typhus, the patient may develop tachypnea and a cough.

Other signs and symptoms include myalgia, chills, hypotension, photophobia, nausea, vomiting, and delirium. Mild splenomegaly and hepatomegaly may be present.

DIAGNOSTIC TESTS

▶ Diagnosis is made mostly by clinical signs and symptoms and the patient history.
▶ Indirect immunofluorescence assay or enzyme immunoassay showing a rise in immunoglobulin M indicates acute primary disease.
▶ Complement fixation testing can detect antibodies to the specific rickettsial organism.
▶ A complete blood count may show leukopenia, especially in early stages of the disease; thrombocytopenia may also be present in later stages. Transaminase may be slightly elevated. Electrolyte levels may be abnormal; hyponatremia is most common.

TREATMENT

Typhus is treated with antimicrobial therapy, with doxycycline (Doryx) as the drug of choice. Alternative drugs include chloramphenicol, azithromycin (Zithromax), fluoroquinolones, and rifampin. If typhus is uncomplicated, antibiotic therapy may be adequate. Antipyretics, such as acetaminophen, and analgesics, such as ibuprofen, may be used to treat fever and myalgia. Complicated typhus requires treatment based on the specific complications. Inpatient therapy is needed, with careful monitoring of body systems, since multisystem organ failure can occur.

Nursing considerations

▶ Maintain standard precautions.
▶ After establishing allergy status, administer medications as ordered and monitor for adverse effects.
▶ Monitor vital signs, including pulse oximetry. Observe for signs and symptoms of complications.
▶ Monitor electrolyte levels, and administer replacement therapy as ordered.
▶ Administer medication to reduce fever and provide comfort, and evaluate the effects after 30 minutes. Provide comfort measures, such as tepid baths, a darkened room, and frequent repositioning.
▶ Refer the patient to social services if circumstances such as inadequate housing, an inability to care for oneself, or homelessness are a concern.

Patient teaching

▶ Teach the patient and family about the infection, including the cause, diagnosis, treatment, and transmission.
▶ Review all prescribed medication, including dosage, administration, and possible adverse effects. Tell the patient to complete the prescription as ordered, even if feeling better.
▶ Discuss signs and symptoms of complications and when to notify the physician.
▶ Review the treatment for lice with the patient and family. Tell them to use the medication as recommended and to boil or avoid infested clothing for at least 5 days.

 PREVENTION Tell the patient that no vaccine exists to prevent typhus; however, potential infection can be minimized by following these measures:
- Avoid rat- or lice-infested areas. If rats are a problem, notify the local sanitation department for assistance.
- Practice good hygiene.
- Use insect repellant when visiting endemic areas, and to apply it to clothing as well as exposed skin.
- Wear protective clothing, such as a long-sleeved shirt, pants securely tucked into laced boots, and a protective head covering such as a cap, when outdoors in areas where ticks are likely to be found.

Urinary tract infection

The two forms of urinary tract infection (UTI) are cystitis (infection of the bladder) and urethritis (infection of the urethra). UTI is nearly 10 times more common in females than in males (except in elderly males) and affects 10% to 20% of all females at least once. UTI is also a prevalent bacterial infection in children, with girls again more commonly affected than boys. In adult males and in children, UTIs are typically associated with anatomic or physiologic abnormalities and therefore need close evaluation. Most UTIs respond readily to treatment, but recurrence and resistant bacterial flare-up during therapy are possible.

CAUSES

Most UTIs result from ascending infection by a single gram-negative, enteric bacterium, such as *Escherichia coli*, *Klebsiella*, *Proteus*, *Enterobacter*, *Pseudomonas*, or *Serratia*. In a patient with neurogenic bladder, an indwelling urinary catheter, or a fistula between the intestine and bladder, UTI may result from simultaneous infection with multiple pathogens.

Studies suggest that infection results from a breakdown in local defense mechanisms in the bladder that allows bacteria to invade the bladder mucosa and multiply. These bacteria can't be readily eliminated by normal urination.

The pathogen's resistance to the prescribed antimicrobial therapy usually causes bacterial flare-up during treatment. Even a small number of bacteria (fewer than 10,000/ml) in a midstream urine specimen collected during treatment casts doubt on the effectiveness of treatment.

In most patients, recurrent UTIs result from re-infection by the same organism or by some new pathogen. In the remaining patients, recurrence reflects persistent infection, usually from renal calculi, chronic bacterial prostatitis, or a structural anomaly that is a source of infection. The high incidence of UTI among females is likely due to the natural anatomic features of females that facilitate infection. (See *UTI risk factors.*)

COMPLICATIONS

Untreated chronic UTI can seriously damage the urinary tract lining. Infection of adjacent organs and structures (for example, pyelonephritis) may also occur. When this happens, the prognosis is poor.

ASSESSMENT FINDINGS

The patient may complain of urinary urgency and frequency, dysuria, bladder cramps or spasms, itching, a feeling of warmth during urination, nocturia, and urethral discharge (in males). Other complaints include low back pain, malaise, nausea, vomiting, pain or tenderness over the bladder, chills, and flank pain. Inflammation of the bladder wall also causes hematuria and fever. The most common initial symptoms of UTI in elderly patients are lethargy and a change in mental status.

 ALERT Having a workup done on all children with proven UTI can exclude an abnormality of the urinary tract that would predispose them to renal damage.

DIAGNOSTIC TESTS

▶ Microscopic urinalysis showing red and white blood cell counts greater than 10 per high-power field suggests UTI. The presence of leukocyte esterase and nitrites may also indicate the presence of bacteria in the urine.
▶ Clean-catch urinalysis revealing a bacterial count of more than 100,000/ml confirms UTI. Lower counts don't necessarily rule out infection, especially if the patient is urinating frequently, because bacteria require 30 to 45 minutes to reproduce in urine.
▶ Sensitivity testing is used to determine the appropriate antimicrobial drug treatment.
▶ Voiding cystourethrography or excretory urography may disclose congenital anomalies that predispose the patient to recurrent UTI.

UTI risk factors

Certain factors increase the risk of UTI. These include natural anatomic variations, trauma or invasive procedures, urinary tract obstructions, and vesicourethral and vesicoureteral reflux, among others.

Natural anatomic variations

Females are more prone to UTIs than males because the female urethra is shorter than the male urethra (about 1 to 2″ [2.5 to 5 cm] compared with 7 to 8″ [18 to 20 cm]). It's also closer to the anus, allowing bacterial entry into the urethra from the vagina, perineum, or rectum or from a sexual partner.

Pregnant females are especially prone to UTIs because of hormonal changes. Also, the enlarged uterus displaces the bladder and exerts greater pressure on the ureters, increasing their length. This restricts urine flow, allowing bacteria to linger longer in the urinary tract.

In men, release of prostatic fluid serves as an antibacterial shield. Males lose this protection around age 50, when the prostate gland begins to grow. This enlargement, in turn, may promote urine retention.

Trauma or invasive procedures

Fecal matter, sexual intercourse, and medical instruments, such as catheters and cystoscopes, can introduce bacteria into the urinary tract to trigger infection.

Urinary tract obstructions

A narrowed ureter or calculi lodged in the ureters or bladder can obstruct urine flow. Slowed urine flow allows bacteria to remain and multiply, risking damage to the kidneys.

Vesicourethral and vesicoureteral reflux

Vesicourethral reflux results when pressure inside the bladder (caused by coughing or sneezing) pushes a small amount of urine from the bladder into the urethra. When pressure in the bladder returns to normal, the urine flows back into the bladder, bringing bacteria from the urethra with it.

In vesicoureteral reflux, urine flows from the bladder back into one or both ureters. The vesicoureteral valve normally shuts off reflux. However, damage can prevent the valve from doing its job.

Other risk factors

Urinary stasis can promote infection. Undetected infection can spread to the entire urinary system. Because urinary tract bacteria thrive on sugars, diabetes is also a risk factor.

TREATMENT

Appropriate antibiotics are the treatment of choice for most initial UTIs. A 7- to 10-day course is standard, but studies suggest that a single dose or a 3- to 5-day regimen may be sufficient to render the urine sterile. (Elderly patients may still need 7 to 10 days of antibiotics to fully benefit from treatment.) A culture that reveals nonsterile urine after 3 days of antibiotic therapy likely indicates bacterial resistance, and a different antibiotic is prescribed.

A single dose of amoxicillin or co-trimoxazole may be effective for females with acute, uncomplicated UTI. A urine culture 1 to 2 weeks later indicates whether the infection has been eradicated. Recurrent infections from infected renal calculi, chronic prostatitis, or structural abnormalities may necessitate surgery. Prostatitis also requires long-term antibiotic therapy. In patients without these predisposing conditions, long-term, low-dose antibiotic therapy is the treatment of choice. Fluoroquinolones aren't used in children because of possible adverse effects on developing cartilage.

NURSING CONSIDERATIONS

❱ Watch for GI disturbances related to antimicrobial therapy. If ordered, administer nitrofurantoin macrocrystals with milk or meals to prevent GI distress.

▌ Assess the need for a urinary catheter daily, and remove the catheter as soon as it is no longer needed.

▌ If sitz baths do not relieve perineal discomfort, apply warm compresses sparingly to the perineum, but be careful not to burn the patient. Apply topical antiseptics on the urethral meatus as necessary.

▌ Be careful and prompt when collecting urine specimens for culture and sensitivity.

▌ Have the patient use a commode rather than a bedpan, if possible, to promote sitting up, which assists in emptying the bladder.

PREVENTION Use strict sterile technique when inserting an indwelling urinary catheter. Do not interrupt the closed drainage system for any reason. Obtain urine specimens with a syringe inserted through the needleless aspirating port of the catheter itself. Clean the catheter insertion site with soap and water at least twice daily. Do not allow the catheter to become encrusted. To prevent accidental urine reflux, keep the drainage bag below the tubing and do not raise the bag above the bed, clamp the tubing, or empty the bag before transferring the patient to a

wheelchair or stretcher. If urine output is considerable, empty the bag more frequently than once every 8 hours because bacteria can multiply in standing urine and migrate up the catheter into the bladder.

Patient teaching

▌ Teach the patient about the infection, including its cause, diagnosis, and treatment.

▌ Explain the nature and purpose of antimicrobial therapy. Emphasize the importance of completing the prescribed course of therapy or, with long-term prophylaxis, of strictly adhering to the ordered dosage.

▌ Familiarize the patient with all prescribed medications, including any possible adverse effects. If antibiotics cause GI distress, explain that taking nitrofurantoin macrocrystals with milk or a meal can help prevent such problems. If therapy includes phenazopyridine, warn the patient that this drug turns urine red-orange and stains clothing.

▌ Explain that an uncontaminated midstream urine specimen is essential for accurate diagnosis. Before collection, teach the female patient to clean the perineum properly

PREVENTION

Preventing recurrent UTIs

Use the following points as a guide to help prevent recurrent UTIs in your patients:

• Teach the female patient to carefully wipe the perineum from front to back after urinating and to thoroughly clean the perineum with soap and water after bowel movements. If the patient is prone to infection, she should urinate immediately after sexual intercourse. Tell her never to postpone urination and to empty her bladder completely.

• Tell the male patient that prompt treatment of predisposing conditions, such as chronic prostatitis, helps prevent recurrent UTIs.

• Urge the patient to drink about 2 qt (2 L; about eight 8-oz glasses) of fluid a day during treatment. More or less than this

amount may alter the antimicrobial's effect. Be aware that the elderly patient may resist this suggestion because it causes him to make frequent trips, possibly up and down the stairs, to urinate.

• Explain that fruit juices, especially cranberry juice, and oral doses of vitamin C may help acidify urine and enhance the action of some medications.

• Tell the female patient that use of deodorant sprays or other feminine products, such as douches and powders, should be avoided because they can irritate the urethra.

• Encourage frequent comfort stops during long car trips.

• Teach proper catheter care if the patient is sent home with a catheter in place.

and to keep the labia separated during urination.

▶ For the patient with vesicoureteral reflux (which may cause UTI), teach the practice of double urinating (urinating once, then again in a few minutes) in order to ensure complete emptying of the bladder. Because the natural urge to urinate may be impaired, advise the patient to urinate every 2 to 3 hours regardless of whether he or she feels the urge.

▶ Review signs and symptoms of complications, such as persistent fever, decreased urine output, and abdominal or flank pain, and when to notify the physician.

▶ Teach the patient measures to prevent recurrence of a UTI. (See *Preventing recurrent UTIs*.)

CONTACT PRECAUTIONS

Vancomycin-resistant *Enterococcus* infection

Vancomycin-resistant *Enterococcus* (VRE) infection is a mutation of a common bacterium normally found in the GI tract. The infection is spread easily by direct person-to-person contact. Facilities in more than 40 states have reported VRE infections. In intensive care units (ICUs), 30% of *Enterococcus* infections have been found to be resistant to vancomycin. In non-ICU settings, resistance to vancomycin has been noted in 25% of *Enterococcus* infections.

Those most at risk for VRE infection include the following:

▶ Immunosuppressed patients, such as transplant recipients, or those with severe underlying disease
▶ Patients with a history of taking vancomycin, third-generation cephalosporins, antibiotics targeted at anaerobic bacteria (such as *Clostridium difficile*), or multiple courses of antibiotics
▶ Patients with indwelling urinary or central venous catheters
▶ Elderly patients, especially those with prolonged or repeated hospital admissions
▶ Patients with cancer or chronic renal failure
▶ Patients undergoing cardiothoracic or intra-abdominal surgery or organ transplantation
▶ Patients with wounds opening into the pelvic or intra-abdominal area, including surgical wounds, burns, and pressure ulcers
▶ Patients with enterococcal bacteremia, typically associated with endocarditis
▶ Patients exposed to contaminated equipment or to another VRE-positive patient, such as health care workers

CAUSES

Although there are 17 types of *Enterococcus* organisms, *E. faecalis* and *E. faecium* are the species most often cultured from humans (approximately 90%). *E. faecium* is most often vancomycin resistant. VRE enters health care facilities through an infected or colonized patient or a colonized health care worker. It can also develop following treatment with vancomycin. VRE spreads through direct contact between the patient and caregiver or between patients. It can also spread through patient contact with contaminated surfaces such as an over-bed table, where the microorganism is capable of living for weeks. VRE has also been detected on patient gowns, bed linens, and handrails.

COMPLICATIONS

VRE can result in sepsis, multisystem organ dysfunction, and death in immunocompromised patients.

ASSESSMENT FINDINGS

The patient who presents with risk factors should be considered for VRE infection. The causative agent may be found incidentally with culture results. Some institutions will routinely culture patients from long-term care facilities on admission. Once colonized, a patient is more than 10 times as likely to become infected with VRE, for example, through a breach in the immune system. The specific signs and symptoms related to VRE infection are associated with the enterococcal infection, such as urinary tract infection, endocarditis, meningitis, or wound infection.

DIAGNOSTIC TESTS

▶ A person with no signs or symptoms of infection is considered colonized if VRE can be isolated from a stool specimen or rectal swab.

TREATMENT

New antimicrobials, such as linezolid (Zyvox), quinupristin, or dalfopristin, are available for treatment of VRE infection. Patients who are already colonized with VRE usually aren't treated with antimicrobials.

Instead, the physician may stop all antibiotics and simply wait for normal bacteria to repopulate and replace the VRE strain. Combinations of various drugs may also be used, depending on the source of infection.

Patients with a positive culture for VRE in stool, blood, or wound drainage must be assigned a private room and placed on contact precautions to prevent transmission to other patients. Strict handwashing with an antimicrobial soap or an alcohol-based hand sanitizer must be emphasized. To prevent the spread of VRE, some facilities perform weekly surveillance cultures on at-risk patients in the ICU and/or oncology unit and on patients who have been transferred from a long-term care facility. Any colonized patient is then placed under contact precautions until he or she tests culture negative or until discharge. Colonization can last indefinitely; no protocol has been established for the length of time a patient should remain under contact precautions.

NURSING CONSIDERATIONS

▶ Hand hygiene before and after care of the patient is crucial. Good hand hygiene is the most effective way to prevent VRE from spreading. Use an antimicrobial soap such as chlorhexidine because bacteria have been cultured from workers' hands after they've washed with milder soap. Alcohol-based hand sanitizers are effective as well.

◗ Use contact precautions when in contact with the patient or the patient's environment. Provide the patient with a private room and dedicated equipment. Disinfect the environment and the equipment frequently.

▶ Change gloves when contaminated or when moving from a "soiled" area of the body to a clean one.

▶ Don't touch potentially contaminated surfaces such as over-bed tables after removing your gown and gloves.

▶ Be particularly prudent in caring for a patient with an ileostomy, colostomy, or draining wound that is not contained by a dressing.

▶ Consider grouping infected or colonized patients together and assigning the same nursing staff to them.

◗ Use dedicated equipment and leave it in the room for the duration of the contact precautions. Otherwise, wipe the equipment with the appropriate disinfectant before leaving the room.

▶ Ensure judicious and careful use of antibiotics. Encourage physicians to limit their use.

Patient teaching

▶ Teach the patient about the infection, including its cause, diagnosis, treatment, and transmission.

▶ Instruct the patient's family and friends regarding proper hand hygiene.

▶ Provide teaching and emotional support to the patient and family members.

▶ Review all prescribed medications, including dosage, administration, and possible adverse effects. Instruct patients to take antibiotics for the full period prescribed, even if feeling better.

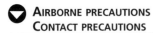

Varicella

Varicella, commonly known as chickenpox, is a common, acute, and very contagious infection. Varicella can occur at any age, but it's most common in children ages 2 to 8. Congenital varicella may affect infants whose mothers had acute infections during their first or early second trimester. Neonatal infection is rare, probably because of transient maternal immunity. However, neonates born to mothers who develop varicella from 5 days before to 2 days after delivery are at risk for developing severe generalized varicella.

Varicella occurs worldwide and is endemic in large cities. Outbreaks occur sporadically, usually in areas with large groups of susceptible children. It affects all races and both genders equally. Seasonal distribution varies; in temperate areas, the incidence is higher during late fall, winter, and spring. Second infections are rare.

Most children recover completely. Potentially fatal complications may affect children who are taking corticosteroids, antimetabolites, or other immunosuppressants and those with leukemia, neoplasms, or immunodeficiency disorders. Congenital and adult varicella may also have severe effects.

Causes

Caused by the herpesvirus varicella zoster—the same virus that, in its latent stage, causes herpes zoster (shingles)—varicella is transmitted by direct contact (primarily with respiratory secretions; less commonly, with skin lesions) or indirect contact (airborne). The incubation period usually lasts 14 to 17 days but can be as short as 10 days and as long as 20 days. (See *Incubation and duration of common rash-producing infections.*) Varicella is probably communicable from 1 day before lesions erupt to 6 days after vesicles form, although it's most contagious in the early stages of eruption of skin lesions.

Complications

Severe pruritus with this rash may provoke persistent scratching, which can lead to infection, scarring, impetigo, furuncles, and cellulitis. Rare complications include pneumonia, myocarditis, fulminating encephalitis (Reye syndrome), bleeding disorders, arthritis, nephritis, hepatitis, and acute myositis. Congenital varicella causes hypoplastic deformity and limb scarring, retarded growth, and central nervous system and eye manifestations.

Assessment findings

The patient's history reveals exposure within the past 2 to 3 weeks to someone with varicella. The infection produces distinctive signs and symptoms, notably a pruritic rash. During the prodromal phase, the patient has slight fever, malaise, and anorexia. Within 24 hours, the rash typically begins as crops of small, erythematous macules on the trunk or scalp. Macules progress to papules and then clear vesicles on an erythematous base (the so-called dewdrop on a rose petal). These vesicles become cloudy and break easily; then scabs form.

The rash spreads to the face and over the trunk, then to the limbs, buccal mucosa, axillae, upper respiratory tract, conjunctivae and, occasionally, the genitalia. New vesicles continue to appear for 3 or 4 days, so the rash contains a combination of red papules, vesicles, and scabs in various stages. Examination reveals a temperature of 101 to 103° F (38.3 to 39.4° C), which usually persists for 3 to 5 days. In progressive varicella, however, an immunocompromised patient may have more lesions and a high fever lasting for more than 7 days. These lesions often are hemorrhagic and take longer to heal.

Diagnostic tests

▶ Diagnosis rests on the characteristic clinical signs and usually doesn't require laboratory tests. However, the virus can be isolated from vesicular fluid within the first 3 or 4 days of the rash; Giemsa stain distinguishes varicella zoster from vaccinia and variola viruses.

Incubation and duration of common rash-producing infections

Infection	Incubation period (days)	Duration (days)
Herpes simplex	2 to 12	7 to 21
Roseola infantum	10 to 15	3 to 7
Rubella	12 to 23	5
Rubeola	10 to 12	3 to 5
Varicella	10 to 20	7 to 14

▶ Serum contains antibodies 7 days after onset.

TREATMENT

The Centers for Disease Control and Prevention recommends airborne and contact precautions until all vesicles and most of the scabs are dry (no new lesions; usually 1 week after the onset of the rash). Children with only a few remaining scabs are no longer contagious and can return to school. Congenital varicella requires no isolation.

In most patients with chickenpox, treatment consists of local or systemic antipruritics: lukewarm oatmeal baths, calamine lotion, and/or diphenhydramine (Benadryl) or another antihistamine. Antibiotics are unnecessary unless bacterial infection develops. Salicylates are contraindicated because of their link to Reye syndrome in children.

Patients who are susceptible to varicella may need special treatment. When given up to 72 hours after exposure to varicella, varicella zoster immune globulin may provide passive immunity. The antiviral agents acyclovir and famciclovir (Famvir) may slow vesicle formation, speed skin healing, and control the systemic spread of infection.

NURSING CONSIDERATIONS

▶ Care is supportive and emphasizes patient and family teaching and preventive measures.

▶ Tell the patient not to scratch the lesions. However, because the need to scratch may be overwhelming, parents should trim the child's fingernails or tie mittens on the hands.

◗ Maintain contact and airborne precautions while the patient is in the contagious stage of the illness.

Patient teaching

▶ Teach the child and family how to apply topical antipruritic medications correctly. Stress the importance of good hand hygiene.

▶ Warn parents to watch for and immediately report signs of complications. Severe skin pain and burning may indicate a serious secondary infection that requires prompt medical attention.

 PREVENTION

- Varicella vaccine, which is part of the recommended childhood immunization schedule, effectively prevents infection. It is also effective if given 5 days postexposure.

- To help prevent varicella, do not admit a child exposed to varicella to a unit that contains children who receive immunosuppressants or who have leukemia or other immunodeficiency disorders. An immune-suppressed child who has been exposed to varicella should be evaluated for administration of varicella zoster immune globulin to lessen the severity of the infection.

Vibriosis

Vibriosis is a bacterial infection acquired from eating raw or undercooked shellfish, particularly those found in warm coastal waters, such as oysters. It can also be acquired by swimming in warm ocean water with an open wound, especially on the fingers, palms of the hands, and soles of the feet, as the bacteria are found naturally in that environment. Vibriosis causes GI illness that can be mild or severe, although severe illness is rare. Infection can be fatal in immunocompromised patients.

CAUSES

Vibrio parahaemolyticus and *Vibrio vulnificus* cause vibriosis. *Vibrio* bacteria cause diarrhea, skin infections, and/or blood infections. The diarrhea-causing *V. parahaemolyticus* is a relatively harmless infection, but *V. vulnificus* infection, although rare, often progresses to blood poisoning and death. These bacteria live in brackish salt water along the coastal areas of the United States and Canada and thrive in the warmer summer months. Vibriosis is a reportable infection. Although underreported because laboratories may not always use the appropriate tests to specifically identify it, the infection is thought to affect approximately 4,500 people annually in the United States.

COMPLICATIONS

Complications of vibriosis include dehydration from severe fluid loss. Compartment syndrome may develop in patients with a wound infection. Patients with liver disease or underlying medical conditions (such as hemochromatosis or thalassemia) may develop disseminated intravascular coagulation, multiple organ dysfunction, or acute respiratory distress syndrome. Patients with diabetes, acquired immunodeficiency syndrome, or other immunosuppressive conditions are at increased risk of complications, including septicemia and death.

ASSESSMENT FINDINGS

Symptoms of vibriosis generally begin within 24 hours of ingestion and may last 2 to 10 days. The patient may present with the complaint of watery diarrhea, which may be accompanied by nausea, vomiting, abdominal pain, fever, and chills. Stools may be bloody. Signs and symptoms of dehydration may be present, such as poor skin turgor, tachycardia, and decreased blood pressure, depending on the severity of fluid loss. A patient with an open wound may present with pain, swelling, redness, and purulent drainage at the wound site, along with fever.

DIAGNOSTIC TESTS

▶ A patient history of ingesting raw shellfish or exposure to warm ocean water, along with signs and symptoms, could indicate infection with *V. parahaemolyticus* or *V. vulnificus*.

▶ Stool, blood, or wound cultures identify the causative organism. The medium needed for isolation contains thiosulfate, citrate, bile salts, and sucrose, and the laboratory should be instructed to use this medium if vibriosis is suspected.

▶ Serum electrolytes may be abnormal in a patient with gastroenteritis.

TREATMENT

Vibriosis is a self-limiting illness, and treatment is usually not necessary. Symptomatic treatment can be provided and includes adequate fluid intake and wound care, as appropriate. Antibiotics, such as doxycycline (Doryx), may be prescribed for patients with wound infections or if the illness is prolonged or severe. Surgical debridement of an infected wound may be necessary; a fasciotomy may be required if compartment syndrome develops.

NURSING CONSIDERATIONS

▶ Follow standard precautions. Report all cases of vibriosis to the local health department within 72 hours of identification.

PREVENTION Timely reporting of vibriosis to the local health department allows for investigation of the source of the infection. Shellfish experts may check harvest areas, such as oyster beds, and close areas that may cause infection to others.

▶ Monitor electrolyte values in the patient with profuse diarrhea. Administer replacement therapy as ordered.

▶ Monitor intake and output. Assess for signs and symptoms of dehydration, and encourage increased oral intake of fluids. If the patient is unable to sustain oral intake, administer I.V. fluids as ordered.

▶ Provide wound care, as indicated. Assess the wound for improvement or deterioration. Observe for compartment syndrome.

▶ Provide supportive care, especially if severe wound infection requires debridement or fasciotomy.

▶ Provide pain medication, as ordered, and evaluate 30 minutes after administration for effect.

Patient teaching

▶ Teach the patient about the infection, including its cause, diagnosis, treatment, and transmission.

▶ If the patient is placed on medication, review its dosage, administration, and possible adverse effects.

▶ Explain the signs and symptoms of complications and when to report them to the physician.

▶ Refer the patient to the Food and Drug Administration's Center for Food Safety and Applied Nutrition for more information regarding seafood consumption and handling.

 PREVENTION Teach the patient how to avoid vibriosis by following these recommendations:

- Do not eat raw or undercooked shellfish. Remember that contaminated seafood cannot be distinguished by smell or taste.
- Cook seafood appropriately: Fry, bake, steam, or boil oysters, mussels, or clams up to 9 minutes or until plump. Note that fish is cooked when the center is opaque.
- Avoid swimming in recreational areas with any open wound.
- Avoid handling food if experiencing diarrhea.
- Seek medical care with prolonged signs and symptoms of gastroenteritis or if a wound becomes inflamed and painful after swimming in warm coastal waters.

Vulvovaginitis

Vulvovaginitis is an inflammation of the vulva (vulvitis) and vagina (vaginitis) that may occur at any age and affects most females at some time. Because of the proximity of these two structures, inflammation of one usually precipitates inflammation of the other. The prognosis is good with treatment.

CAUSES

Common causes of vaginitis (with or without consequent vulvitis) include the following:

▶ Infection with *Trichomonas vaginalis*, a protozoan flagellate that is usually transmitted through sexual intercourse
▶ Infection with *Candida albicans*, a fungus that requires glucose for growth
▶ Bacterial vaginosis (previously known by various names such as *Gardnerella vaginalis*, *Haemophilus vaginalis*, and nonspecific vaginitis), which is characterized by a decrease in lactobacilli with a concomitant increase in anaerobic bacteria
▶ Venereal infection with *Neisseria gonorrhoeae* (gonorrhea), a gram-negative diplococcus
▶ Viral infection with genital warts (*Condylomata acuminata*) or herpes simplex virus type 2, which are usually transmitted by intercourse

Common causes of vulvitis (with or without consequent vaginitis) include the following:

▶ Parasitic infection (*Pthirus pubis*, or crab lice), traumatic injury, or poor personal hygiene
▶ Chemical irritations or allergic reactions to hygiene sprays, douches, detergents, clothing, or toilet paper
▶ Retention of a foreign body such as a tampon

Vaginal mucosal atrophy in menopausal women increases the risk for bacterial invasion because of decreasing estrogen levels.

COMPLICATIONS

Inflammation and edema may affect the perineum. Skin breakdown may lead to secondary infection.

ASSESSMENT FINDINGS

Signs and symptoms may vary according to the infecting organism:

▶ A patient with trichomonal vaginitis may have vaginal irritation and itching along with urinary symptoms, such as burning and frequency. Inspection may reveal vaginal discharge that's thin, bubbly, green tinged, and malodorous.
▶ A patient with candidal vaginitis may report intense vaginal itching and a thick, white, cottage-cheese-like discharge. Red, edematous mucous membranes with white flecks may be seen on the vaginal wall.
▶ In a patient with bacterial vaginosis, inspection may disclose a gray, foul, fishy-smelling discharge, although some patients may be asymptomatic.
▶ Gonorrhea may produce no symptoms, or inspection may reveal a profuse, purulent discharge; the patient may complain of dysuria.
▶ A patient with acute vulvitis may report vulvar burning, pruritus, severe dysuria, and dyspareunia. Inspection may reveal vulvar edema and erythema.
▶ In a patient with herpesvirus infection, ulceration or vesicle formation may be noted on the perineum during the active phase; in a patient with chronic infection, severe edema may involve the entire perineum.

DIAGNOSTIC TESTS

▶ Wet slide preparation of vaginal exudate identifies the infectious organism. With trichomonal infection, the presence of motile, flagellated trichomonads confirms the diagnosis.
▶ With monilial vaginitis, 10% potassium hydroxide is added to the slide; diagnosis requires identification of *C. albicans* fungus.

With bacterial vaginosis, a saline wet mount shows the presence of clue cells (epithelial cells with bacteria adherent to the cell wall), giving a stippled appearance.

Diagnosis of gonorrhea requires a culture of vaginal exudate.

Diagnosis of vulvitis or a suspected sexually transmitted infection (STI) may require a complete blood count, urinalysis, cytology screening, biopsy of chronic lesions (to rule out cancer), and culture of exudate from acute lesions.

TREATMENT

Common therapeutic measures in vulvovaginitis include the following:

Oral metronidazole (Flagyl) for a patient with trichomonal vaginitis; all sexual partners should also be treated (if possible) because recurrence commonly results from reinfection by an infected, asymptomatic male

Topical miconazole 2% or clotrimazole 1% for candidal infection

Metronidazole for bacterial vaginosis

Systemic antibiotic for a patient with gonorrhea and all sexual partners

Doxycycline (Doryx) or erythromycin (E-mycin) for a concurrent chlamydial infection

Cold compresses or cool sitz baths to relieve pruritus in patients with acute vulvitis; severe inflammation may require warm compresses. Other therapies include avoiding drying soaps, wearing loose-fitting clothing to promote air circulation, and applying a topical corticosteroid to reduce inflammation.

Chronic vulvitis may respond to topical hydrocortisone or an antipruritic and good hygiene (especially in elderly or incontinent patients). Topical estrogen ointments may be used to treat atrophic vulvovaginitis. There's no cure for herpesvirus infections; however, oral and topical acyclovir reduce the duration of infection and severity of symptoms in patients with active lesions. Local treatment of genital warts usually consists of the application of trichloroacetic acid.

NURSING CONSIDERATIONS

Provide comfort measures, such as cool or warm compresses, to alleviate pain, burning, and pruritus.

Use meticulous handwashing technique. If necessary, use wound and skin precautions.

 SAFETY Report cases of STI to public health authorities.

Patient teaching

 PREVENTION Teach the patient about the correlation between sexual contact and the spread of vaginal infections. Provide information about the use of condoms to prevent or decrease the spread of STIs. Advise the patient to notify her sexual partners of the need for treatment and to abstain from sexual intercourse until the infection resolves.

Instruct the patient to take the entire course of prescribed medication, as ordered, even if symptoms subside.

Teach the patient how to insert vaginal ointments and suppositories. Emphasize the need for meticulous handwashing before and after drug administration. Advise her that scratching can cause skin breakdown and secondary infections.

Encourage good hygiene. Advise the patient with a history of recurrent vulvovaginitis to wear all-cotton underpants. Tell her to avoid wearing tight-fitting pants and pantyhose.

Warn the patient on metronidazole therapy to abstain from alcoholic beverages because alcohol may provoke a disulfiram-type reaction.

West Nile virus infection

West Nile virus (WNV) is a flavivirus commonly found in humans, birds, and other vertebrates in Africa, West Asia, and the Middle East. The disease is part of a family of vector-borne diseases that also includes malaria, yellow fever, and Lyme disease.

WNV occurs mainly in late summer and early fall. In climates where temperatures are milder, West Nile encephalitis (which stems from WNV) can occur year-round.

The risk of contracting WNV is greater for residents of areas where active cases have been identified. Individuals older than age 50 and those with compromised immune systems are at greatest risk. A number of studies have described the transmission of WNV in utero with subsequent fetal damage. There have also been documented cases of WNV transmission to infants through breast milk. The mortality rate for WNV in the general population ranges from 3% to 15%; it is higher in the elderly.

CAUSES

Birds serve as the reservoir for WNV; mosquitoes are the vector. The virus is transmitted to birds and humans through the bite of an infected mosquito (primarily *Culex*). Mosquitoes acquire WNV by feeding on birds infected with the virus. The mosquitoes may then transmit the virus to humans and animals when taking a blood meal.

Ticks infected with WNV have been found only in Africa and Asia. The role of ticks in the transmission and maintenance of the virus remains uncertain; to date, ticks have not been considered a vector for transmission in the United States.

The Centers for Disease Control and Prevention has reported that there is no evidence that a person can contract the virus by handling live or dead infected birds. However, people should be instructed to use gloves or double plastic bags to place the carcass of any dead bird or animal in a garbage can; the finding should be reported to the local health department.

COMPLICATIONS

Complications of WNV include progression to tremors, occasional convulsions, paralysis, coma, and (rarely) death.

ASSESSMENT FINDINGS

The incubation period for WNV is 5 to 15 days after exposure. Most patients bitten by an infected mosquito develop no symptoms at all. Only 1 in 300 people who are bitten by an infected mosquito actually get sick.

Mild infections with fever, headache, and body aches, often accompanied by rash and swollen lymph glands, are most common. Headache, high fever, neck stiffness, stupor, and disorientation can occur in patients with severe infections.

DIAGNOSTIC TESTS

▶ The immunoglobulin M antibody-capture enzyme-linked immunosorbent assay (MAC-ELISA) is the test of choice for obtaining a rapid definitive diagnosis of WNV infection.
▶ An accurate diagnosis is possible only when serum or CSF specimens are obtained while the patient is still hospitalized with acute illness.

TREATMENT

No specific therapeutic strategy has been established for WNV, and there is no known cure. Treatment is generally aimed at controlling the specific symptoms. Supportive measures, such as I.V. fluids, fever control, and respiratory support, are rendered when necessary. No vaccine exists at present to prevent the transmission of WNV.

NURSING CONSIDERATIONS

▶ Obtain an extensive patient travel history for the previous 2 to 3 weeks (especially around bodies of water, such as lakes and ponds), noting the presence of dead birds and mosquito bites.

▶ Perform a comprehensive physical assessment, and report signs of fever, headache, lymphadenopathy, and maculopapular rash.
▶ Perform a complete neurologic examination, and report any signs of confusion, lethargy, weakness, or slurred speech.
▶ Strictly monitor strict intake and output. Maintain adequate hydration with I.V. fluids.
▶ Administer fever-control measures.
▶ Provide respiratory support measures when applicable.
▶ Although WNV is not transmitted from person to person, employ standard precautions when handling the blood or other body fluids of an infected person.
▶ Report suspected cases of WNV to the state health department.

Patient teaching

▶ Teach the patient about the infection, including its cause, diagnosis, and treatment.
▶ Review all prescribed medication, including dosage, administration, and possible adverse effects.

 PREVENTION To reduce their risk of becoming infected with WNV, advise patients as follows:
- Stay indoors at dawn, dusk, and in the early evening.
- Wear long-sleeved shirts and long pants when outdoors.
- Apply insect repellent sparingly to exposed skin and clothing. Effective repellents contain 20% to 30% DEET (N,N-diethyltoluamide). DEET in high concentrations (more than 30%) can cause adverse effects, particularly in children; avoid products containing more than 30% DEET.

- Insect repellents can irritate the eyes and mouth, so avoid applying them to the hands of children. Insect repellents should not be applied to children younger than age 3.
- Whenever you use an insecticide or insect repellent, be sure to read and follow the manufacturer's directions for use, as printed on the product.
- Note that vitamin B and ultrasonic devices are not effective in preventing mosquito bites.

Whipple disease

Whipple disease is a rare systemic infection that affects the small intestine, joints, central nervous system (CNS), and cardiovascular system. Typically beginning as gastroenteritis, it is slowly progressive, with relapsing signs and symptoms. Fewer than 1,000 cases have been reported worldwide, mostly in North America and Western Europe. Whipple disease has been found primarily to affect white men over the age of 40. Recent studies have shown that the causative bacterium, *Tropheryma whippleii*, is present in fecal samples from healthy adults in Europe (1% to 11%) and in children from Senegal (44%). Diagnosis is sometimes difficult, as this is a rare disease. Without proper treatment, however, Whipple disease is fatal.

CAUSES

In patients with Whipple disease, *T. whippleii* bacteria infiltrate the tissue of various body systems, such as the lamina propria of the small bowel, synovial tissue in the joints, heart valves, and CNS. The exact method by which Whipple disease is acquired has not been established.

COMPLICATIONS

Irreversible CNS complications may occur in Whipple disease, such as seizures or dementia. Left untreated, Whipple disease is always fatal.

ASSESSMENT FINDINGS

Patients with Whipple disease usually present with GI complaints of chronic watery or fatty diarrhea, abdominal pain that is usually more severe after eating, and weight loss. Other initial complaints may include joint pain, fever, blurry vision or night blindness, and chest pain. Inspection may reveal a patient who appears cachetic with a distended abdomen. Peristalsis may be visible and hyperactive bowel sounds audible. Chvostek

and Trousseau signs may be elicited. Gingivitis may be present. Abdominal palpation may reveal tenderness and detect an ill-defined mass. With CNS involvement, ataxia or clonus may be noted, and signs of meningoencephalitis may be present. The family may also report cognitive or personality changes in the patient or an altered mental status.

Many patients may have symptoms for up to 5 years before seeking care because of the vagueness of the initial symptoms. A proposed staging of Whipple disease follows:
▶ Nonspecific: Lasting approximately 5 years, this stage includes joint pain, low-grade fever, a feeling of abdominal fullness, and cough.
▶ Abdominal: Lasting approximately 10 to 20 years, this stage includes chronic diarrhea, anorexia, weight loss, and abdominal pain.
▶ Generalized: Possibly lasting 5 years until death, if left untreated, this stage includes cachexia, fatty stools, and cardiovascular and neurologic involvement.

DIAGNOSTIC TESTS

▶ Results of upper GI computed tomography and a small-bowel series are abnormal in patients with Whipple disease, showing bowel dilation with flocculation and segmentation of barium, although these findings may be nonspecific.
▶ GI biopsy reveals foamy macrophages containing periodic-acid-Schiff-positive, gram-positive bacilli in the mucosal lamina of the small intestine.
▶ Culture of saliva, intestinal fluid, or tissue identifies *T. whippleii*.
▶ Cerebrospinal fluid (CSF) analysis may confirm Whipple disease if the CNS is involved.
▶ Seventy-two-hour fecal fat determination may identify malabsorption but is not specific for Whipple disease.
▶ Magnetic resonance imaging of the brain may be abnormal in a patient with Whipple disease but is not specific for CNS involvement.

TREATMENT

The treatment for Whipple disease is a prolonged course of antibiotics with trimethoprim-sulfamethoxazole (Bactrim). The course is prolonged because relapse has occurred with the usual 2-week course. Penicillin may be used as an alternative therapy but should be followed by 1 year of treatment with trimethoprim-sulfamethoxazole. If a relapse occurs, patients are treated with a 2-week course of parenteral antibiotics followed by another 1 to 2 years of treatment with trimethoprim-sulfamethoxazole. Other symptoms, such as fever and joint pain, may be treated with antipyretics, such as acetaminophen (Tylenol), or analgesics, such as ibuprofen (Motrin).

NURSING CONSIDERATIONS

▶ After establishing allergies, administer medication as ordered and monitor for adverse effects.

▶ The mode of transmission has not been established for Whipple disease; therefore, use standard precautions.

▶ Offer comfort measures, such as tepid baths or frequent repositioning. Administer antipyretics or analgesics as needed, and monitor their effects after 30 minutes.

▶ Provide skin and perineal care, especially to the incontinent patient.

▶ Monitor nutritional status. Encourage fluid intake, and administer I.V. fluids if ordered. Record daily weight.

▶ Monitor neurologic status. Report any change in mental status or seizure activity. Initiate seizure precautions, if indicated.

▶ Monitor laboratory values of the patient with frequent diarrhea. Administer electrolyte replacement therapy as indicated.

▶ Provide emotional support to the patient and family.

Patient teaching

▶ Unfortunately, Whipple disease is sometimes challenging to diagnose; therefore, educating the patient about the specific disease may be delayed until the diagnosis is established. Once the diagnosis is confirmed, teach the patient and family about the cause, diagnosis, and treatment of Whipple disease. If the patient has advanced disease, be sure to explain the prognosis and supportive care that will be provided.

▶ Review all prescribed medication, including dosage, administration, and possible adverse effects. Emphasize the importance of adhering to the prescribed treatment plan in order to avoid relapse or worsening of condition.

▶ Discuss signs and symptoms of complications, such as increasing CNS deterioration or a relapse of symptoms, and when to notify the physician.

▶ Encourage regular follow-up to monitor response to treatment. Repeat testing of saliva, stool, blood, or CSF may be needed to monitor treatment response and detect a possible relapse.

▶ Review end-of-life care with the family of the patient with advanced disease, if they are open to the discussion. Refer the patient and family to social services and hospice care, as appropriate.

CONTACT PRECAUTIONS

Yaws

Yaws, also known as pian, parangi, paru, and frambesia tropica, is a chronic, relapsing skin infection characterized by bumps on the hands, feet, face, and genital area. Following the initial skin infection, the joints and bones may also become affected.

Yaws occurs mainly in warm, humid regions and mostly affects children under age 15. Risk factors include overcrowded living conditions and poor hygiene. Yaws is not typically seen in the United States; the incidence is highest in tropical areas of Africa, Asia, South and Central America, and the Pacific Islands. According to the World Health Organization, approximately 460,000 new cases of yaws are diagnosed annually.

CAUSES

Yaws is caused by the spirochete *Treponema pertenue*, which penetrates an area of broken skin, such as an insect bite, scrape, cut, or abrasion. The initial lesion, called the mother yaw, is a painless ulceration that takes 2 to 8 weeks to grow. It contains a large amount of spirochetes that can be transmitted from person to person via skin contact. In late yaws, the lesions are no longer contagious.

COMPLICATIONS

Complications of yaws include secondary bacterial infection and scarring. Similar to tertiary syphilis, bone, cartilage, skin, and soft tissue may be affected in untreated patients after 5 to 10 years. Resulting conditions may include gangosa (destructive ulcerations of the nasopharynx, palate, and nose); painful skeletal deformities, especially of the legs (termed saber shins); and other soft-tissue changes (gummas, inflammatory cell infiltration).

ASSESSMENT FINDINGS

Yaws has four stages. In the primary stage, a large bump lesion develops up to 3 weeks after inoculation. Called the mother yaw, this lesion is also known as buba, buba madre, or primary frambesioma. It is slightly elevated with a crust that sheds, leaving an area that resembles the texture of a raspberry or strawberry. The lesion is painless, although lymph nodes in the area may be swollen. A light-colored scar remains when the lesion heals, usually in 2 to 9 months. Bone and joint pain and swelling may occur in early disease. Other symptoms include fatigue, general malaise, and anorexia.

About 6 to 16 weeks after the primary stage, secondary lesions, called daughter yaws, develop. The lesions in this secondary stage appear either near the initial lesion or elsewhere on the body, frequently near body orifices, such as the mouth and nose. Crab yaws, which are thick hyperkeratotic plaques, may appear on the palms of the hands and soles of the feet. These lesions are painful and cause the patient to have a crablike gait, hence the name. Lymph nodes may again be swollen, and the lesions may be filled with pus. After the lesions open, they ulcerate. The patient may complain of anorexia and malaise. Secondary lesions may take up to 6 months to heal.

The latent stage occurs when the patient no longer experiences symptoms, although skin lesions may develop occasionally. These skin lesions may recur for 5 years after the infection.

Only 10% of untreated patients with yaws experience the tertiary stage; most continue in the latent stage for the rest of their lives. During the tertiary stage, painless subcutaneous nodules develop and progressively enlarge. These lesions become abscessed, necrotic, and ulcerated. They may become infected and affect underlying structures, such as bones and joints. The lesions may cause deformities and contractures by forming serpiginous tracts that heal with keloid formation.

DIAGNOSTIC TESTS

▶ Clinical features, a history of living in an area where yaws occurs, or contact with someone who has yaws is usually sufficient for diagnosis.

▶ Confirmatory treponemal tests may be helpful but are not always practical based on the area of occurrence.

TREATMENT

A single dose of penicillin G benzathine given by I.M. injection is enough to cure yaws in the primary, secondary and, usually, the latent phase. Erythromycin (E-Mycin), doxycycline (Doryx), and tetracycline are alternative drugs for patients who are allergic to penicillin. Oral therapy may be prescribed but is not as reliable. The patient is no longer contagious 24 hours after treatment. Lesions usually heal within 1 to 2 weeks after treatment.

Patients in the tertiary stage are treated symptomatically, although antibiotics may not be as effective during this stage. A vaccine has not been developed to prevent yaws. After treatment, yaws does not normally recur.

NURSING CONSIDERATIONS

◉ Follow standard and contact precautions. Yaws is transmitted skin to skin, so be sure to wear personal protective equipment.

▶ After checking for allergies, administer medication as ordered. Observe for adverse effects.

▶ Provide appropriate skin care to existing lesions.

▶ If a patient in the tertiary stage has resulting deformities, assist with passive or active range-of-motion exercises.

▶ Provide emotional support for the patient and family if the patient is experiencing any deformities from late yaws.

Patient teaching

▶ Teach the patient and family about the infection, including its cause, diagnostic tests, and treatment.

 SAFETY Be sure to explain how yaws is transmitted, and emphasize to family members that they should avoid contact with the patient's lesions, especially if the family member has any break in skin integrity.

▶ Discuss treatment if other family members develop lesions.

Yellow fever

Throughout history, yellow fever has been a devastating viral hemorrhagic infection. It is a flavivirus whose symptoms range from none to hemorrhagic fever. In the past, the incidence of yellow fever was controlled by vaccination along with mosquito control; however, the incidence is on the rise in poorer countries, such as tropical Africa and Central and South America. The rare occurrence in the United States has been related to international travel. Worldwide, an estimated 200,000 cases are diagnosed annually.

CAUSES

Yellow fever is a virus transmitted by *Aedes aegypti* mosquitoes worldwide, by *Haemagogus* mosquitoes in South America, and by *Aedes africanus* mosquitoes in Africa. The mosquitoes bite monkeys, which act as hosts for the virus, and then the mosquitoes bite humans, transmitting the disease via saliva. The virus can also be transmitted directly by mosquitoes to humans, especially in urban areas. People who work in or near mosquito-infested areas are at increased risk for contracting yellow fever. A successfully treated bout of yellow fever confers lasting immunity.

 PREVENTION The yellow fever vaccine has been in use for several decades and confers immunity for approximately 10 years. It should be obtained by people traveling to or living in areas where yellow fever has been reported, such as parts of South America and Africa. Some countries require proof of vaccination. The vaccine should also be given to laboratory personnel who are exposed to the yellow fever virus. Four groups of persons who should not take the vaccine include infants under age 6 months, pregnant women, persons who are allergic to eggs, and persons who are immune suppressed.

COMPLICATIONS

Complications of yellow fever include coagulopathy and bleeding problems, liver failure and, possibly, renal failure. Secondary infections may lead to respiratory failure. Delirium and coma may occur. Yellow fever is fatal in 15% to more than 50% of patients, primarily in those who progress to the toxic phase.

ASSESSMENT FINDINGS

The patient who develops yellow fever will have a history of travel to an endemic area or live in a mosquito-infested area with a low immunization history. Symptoms begin approximately 3 to 6 days after inoculation and include mild flu-like symptoms of fever, malaise, headache, and myalgia.

During the acute phase, the patient may complain of fever, nausea, bilious vomiting, Faget sign (a slow heart rate despite fever), anorexia, and conjunctival injection. The patient may have a red face or tongue. A short "period of intoxication," or remission, may then occur, during which the patient is asymptomatic. The return of signs and symptoms marks the toxic phase, during which the patient may again experience fevers along with profound weakness, somnolence, jaundice, headache, and lumbosacral pain. Signs of bleeding develop due to hepatic coagulopathy and may include epistaxis, hematemesis (bloody emesis), bleeding gums, oozing from venipuncture sites, petechiae, and bruising. In later stages, the patient may show signs of shock (hypotension, altered level of consciousness, seizures) as well as metabolic acidosis, cardiac arrhythmias, and acute renal failure.

DIAGNOSTIC TESTS

▶ A presumptive diagnosis may be made based on the patient's history and symptoms.
▶ Enzyme immunoassay detects yellow fever antigen.
▶ Immunoglobulin (Ig) M antibody-capture enzyme-linked immunosorbent assay (MAC-ELISA) detects specific IgM for yellow fever.

▶ Liver biopsy may reveal mottled yellow color and friable texture; however, liver biopsy is contraindicated due to the risk of hemorrhage.

▶ A complete blood count shows ÿeucopenia, thrombocytopenia, and decreased hemoglobin and hematocrit levels, with bleeding. Prothrombin time is increased, and clotting time may be prolonged; fibrinogen maybe decreased, and the presence of fibrin split products may indicate disseminated intravascular coagulation. Liver function tests may be abnormal.

TREATMENT

Yellow fever has no specific treatment, other than supportive. Severely ill patients will need treatment in an intensive care unit. Ventilator support may be needed for respiratory failure. Fluids and vasopressors should be administered as indicated. Blood products, such as fresh-frozen plasma and packed red blood cells, may be required if coagulopathy and bleeding occur. Nutritional support may be provided by tube feedings or parenteral nutrition. Dialysis may be required in patients with renal failure.

NURSING CONSIDERATIONS

▶ Maintain standard precautions. Be sure to keep mosquitoes away from patients, as a mosquito can transmit infection from the patient to another person. Use mosquito netting around the patient if appropriate.

▶ Monitor vital signs, including pulse oximetry.

▶ Monitor neurologic status for changes in mental state or level of consciousness.

▶ Monitor cardiac function continuously, including for arrhythmias.

▶ Assist with endotracheal intubation and ventilator management if the patient develops respiratory failure.

▶ Monitor laboratory values, and report abnormalities to the physician. Administer blood products, as indicated.

▶ Provide emotional support to the patient and family.

Patient teaching

▶ Teach the patient and family about the infection, including its cause, diagnosis, and treatment.

▶ Review all prescribed medication, including dosage, administration, and possible adverse effects.

▶ Discuss signs and symptoms of complications and when to notify the physician.

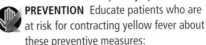 **PREVENTION** Educate patients who are at risk for contracting yellow fever about these preventive measures:

- Apply insect repellent when outdoors, both to exposed skin and to clothing. Use an insect repellent that is registered with the Environmental Protection Agency, such as one containing DEET (N,N-diethyltoluamide).

- When possible, wear long sleeves, long pants, and socks.

- Stay indoors during peak mosquito biting hours—from dusk to dawn. However, *A. aegypti* mosquitoes feed during the day, so in areas where this mosquito dwells, wear mosquito repellent when going outdoors.

- Obtain the yellow fever vaccine if traveling to or living in an area with known cases of yellow fever.

CONTACT PRECAUTIONS

Yersiniosis

Yersiniosis is a rare infectious disease that causes bacterial gastroenteritis. Symptoms vary according to the age of the infected person. It mostly affects young children, predominantly those under age 12 months. Yersiniosis occurs more frequently in cooler climates. The Centers of Disease Control and Prevention (CDC) estimates that 17,000 cases occur in the United States each year. The disease is more common in Japan, Scandinavia, and Europe.

CAUSES

Yersinia enterocolitica, a rod-shaped bacterium, causes yersiniosis. Pigs are a reservoir for some strains of this bacterium, with other strains being found in rodents, rabbits, sheep, cattle, horses, dogs, and cats. Transmission is through ingestion of contaminated food, especially raw or undercooked pork products, including chitterlings (pig intestines), as well as tofu, meats, oysters, and fish. It may also be transmitted after handling contaminated food, not cleaning the hands properly, and then touching toys, bottles, or pacifiers. Transmission may also occur through drinking contaminated unpasteurized milk or untreated water. Rarely, yersiniosis can be transmitted by the fecal-oral route as a result of poor handwashing after defecation. Blood transfusion can cause direct inoculation of the bacteria.

 PREVENTION The Foodborne Diseases Active Surveillance Network (FoodNet) conducts investigations of yersiniosis outbreaks. Their results are also monitored by the CDC. Together, FoodNet and the CDC look for ways to control and prevent outbreaks. An educational campaign has been instituted to increase awareness of preventive measures the public can follow to prevent *Y. enterocolitica* infection.

Other U.S. government agencies that monitor food safety include the Food and Drug Administration, which inspects imported food and milk pasteurization plants; the Department of Agriculture, which monitors the health of food animals and the quality of slaughtered and processed meat; and the Environmental Protection Agency, which monitors the safety of drinking water.

COMPLICATIONS

Complications of yersiniosis are rare but may include joint pain, most commonly in the knees, ankles, or wrists, which usually resolves within 6 months. Erythema nodosum, a rash, may develop on the legs and trunk and resolves within a month. More serious complications include bacteremia, enterocolitis, pseudoappendicitis, mesenteric adenitis, reactive arthritis, septicemia, pharyngitis, dermatitis, myocarditis, and glomerulonephritis. Death may occur as a result of bacteremia, which affects older patients more often than younger patients.

ASSESSMENT FINDINGS

In children, the symptoms of yersiniosis develop 4 to 7 days after exposure and include low-grade fever, abdominal pain, diarrhea and, occasionally, vomiting. These symptoms may last 2 to 3 weeks. With severe illness, diarrhea may become bloody. In adults and older children, signs and symptoms of yersiniosis often mimic those of appendicitis, with right-sided abdominal pain, fever, and leukocytosis.

DIAGNOSTIC TESTS

▶ Stool culture identifies the organism, but the laboratory may need to be asked to test specifically for *Y. enterocolitica*.
▶ Throat, lymph node, synovial fluid, urine, bile, and blood cultures may identify *Y. enterocolitica*.
▶ Stool samples are positive for leukocytes.
▶ Computed tomography or ultrasonography of the abdomen may rule out appendicitis.

▶ Colonoscopy may show exudates and left-sided colitis, but findings are usually nonspecific.

TREATMENT

Although most cases of yersiniosis resolve without treatment, more severe cases may be treated with antibiotics, such as aminoglycosides, doxycycline (Doryx), trimethoprim-sulfamethoxazole (Bactrim), or fluoroquinolones. Fluids and electrolytes should be provided as needed. Complications should be treated symptomatically. Analgesia may be administered for pain. Skin care should be provided.

NURSING CONSIDERATIONS

⬇ Initiate contact precautions for patients who are diapered or incontinent; for all other patients, use standard precautions.
▶ Be sure to wash hands thoroughly after contact with an infected patient.
▶ Administer pain medications as ordered, and evaluate their effects after 30 minutes.
▶ Send stool specimens to the laboratory as ordered for testing. Assist with acquiring other samples, such as synovial fluid via joint aspiration, as appropriate.
▶ Provide good skin care, especially in patients with frequent diarrhea.
▶ Monitor laboratory values. Administer electrolyte replacement therapy as ordered.
▶ Encourage oral fluids. If the patient is unable to tolerate oral fluids, administer I.V. fluids as ordered.

Patient teaching
▶ Teach the patient and family about the infection, including its cause, diagnosis, and treatment.
▶ Review how the infection is transmitted. Stress the importance of proper handwashing.

PREVENTION To prevent yersiniosis, tell the patient and family to avoid eating raw or undercooked pork as well as unpasteurized milk or milk products. Stress the importance of washing hands with soap and water before handling food, including raw meat; after using the bathroom; and after contact with animals. Be sure to clean all surfaces with hot, soapy water after preparing raw meat.

After preparing chitterlings (pig intestines), be sure to wash hands thoroughly, including under the fingernails, before touching infants or their belongings.

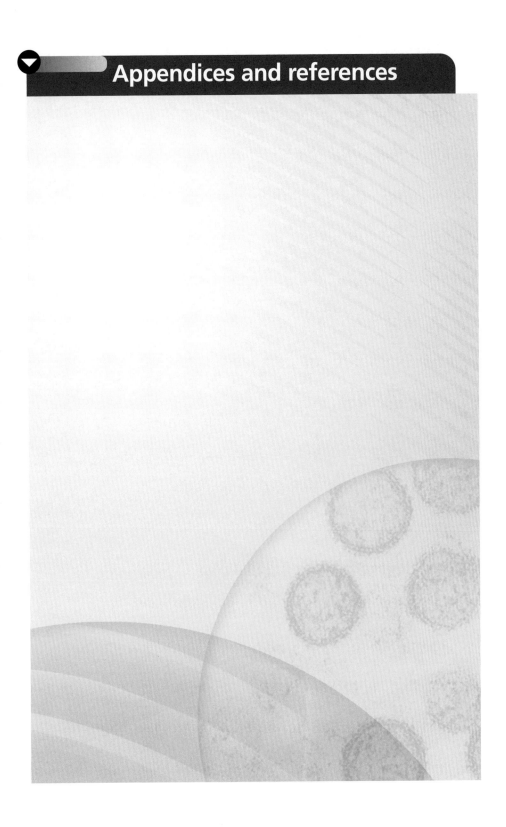

Appendices and references

Guide to anti-infective drugs

Drug classes & examples	Pharmacodynamics	Pharmacotherapeutics
Antibacterial drugs		
Aminoglycosides • Amikacin • Gentamicin • Neomycin • Paromomycin • Streptomycin • Tobramycin	Have bactericidal action against susceptible organisms by binding to the bacterium's 30S subunit, a specific ribosome, thereby interrupting protein synthesis and causing the bacterium to die.	• Many gram-negative (such as *Pseudomonas*) and some gram-positive (such as *Enterococcus*) bacilli • Serious health care–associated infections (gram-negative bacteremia, peritonitis, pneumonia) • Urinary tract infection (UTI) caused by enteric bacilli resistant to less toxic antibiotics (penicillin, cephalosporin) • Central nervous system and eye infections • Used in combination with penicillin to treat gram-positive organisms
Penicillins • Penicillin G benzathine • Penicillin V potassium • Amoxicillin • Ampicillin	Have bactericidal action by binding reversibly to several enzymes outside the bacterial cytoplasmic membrane. Interference with the enzymes inhibits cell-wall synthesis, causing rapid destruction of the cell.	• Gram-positive infections (such as *Listeria*) • Gram-negative infections (such as *Neisseria gonorrhoeae*)
Cephalosporins • Cefazolin • Cephalexin • Cefoxitin • Cefuroxime • Cefixime • Cefotaxime • Ceftriaxone	Inhibit cell-wall synthesis by binding to the bacterial enzymes located on the cell membrane. The body's natural defense mechanisms can then destroy the bacteria.	• First and second generations act against gram-positive organisms (such as *Streptococcus*) and are also used as an alternative to penicillin • Third generation acts against gram-negative organisms (such as *Neisseria meningitidis*) • Fourth generation acts against many gram-positive and gram-negative bacteria and is the drug of choice for treating *Pseudomonas aeruginosa* infection
Tetracyclines • Demeclocycline hydrochloride • Doxycycline	Have bacteriostatic action by inhibiting the growth or multiplication of bacteria. They penetrate the bacterial cell wall by an energy-dependent process. Within the cell, they bind primarily to a subunit of the ribosome, inhibiting the protein synthesis needed to maintain the bacterial cell.	• Gram-positive (such as *Actinomyces israelii*) and gram-negative (such as *Bordetella pertussis*) bacteria • Rickettsiae • Some protozoa

Drug classes & examples	Pharmacodynamics	Pharmacotherapeutics
Lincomycin derivative • Clindamycin	Inhibits bacterial protein synthesis by inhibiting the binding of bacterial ribosomes. Clindamycin is primarily bacteriostatic against most organisms.	• Aerobic gram-positive organisms (such as *Staphylococcus*) • Most anaerobes; anaerobic intra-abdominal, pleural, or pulmonary infections caused by *Bacteroides fragilis* • Clindamycin and lincomycin are alternatives to penicillin for staphylococcal infections
Macrolides • Erythromycin • Azithromycin • Clarithromycin	Inhibit RNA-dependent protein synthesis by acting on a small portion of the ribosome.	• Gram-positive and gram-negative bacteria • Drug of choice for treating *Mycoplasma pneumoniae* infections and pneumonia caused by *Legionella pneumophila* • Alternative to penicillin for infections caused by group A beta-hemolytic streptococci or *Streptococcus pneumoniae*; gonorrhea and syphilis in those intolerant to penicillin G or tetracyclines • Minor staphylococcal infections of the skin • Used in combination with antacids, histamine-2 blockers, and proton pump inhibitors to treat *Helicobacter pylori*–induced duodenal ulcer disease
Vancomycin	Inhibits cell wall synthesis, damaging the bacterial plasma membrane. The body's natural defenses then attack the organism.	• Gram-positive organisms, such as *Staphylococcus aureus*, *Staphylococcus epidermidis*, *Streptococcus pyogenes*, *Enterococcus*, and *S. pneumoniae* • Used in combination with aminoglycosides for treating *Enterococcus faecalis* endocarditis in those allergic to penicillin
Carbapenems • Ertapenem • Imipenem-cilastatin • Meropenem	Beta-lactam antibiotics are bactericidal and exert antibacterial activity by inhibiting bacterial cell-wall synthesis.	• Aerobic gram-positive bacteria (such as *Streptococcus*, *S. aureus*, and *S. epidermidis*); most anaerobic bacteria, (such as *B. fragilis*) • Most *Enterobacter* species • Health care–associated infections and infections in immunocompromised patients caused by mixed aerobic and anaerobic organisms • Bacterial meningitis caused by susceptible organisms • Intra-abdominal, skin, urinary tract, and gynecologic infections

Drug classes & examples	Pharmacodynamics	Pharmacotherapeutics
Monobactam • Aztreonam	Bactericidal activity results from inhibition of bacterial cell-wall synthesis. It binds to the penicillin-binding protein 3 of susceptible gram-negative bacterial cells, inhibiting cell wall division and resulting in lysis.	• Gram-negative bacteria (such as *Escherichia coli*) • Complicated and uncomplicated UTIs, septicemia, and lower respiratory tract, skin and skin-structure, intra-abdominal, and gynecologic infections caused by susceptible gram-negative bacteria
Fluoroquinolones • Ciprofloxacin • Levofloxacin • Moxifloxacin • Norfloxacin • Ofloxacin	Interrupt DNA synthesis during bacterial replication by inhibiting DNA gyrase, an essential enzyme of replicating DNA. As a result, the bacteria can't reproduce.	• Aerobic gram-positive (such as *S. aureus*) and aerobic gram-negative (such as *N. meningitidis*) bacteria • Lower respiratory tract infections • Infectious diarrhea • Acute bacterial sinusitis • Prostatitis • UTI • Selected sexually transmitted infections • Skin and skin-structure infections
Sulfonamides • Sulfadiazine • Trimethoprim-sulfamethozaxole	Bacteriostatic drugs prevent the growth of microorganisms by inhibiting folic acid production. The decreased folic acid synthesis decreases the number of bacterial nucleotides and inhibits bacterial growth.	• Gram-negative (such as *Haemophilus influenzae*) and gram-positive (such as *Nocardia* species) bacteria • UTI susceptible to sulfonamides • Trimethoprim-sulfamethoxazole also used for *Pneumocystis carinii* pneumonia, acute otitis media, and acute exacerbations of chronic bronchitis
Nitrofurantoin	Usually bacteriostatic; may become bactericidal depending on its urinary concentration and susceptibility of the infecting organism. Inhibits formation of acetyl coenzyme A from pyruvic acid, inhibiting the energy production of the infecting organism. It may also disrupt bacterial cell-wall function.	• UTI

Antiviral drugs

Synthetic nucleosides • Acyclovir • Famciclovir • Ganciclovir • Valacyclovir • Valganciclovir	Acyclovir, famciclovir, and ganciclovir are metabolized into their active forms and inhibit DNA synthesis. Valacyclovir converts to acyclovir and valganciclovir is converted to ganciclovir before inhibiting viral DNA synthesis.	• Herpes simplex viruses, including types 1 and 2, and varicella-zoster virus • Cytomegalovirus (CMV) retinitis in immunocompromised patients • Genital herpes • Herpes labialis

Drug classes & examples	Pharmacodynamics	Pharmacotherapeutics
Pyrophosphate analogue • Foscarnet	Prevents viral replication by selectively inhibiting DNA polymerase.	• CMV retinitis in patients with acquired immunodeficiency syndrome • Used in combination with ganciclovir for those who relapsed with either drug
Influenza A and syncytial virus drugs • Amantadine • Rimantadine • Ribavirin	Amantadine inhibits an early stage of viral replication. Rimantadine inhibits viral RNA and protein synthesis. Ribavirin inhibits viral DNA and RNA synthesis, halting viral replication.	• Prevent and treat respiratory tract infections caused by strains of influenza A • Severe respiratory syncytial virus in children • In adults, used in combination with interferon alfa-2B for chronic hepatitis C
Non-nucleoside reverse transcriptase inhibitors • Delavirdine • Efavirenz • Nevirapine	Nevirapine and delavirdine bind to reverse transcriptase enzyme, preventing it from exerting its effect and preventing human immunodeficiency virus (HIV) replication. Efavirenz competes for the enzyme through noncompetitive inhibition.	Used in combination with other antiretrovirals in HIV treatment; nevirapine is indicated for patients whose clinical condition and immune status have deteriorated
Protease inhibitors • Amprenavir • Fosamprenavir • Indinavir • Ritonavir • Tipranavir	Inhibit the activity of HIV protease and prevent the cleavage of viral polyproteins.	Used in combination with other antiretroviral agents to treat HIV infection
Antitubercular drugs		
• Isoniazid • Rifampin • Pyrazinamide • Ethambutol	Ethambutol and isoniazid are tuberculostatic, inhibiting the growth of *Mycobacterium tuberculosis*. Rifampin is tuberculocidal, destroying the mycobacteria. Pyrazinamide is converted into an active metabolite, which creates an acidic environment where mycobacteria cannot replicate.	• Usually used in combinations to prevent or delay the development of resistance • Ethambutol is also used to treat infections resulting from *Mycobacterium bovis* and *Mycobacterium kansasii* • Rifampin is also used to treat asymptomatic carriers of *N. meningitidis* when the risk of meningitis is high
Antimycotic drugs		
Polyenes • Amphotericin B • Nystatin	Bind to sterol (a lipid) in the fungal cell membrane, altering cell permeability and producing fungistatic and fungicidal actions.	• Amphotericin B treats life-threatening, systemic fungal infections and meningitis caused by fungi sensitive to the drug • Nystatin treats candidal skin infections topically and GI infections orally

Drug classes & examples	Pharmacodynamics	Pharmacotherapeutics
Fluorinated pyrimidine • Flucytosine	Penetrates fungal cells and is converted into an active metabolite (fluorouracil), which is then incorporated into the RNA of fungal cells, altering protein synthesis and causing cell death.	• Used in combination with amphotericin B to treat candidal and cryptococcal meningitis • *Candida* infections of the lower urinary tract • Effective against *Candida glabrata, Phialophora, Aspergillus*, and *Cladosporium*
Imidazole • Ketoconazole	Interferes with sterol synthesis, damaging cell membranes and increasing their permeability; this leads to a loss of intracellular elements and inhibits cell growth. Produces fungistatic and fungicidal effects.	• Topical and systemic infections caused by susceptible fungi, including dermatophytes
Synthetic triazoles • Fluconazole • Itraconazole • Voriconazole	Fluconazole inhibits fungal cytochrome P-450, an enzyme responsible for fungal sterol synthesis, causing fungal cell walls to weaken. Itraconazole and voriconazole interfere with fungal cell-wall synthesis by inhibiting formation of ergosterol and increasing cell-wall permeability, making fungus susceptible to osmotic instability.	• Serious systemic candidal infections, including UTIs, peritonitis, and pneumonia • Cryptococcal meningitis • Blastomycosis • Nonmeningeal histoplasmosis • Candidiasis • Aspergillosis • Fungal nail disease • Invasive aspergillosis
Glucan synthesis inhibitor • Caspofungin	Inhibits synthesis of beta (1,3) D-glucan, an integral component of the fungal cell wall.	Invasive aspergillosis in those unresponsive or intolerant of other antifungals
Synthetic allylamine derivative • Terbinafine	Inhibits squalene epoxidase, which blocks the biosynthesis of ergosterol, an essential component of fungal cell membranes.	• Tinea unguium (fungal infections of the fingernail or toenail)

Recombinant human activated protein C (rhAPC) drug

• Drotrecogin alfa	Has antithrombotic, anti-inflammatory, and fibrinolytic properties. Possibly produces dose-dependent reductions in D-dimer and interleukin-6. Activated protein C exerts an antithrombotic effect by inhibiting factors Va and VIIIa.	• Severe sepsis associated with acute organ dysfunction and high risk of death

CDC isolation precautions

Standard precautions are generally always used unless otherwise indicated, or they are used in conjunction with other precaution measures. The length of time for isolation precautions will vary depending on the nature and seriousness of the patient's infection or disease. Check with the facility's infection control department, local and state health departments, and the Centers for Disease Control and Prevention, as recommendations can change for individual diseases or for new and emerging infections.

Precautions	Equipment needed
Standard precautions: Used for all patients regardless of diagnosis or presumed infection	• Gloves are indicated for use with all patients when touching blood and body fluids, mucous membranes, or broken skin; when handling items or touching surfaces soiled with blood or body fluids; and when performing venipuncture and other vascular access procedures. • Masks and protective eyewear or a face shield are needed to protect mucous membranes of the mouth, nose, and eyes during procedures that may generate drops of blood or other body fluids. • A gown or apron is indicated during procedures that are likely to generate splashing of blood or other body fluids.
Airborne precautions (used in addition to standard precautions): Used when microorganisms may be carried through air and dispersed widely by air currents, resulting in inhalation or deposition on a susceptible host	• Special air handling and ventilation procedures are needed to prevent the spread of infection. • Use of an N95 particulate respirator is indicated when entering an infected patient's room.
Droplet precautions (used in addition to standard precautions): Used when infectious agents may be transmitted through large-particle droplets (>5 μm) traveling short distances of 3′ or less and/or when those droplets may come in contact with the conjunctivae or nasal or oral mucous membranes of a susceptible person	• A mask is indicated to protect the mucous membranes.

Indications

Apply when coming in contact with:
- Blood
- All body fluids, secretions, and excretions, except sweat, regardless of whether they contain visible blood
- Skin that is not intact
- Mucous membranes

Patients known to have or suspected of having a serious illness transmitted by airborne droplet nuclei, such as:
- Herpes zoster virus
- Influenza virus (H1N1 strain)
- Monkeypox virus
- Rubeola (measles)
- Severe acute respiratory syndrome
- Smallpox (variola)
- Tuberculosis, mycobacterial infection
- Varicella-zoster virus

Patients known to have or suspected of having a serious illness transmitted by large-particle droplets, such as:
- Epiglottiditis (due to *Haemophilus influenzae* type b)
- Diphtheria (pharyngeal)
- Influenza virus (human seasonal, pandemic)
- Meningitis (*H. influenzae* type b)
- Meningococcal disease (sepsis, meningitis, pneumonia)
- Mumps (infectious parotitis)
- *Mycoplasma* pneumonia
- Parvovirus B19 (erythema infectiosum)
- Pertussis (whooping cough)
- Pneumonic plague (*Yersinia pestis*)
- Pneumonia (adenovirus; *H. influenzae* type b in infants and children; meningococcal; group A *Streptococcus*)
- Rhinovirus
- Rubella (German measles)
- Rubeola
- Severe acute respiratory syndrome
- Streptococcal disease (group A major skin disease, wound, or burn; pharyngitis or scarlet fever in infants and young children; pneumonia; serious invasive disease)
- Viral hemorrhagic fever viruses (Lassa, Ebola, Marburg, Crimean-Congo)

Precautions	Equipment needed
Contact precautions (used in addition to standard precautions): Used to reduce the risk of transmitting infectious agents by direct or indirect contact (direct contact transmission can occur through patient care activities that require physical contact; indirect contact transmission involves a susceptible host coming in contact with a contaminated, usually inanimate, object in the patient's environment)	• A gown and gloves are indicated, and dedicated equipment (thermometer, stethoscope, and blood pressure cuff) is used for each patient.

Data from Siegel, J. D. , Rhinehart, E., Jackson, M., Chiarello, L. & the Healthcare Infection Control Practices Advisory Committee. *2007 Guideline for Isolation Precautions: Preventing Transmission of Infectious Agents in Healthcare Settings.* Retrieved from http://www.cdc.gov/hicpac/pdf/isolation/Isolation2007.pdf.

Indications

Patients known to have or suspected of having a serious illness easily transmitted by direct patient contact or by contact with items in the patient's environment, such as:

- Bronchiolitis
- *Clostridium difficile* gastroenteritis
- Congenital rubella
- Conjunctivitis (acute viral/acute hemorrhagic)
- Cutaneous diphtheria
- Furunculosis, staphylococcal infection (infants and young children)
- Hepatitis A virus (diapered or incontinent patients)
- Herpes simplex virus (herpesvirus hominis): mucocutaneous (disseminated or primary severe) or neonatal
- Herpes zoster virus
- Human metapneumovirus
- Impetigo
- Influenza, avian virus (H5N1, H7, and H9 strains)
- Pediculosis (head lice)
- Monkeypox
- Multidrug-resistant organisms, infection, or colonization (methicillin-resistant *Staphylococcus aureus*, vancomycin-resistant *Enterococcus*, vancomycin-intermediate and vancomycin-resistant *S. aureus*, extended-spectrum beta-lactamase–resistant *S. pneumoniae*)
- Parainfluenza virus infection, respiratory infection in infants and young children
- Pneumonia (adenovirus, *Burkholderia cepacia*)
- Poliomyelitis
- Pressure ulcer (major, infected)
- Respiratory infectious disease (acute in infants and children)
- Respiratory syncytial virus (infants, young children, and immunocompromised adults)
- Rotavirus (gastroenteritis)
- Scabies
- Severe acute respiratory syndrome
- Shigellosis
- Smallpox (variola)
- Staphylococcal disease (major)
- Streptococcal disease (group A major skin, wound, or burn)
- Vaccinia virus (vaccination-site infection with eczema vaccinatum; fetal, generalized or progressive vaccinia)
- Varicella-zoster virus
- Viral hemorrhagic fever viruses (Lassa, Ebola, Marburg, Crimean-Congo)
- Wound infections (major)

Selected references

American Academy of Pediatrics. (2009). *2009 Report of the committee on infectious diseases* (28th ed.). Elk Grove Village, IL: Author.

Brooks, K. (Ed.). (2007). *Ready reference to microbes* (2nd ed.). Washington DC: Association for Professionals in Infection Control and Epidemiology.

Carrico, R. (Ed.). (2009). *APIC test of infection control and epidemiology* (3rd ed.). Washington DC: Association for Professionals in Infection Control and Epidemiology.

Centers for Disease Control and Prevention. (2007). *2007 Guideline for isolation precautions: Preventing transmission of infectious agents in healthcare settings.* Atlanta: Author.

Diseases: A nursing process approach to excellent care (4th ed.). (2006). Philadelphia: Lippincott Williams & Wilkins.

Fenollar, F., Puéchal, X., & Raoult, D. (2007). Whipple's disease. *The New England Journal of Medicine, 356,* 55–66.

Gould, C. V., Umscheid, C. A., Agarwal, R. K., Kuntz, G., Pegues, D. A., & the Healthcare Infection Control Practices Advisory Committee. (2009). *Guideline for prevention of catheter-associated urinary tract infections.* Atlanta: Centers for Disease Control and Prevention.

Heymann, D. (Ed.). (2008). *Control of communicable diseases manual* (19th ed.). Washington DC: American Public Health Association.

Lashley, F., & Durham, J. (2007). *Emerging infectious diseases* (2nd ed.). New York: Springer.

The Merck Manuals Online Medical Library: Actinomycosis [reviewed/revised September 2008]. Retrieved September 2, 2009, from http://www.merck.com/mmhe/sec17/ch190/ch190b.html

Murray, P. R., Rosenthal, K. S., & Pfaller, M. A. (2009). *Medical microbiology* (6th ed.). St. Louis: Mosby.

Professional guide to diseases (9th ed.). (2009). Philadelphia: Lippincott Williams & Wilkins.

Understanding diseases. In *Nursing, the series for clinical excellence.* (2008). Philadelphia: Lippincott Williams & Wilkins.

Index

f figure

---

f figure

---

f figure